Advanced Imaging Techniques in Brain Tumors

Guest Editor

PIA C. SUNDGREN, MD, PhD

NEUROIMAGING CLINICS OF NORTH AMERICA

www.neuroimaging.theclinics.com

Consulting Editor

SURESH K. MUKHERJI, MD

November 2009 • Volume 19 • Number 4

SAUNDERS an imprint of ELSEVIER, Inc.

W.B. SAUNDERS COMPANY
A Division of Elsevier Inc.

1600 John F. Kennedy Boulevard ● Suite 1800 ● Philadelphia, Pennsylvania 19103-2899

http://www.theclinics.com

NEUROIMAGING CLINICS OF NORTH AMERICA Volume 19, Number 4
November 2009 ISSN 1052-5149, ISBN 13: 978-1-4377-1837-9

Editor: Joanne Husovski
Developmental Editor: Donald Mumford

Neuroimaging Clinics of North America (ISSN 1052-5149) is published quarterly by Elsevier Inc., 360 Park Avenue South, New York, NY 10010-1710. Months of issue are February, May, August, and November. Business and editorial offices: 1600 John F. Kennedy Blvd., Suite 1800, Philadelphia, PA 19103-2899. Periodicals postage paid at New York, NY, and additional mailing offices. Subscription prices are USD 293 per year for US individuals, USD 415 per year for US institutions, USD 150 per year for US students and residents, USD 339 per year for Canadian individuals, USD 520 per year for Canadian institutions, USD 431 per year for international individuals, USD 520 per year for international institutions and USD 215 per year for Canadian and foreign students and residents. To receive student/resident rate, orders must be accompanied by name of affiliated institution, date of term, and the *signature* of program/residency coordinator on institution letterhead. Orders will be billed at individual rate until proof of status is received. Foreign air speed delivery is included in all *Clinics* subscription prices. All prices are subject to change without notice. POSTMASTER: Send address changes to *Neuroimaging Clinics of North America*, Elsevier Health Sciences Division, Subscription Customer Service, 3251 Riverport Lane, Maryland Heights, MO 63043. Telephone: 1-800-654-2452 (U.S. and Canada); 314-447-8871 (outside U.S. and Canada). Fax: 314-447-8029. E-mail: journalscustomerservice-usa@elsevier.com (for print support); journalsonlinesupport-usa@elsevier.com (for online support).

Reprints. For copies of 100 or more of articles in this publication, please contact the Commercial Reprints Department, Elsevier Inc., 360 Park Avenue South, New York, NY 10010-1710. Tel.: 212-633-3812; Fax: 212-462-1935; E-mail: reprints@elsevier.com.

Neuroimaging Clinics of North America is covered by *Excerpta Medical/EMBASE*, the RSNA Index of Imaging Literature, *MEDLINE/PubMed (Index Medicus)*, MEDLINE/MEDLARS, SciSearch, Research Alert, and Neuroscience Citation Index.

Printed and bound in the United Kingdom
Transferred to Digital Print 2011

Cover image © Lydia Gregg 2009.

GOAL STATEMENT

The goal of *Neuroimaging Clinics of North America* is to keep practicing radiologists and radiology residents up to date with current clinical practice in radiology by providing timely articles reviewing the state of the art in patient care.

ACCREDITATION

The *Neuroimaging Clinics of North America* is planned and implemented in accordance with the Essential Areas and Policies of the Accreditation Council for Continuing Medical Education (ACCME) through the joint sponsorship of the University of Virginia School of Medicine and Elsevier. The University of Virginia School of Medicine is accredited by the ACCME to provide continuing medical education for physicians.

The University of Virginia School of Medicine designates this educational activity for a maximum of 15 *AMA PRA Category 1 Credits*™ for each issue, 60 credits per year. Physicians should only claim credit commensurate with the extent of their participation in the activity.

The American Medical Association has determined that physicians not licensed in the US who participate in this CME activity are eligible for a maximum of 15 *AMA PRA Category 1 Credits*™ for each issue, 60 credits per year.

Credit can be earned by reading the text material, taking the CME examination online at http://www.theclinics.com/home/cme, and completing the evaluation. After taking the test, you will be required to review any and all incorrect answers. Following completion of the test and evaluation, your credit will be awarded and you may print your certificate.

FACULTY DISCLOSURE/CONFLICT OF INTEREST

The University of Virginia School of Medicine, as an ACCME accredited provider, endorses and strives to comply with the Accreditation Council for Continuing Medical Education (ACCME) Standards of Commercial Support, Commonwealth of Virginia statutes, University of Virginia policies and procedures, and associated federal and private regulations and guidelines on the need for disclosure and monitoring of proprietary and financial interests that may affect the scientific integrity and balance of content delivered in continuing medical education activities under our auspices.

The University of Virginia School of Medicine requires that all CME activities accredited through this institution be developed independently and be scientifically rigorous, balanced and objective in the presentation/discussion of its content, theories and practices.

All authors/editors participating in an accredited CME activity are expected to disclose to the readers relevant financial relationships with commercial entities occurring within the past 12 months (such as grants or research support, employee, consultant, stock holder, member of speakers bureau, etc.). The University of Virginia School of Medicine will employ appropriate mechanisms to resolve potential conflicts of interest to maintain the standards of fair and balanced education to the reader. Questions about specific strategies can be directed to the Office of Continuing Medical Education, University of Virginia School of Medicine, Charlottesville, Virginia.

The faculty and staff of the University of Virginia Office of Continuing Medical Education have no financial affiliations to disclose.

The authors/editors listed below have identified no professional/financial affiliations for themselves or their spouse/partner:
Abass Alavi, MD, PhD (Hon), DSc (Hon); Ian C. Atkinson, PhD; Sandip Basu, MBBS (Hons), DRM, DNB, MNAMS; Lorenzo Bello, MD; Giulio Bertani, MD; Alberto Bizzi, MD; Alexandra Borges, MD; Giorgio Carrabba, MD; Giuseppe Casaceli, MD; Fred Damen, MS; Andrea Falini, MD; Enrica Fava, MD; Sergio M. Gaini, MD; Craig J. Galbán, PhD; Joanne Husovski (Acquisitions Editor); Deepak Kunthia, MD; Saulo P. Lacerda, MD; Aiming Lu, PhD; Bradford A. Moffat, PhD; Costanza Papagno, MD; H. Ian Robins, MD, PhD; Lubda M. Shah, MD (Test Author); Pia C. Sundgren, MD, PhD (Guest Editor); and John Villano, MD, PhD.

The authors listed below have identified the following professional/financial affiliations for themselves or their spouse/partner:
Yue Cao, PhD is on the Advisory Committee/Board of Calypso Medical Technologies.
Thomas L. Chenevert, PhD serves on the Advisory Committee/Board for Philips Healthcare, and is a Co-inventor on diffusion-related patent for the University of Michigan.
Andrew B. Lassman, MD is a consultant for Cephalon, Eisai, Imclone, and is an industry funded research/investigator and a consultant, and serves on the Speakers Bureau and Advisory Committee/Board, for Schering Plough and Genentech.
Meng Law, MD, MBBS, FRACR serves as a speaker for Siemens Medical Solutions and Bayer Healthcare, is a consultant for Bracco Diagnostics, and owns stock in Prism Clinical Imaging.
Suresh K. Mukherji, MD, FACR (Consulting Editor) is a consultant for Phillips Medical and Bracco.
Alnawaz Rehemtulla, PhD owns stock in ImBio, LLC.
Brian D. Ross, PhD owns stock in ImBio, LLC.
Keith R. Thulborn, MD, PhD is a research/investigator for GE Healthcare.

Disclosure of Discussion of Non-FDA Approved Uses for Pharmaceutical Products and/or Medical Devices.
The University of Virginia School of Medicine, as an ACCME provider, requires that all faculty presenters identify and disclose any off-label uses for pharmaceutical and medical device products. The University of Virginia School of Medicine recommends that each physician fully review all the available data on new products or procedures prior to clinical use.

TO ENROLL

To enroll in the Neuroimaging Clinics of North America Continuing Medical Education program, call customer service at 1-800-654-2452 or sign up online at **http://www.theclinics.com/home/cme**. The CME program is available to subscribers for an additional annual fee of USD 175.

Neuroimaging Clinics of North America

THE CLINICS ARE NOW AVAILABLE ONLINE!

Access your subscription at:
www.theclinics.com

Contributors

CONSULTING EDITOR

SURESH K. MUKHERJI, MD, FACR
Professor and Chief of Neuroradiology
and Head & Neck Radiology, Professor
of Radiology, Otolaryngology, Head & Neck
Surgery & Radiation Oncology, University
of Michigan Health System, Ann Arbor,
Michigan

GUEST EDITOR

PIA C. SUNDGREN, MD, PhD
Professor, Diagnostic Centre for Imaging
and Functional Medicine, Malmö University
Hospital, University of Lund, Malmö,
Sweden; Professor, Department of Radiology,
University of Michigan, Ann Arbor, Michigan

AUTHORS

ABASS ALAVI, MD, PhD (Hon), DSc (Hon)
Division of Nuclear Medicine, Department
of Radiology, University of Pennsylvania
School of Medicine, Hospital of the
University of Pennsylvania, Philadelphia,
Pennsylvania

IAN C. ATKINSON, PhD
Center for Magnetic Resonance Research,
University of Illinois at Chicago, Chicago,
Illinois

**SANDIP BASU, MBBS (Hons) DRM, DNB,
MNAMS**
Radiation Medicine Centre (BARC), Tata
Memorial Hospital Annexe, Parel, Bombay,
India

LORENZO BELLO, MD
Neurosurgery, Department of Neurological
Sciences, Università degli Studi di Milano,
Milano, Italy

GIULIO BERTANI, MD
Neurosurgery, Department of Neurologic
Sciences, Università degli Studi di Milano,
Milano, Italy

ALBERTO BIZZI, MD
Eccellenza Professionale in Tecniche Avanzate
di RM [Professional Excellence in Advanced
Magnetic Resonance Technique],
Neuroradiology Unit, Fondazione IRCCS
Istituto Neurologico Carlo Besta, Via Celoria,
Milan, Italy

ALEXANDRA BORGES, MD
Department of Radiology, Instituto Português
de Oncologia de Francisco Gentil, Centro de
Lisboa, Portugal

YUE CAO, PhD
Associate Professor, Department
of Radiation Oncology and Radiology,
University of Michigan, Ann Arbor, Michigan

GIORGIO CARRABBA, MD
Neurosurgery, Department of Neurologic
Sciences, Università degli Studi di Milano,
Milano, Italy

GIUSEPPE CASACELI, MD
Neurosurgery, Department of Neurological
Sciences, Università degli Studi di Milano,
Milano, Italy

THOMAS L. CHENEVERT, PhD
Professor of Radiology, Department of
Radiology, University of Michigan Medical
Center, Ann Arbor, Michigan

FRED DAMEN, MS
Center for Magnetic Resonance Research,
University of Illinois at Chicago, Chicago, Illinois

ENRICA FAVA, MD
Neurosurgery, Department of Neurological
Sciences, Università degli Studi di Milano,
Milano, Italy

ANDREA FALINI, MD
Department of Neuroradiology, Università
Vita e Salute, Istituto Scientifico San Raffaele;
Neuroradiology, Ospèdale San Raffaele,
Milano, Italy

SERGIO M. GAINI, MD
Neurosurgery, Department of Neurologic
Sciences, Università degli Studi di Milano,
Milano, Italy

CRAIG J. GALBÁN, PhD
Assistant Professor, Department of Radiology,
University of Michigan, Ann Arbor, Michigan

DEEPAK KHUNTIA, MD
Associate Professor, Department of Human
Oncology, University of Wisconsin School of
Medicine and Public Health, Madison,
Wisconsin

SAULO LACERDA, MD
Department of Radiology, Mount Sinai Medical
Center, New York; Professor of Radiology and
Neurosurgery, Director of Neuroradiology,
MedImagem-Hospital Beneficencia
Portuguesa, Sao Paulo, Brazil

ANDREW B. LASSMAN, MD
Assistant Member, Department of Neurology
and the Brain Tumor Center, Memorial
Sloan-Kettering Cancer Center, New York,
New York

MENG LAW, MD
University of Southern California Medical
Center and LA County Hospitals, Keck School
of Medicine, Los Angeles, California

AIMING LU, PhD
Center for Magnetic Resonance Research,
University of Illinois at Chicago, Chicago,
Illinois

BRADFORD A. MOFFAT, PhD
Senior Research Fellow, Department of
Radiology, The Royal Melbourne Hospital,
University of Melbourne, Parkville, Victoria,
Australia

COSTANZA PAPAGNO, MD
Department of Psychology, Università Milano
Bicocca, Milano, Italy

ALNAWAZ REHEMTULLA, PhD
Professor, Department of Radiation Oncology,
University of Michigan; Professor, Department
of Radiology, University of Michigan,
Ann Arbor, Michigan

H. IAN ROBINS, MD, PhD
Professor, Department of Medicine,
University of Wisconsin School of Medicine
and Public Health; Department of Neurology,
University of Wisconsin School of Medicine
and Public Health; Department of Human
Oncology, University of Wisconsin School of
Medicine and Public Health, Madison,
Wisconsin

BRIAN D. ROSS, PhD
Professor of Radiology, Department of
Radiology, University of Michigan Medical
Center, Ann Arbor, Michigan

PIA C. SUNDGREN, MD, PhD
Professor, Diagnostic Centre for Imaging and
Functional Medicine, Malmö University
Hospital, University of Lund, Malmö, Sweden;
Department of Radiology, University of
Michigan, Ann Arbor, Michigan

KEITH R. THULBORN, MD, PhD
Center for Magnetic Resonance Research,
University of Illinois at Chicago, Chicago,
Illinois

JOHN L. VILLANO, MD, PhD
Center for Magnetic Resonance Research,
University of Illinois at Chicago, Chicago,
Illinois

Contents

> Advanced magnetic resonance imaging (MRI) techniques, such as magnetic reso-
> nance spectroscopy, diffusion MRI, and perfusion MRI, allow for a diverse range
> of multidimensional information regarding brain tumor physiology to be obtained
> in addition to the traditional anatomic images. Although it is well documented that
> MRI of rodent brain tumor models plays an important role in the basic research
> and drug discovery process of new brain tumor therapies, the role that animal
> models have played in translating these methodologies is rarely discussed in such
> articles. Even in consensus reports outlining the pathway to validation of these tech-
> niques, the use of animal models is given scant regard. This is despite that the use
> of rodent cancer models to test advanced MRI techniques predates and was integral
> to the development of clinical MRI. This article highlights just how integral preclinical
> imaging is to the discovery, development, and validation of advanced MRI tech-
> niques for imaging brain neoplasms.

> Recent evidence suggests that vascular permeability and the presence of vascular
> endothelial growth factor/vascular permeability factor (VEGF/VPF) are important
> mediators of brain tumor growth in addition to angiogenesis. Perfusion and perme-
> ability magnetic resonance (MR) imaging can now measure parameters such as
> cerebral blood volume and vascular permeability, which can be directly correlated
> with these histopathologic changes as well as molecular markers such as VEGF.
> The major techniques currently used in both the clinical and research settings are
> T1-weighted steady-state dynamic contrast-enhanced MR imaging (DCE MR imag-
> ing) and T2*-weighted first-pass, dynamic susooptibility contrast MR imaging (DSC
> MR imaging). The advantages and disadvantages of each technique with regard to
> characterizing tumor biology are discussed in this article. Most clinicians and inves-
> tigators are currently using the DSC MR imaging T2*-weighted technique for brain
> tumor perfusion MR imaging. The existence of multiple approaches to pathologic
> classification of human glioma implies that there is a lack of consensus among
> experts as to which is the single best approach. These multiple grading systems
> do, however, agree on the histologic parameters that are important in the deter-
> mination of glioma biology, namely hypercellularity, pleomorphism, vascular
> endothelial proliferation, mitotic activity, and necrosis.

Advanced imaging provides insight into biophysical, physiologic, metabolic, or functional properties of tissues. Because water mobility is sensitive to cellular homeostasis, cellular density, and microstructural organization, it is considered a valuable tool in the advanced imaging arsenal. This article summarizes diffusion imaging concepts and highlights clinical applications of diffusion MR imaging for oncologic imaging. Diffusion tensor imaging and its derivative maps of diffusion anisotropy allow assessment of tumor compression or destruction of adjacent normal tissue anisotropy and may aid to assess tumor infiltration and aid presurgical planning.

Functional magnetic resonance (fMR) imaging and diffusion MR tractography have emerged as valuable tools in the evaluation of verbal language in brain tumor patients, and have changed the way neurosurgeons look at patients with a mass in the dominant hemisphere. The techniques have obtained recognition as valuable presurgical clinical tools in the determination of hemispheric dominance and in the selection of candidates who may benefit from awake craniotomy. In the near future fMRI and diffusion MR Tractography may contribute to elucidate mechanisms of brain plasticity and may provide predictors of favorable postoperative clinical outcome. The functional anatomy of the language network and the role of fMR imaging and diffusion MR tractography in the evaluation of patients with a brain tumor are the focus of this article.

This article describes the rationale, indications, and modality for intraoperative brain mapping for safe and effective surgical removal of tumors located within functional brain areas.

Treatment of high-grade primary brain tumors is based on experience from multicenter trials. However, the prognosis has changed little in 3 decades. This suggests that there is a fundamental oversight in treatment. This article provides an imaging perspective of how regional responses of primary brain tumors may be examined to guide a flexible treatment plan. Sodium imaging provides a measurement of cell density that can be used to measure regional cell kill. Such a bioscales of regionally and temporally sensitive biologic-based parameters may be helpful to guide tumor treatment. These suggestions are speculative and still being examined, but are presented to challenge the medical community to be receptive to changes in the standard of care when that standard continues to fail.

Despite the recognized limitations of ^{18}Fluorodeoxyglucose positron emission tomography (FDG-PET) in brain tumor imaging due to the high background of normal gray matter, this imaging modality provides critical information for the management of patients with cerebral neoplasms with regard to the following aspects: (1) providing a global picture of the tumor and thus guiding the appropriate site for stereotactic biopsy, and thereby enhancing its accuracy and reducing the number of biopsy samples; and (2) prediction of biologic behavior and aggressiveness of the tumor, thereby aiding in prognosis. Another area, which has been investigated extensively, includes differentiating recurrent tumor from treatment-related changes (eg, radiation necrosis and postsurgical changes). Furthermore, FDG-PET has demonstrated its usefulness in differentiating lymphoma from toxoplasmosis in patients with acquired immune deficiency syndrome with great accuracy, and is used as the investigation of choice in this setting. Image coregistration with magnetic resonance imaging and delayed FDG-PET imaging are 2 maneuvers that substantially improve the accuracy of interpretation, and hence should be routinely employed in clinical settings. In recent years an increasing number of brain tumor PET studies has used other tracers (like labeled methionine, tyrosine, thymidine, choline, fluoromisonidazole, EF5, and so forth), of which positron-labeled amino acid analogues, nucleotide analogues, and the hypoxia imaging tracers are of special interest. The major advantage of these radiotracers over FDG is the markedly lower background activity in normal brain tissue, which allows detection of small lesions and low-grade tumors. The promise of the amino acid PET tracers has been emphasized due to their higher sensitivity in imaging recurrent tumors (particularly the low-grade ones) and better accuracy for differentiating between recurrent tumors and treatment-related changes compared with FDG. The newer PET tracers have also shown great potential to image important aspects of tumor biology and thereby demonstrate ability to forecast prognosis. The value of hypoxia imaging tracers (such as fluoromisonidazole or more recently EF5) is substantial in radiotherapy planning and predicting treatment response. In addition, they may play an important role in the future in directing and monitoring targeted hypoxic therapy for tumors with hypoxia. Development of optimal image segmentation strategy with novel PET tracers and multimodality imaging is an approach that deserves mention in the era of intensity modulated radiotherapy, and which is likely to have important clinical and research applications in radiotherapy planning in patients with brain tumor.

This article reviews the current status and trends in the treatment of primary gliomas, focusing predominantly on glioblastoma. It also discusses the current standard of care and new targeted agents currently under investigation. Furthermore, the concepts of pseudoprogression and pseudoresponse are introduced, which are new imaging correlates that have significant impact on understanding of the disease.

Radiation therapy is a major treatment modality for malignant and benign brain tumors. Concerns of radiation effects on the brain tissue and neurocognitive function and quality of life increase as survival of patients treated for brain tumors improves. In this article, the clinical and neurobehavioral symptoms and signs of radiation-induced brain injury, possible histopathology, and the potential of functional, metabolic, and molecular imaging as a biomarker for assessment and prediction of neurotoxicity after brain irradiation and imaging findings in radiation necrosis are discussed.

The central skull base (CSB) constitutes a frontier between the extracranial head and neck and the middle cranial fossa. The anatomy of this region is complex, containing most of the bony foramina and canals of the skull base traversed by several neurovascular structures that can act as routes of spread for pathologic processes. Lesions affecting the CSB can be intrinsic to its bony-cartilaginous components; can arise from above, within the intracranial compartment; or can arise from below, within the extracranial head and neck. Crosssectional imaging is indispensable in the diagnosis, treatment planning, and follow-up of patients with CSB lesions. This review focuses on a systematic approach to this region based on an anatomic division that takes into account the major tissue constituents of the CSB.

Foreword

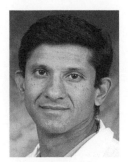

Suresh K. Mukherji, MD, FACR
Consulting Editor

It is my distinct pleasure to have Pia Sundgren as our guest editor for this issue of *Neuroimaging Clinics of North America*. As many of you may know, Pia and I worked together for 8 years at the University of Michigan. She is now Professor of Radiology at the University of Lund. Pia is a very accomplished individual and is one of the hardest working individuals with whom I have ever been associated. All of her accolades and accomplishments are extremely deserved.

The title of her issue is "Advanced Imaging Techniques in Brain Tumors." She has assembled world-renowned authors to cover the topics of advanced imaging techniques in brain tumors, including magnetic resonance (MR) diffusion–weighted and tensor imaging, MR tractography, MR spectroscopy, MR perfusion, functional MR imaging and other imaging techniques complementary to MR

imaging, such as positron emission tomography. There is also coverage of current concepts regarding brain tumor classification, current status, and trends for the treatment of gliomas.

As her prior neuroradiology division director, I am very proud of Pia and all that she has accomplished. She is one of the brightest minds in our field and I am very honored that she accepted our invitation to edit this issue of *Neuroimaging Clinics of North America*.

Suresh K. Mukherji, MD, FACR
University of Michigan Health System
1500 E., Medical Center Drive
Ann Arbor, MI 48109-0030, USA

E-mail address:
mukherji@med.umich.edu

Neuroimag Clin N Am 19 (2009) xi
doi:10.1016/j.nic.2009.10.002
1052-5149/09/$ – see front matter

Preface

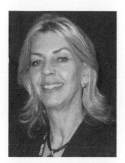

Pia C. Sundgren, MD, PhD
Guest Editor

Over the past decade we have seen a shift in brain tumor imaging from merely providing anatomical information toward providing information about individual tumor biology and pathophysiology. Despite the emergence of new treatment strategies and, successful management of brain tumors in adults and children remains largely unsatisfactory.

The recent advances in brain tumor imaging offer unique anatomical as well as pathophysiological information that provides new insights into brain tumor biology and behavior. Currently this information is used to facilitate therapeutic decisions, provide information regarding prognosis, and monitor therapy response. The advanced neuroimaging methods also provide morphological, metabolic, and functional measurements that have the potential of guiding and refining surgical treatment.

With this issue of *Neuroimaging Clinics of North America* we would like to update the reader about the current and the new advanced imaging techniques. We will not only focus on MR imaging such as diffusion-weighted and tensor imaging and MR tractography, MR spectroscopy, MR perfusion with different techniques, and functional MRI, but also on other imaging techniques such as positron emission tomography (PET), which is complementary to MRI. For example, new radiolabeled PET tracers have allowed more specific interrogation of glioma physiology such as hypoxia assessment or tumor proliferation rate and will likely yield important information on tumor response to therapy. This issue of *Neuroimaging Clinics of North America* is not only focusing on new advanced imaging techniques in brain tumors but we are also presenting the current concept for brain tumor classification and current status and trends for the treatment of gliomas, as well as some of the difficulties and controversies alluded to here, illustrating the negative effects of radiation on normal brain tissue, and giving the reader some insight into the continued important focus on translational research.

Both in clinical practice as well as in research there is an ongoing search and interest in refining different imaging methods and techniques so that imaging will continue to provide new and unique insights into brain tumor pathophysiology and behavior. In the future these techniques may allow development of patient-specific therapy to improve outcome in patients with brain tumors.

I hope the reader will find the same pleasure reading this issue as I did and that they will find this issue to be helpful, informative, and educational about new advances in brain tumor imaging methods and techniques.

I would like to express my sincere gratitude to all the authors for their time, their effort, and their expertise in preparing their manuscripts for this issue. The success of this issue is largely a result of their efforts. I would also like to thank Ms Joanne Husovski from Elsevier for her encouraging support and assistance during this process, and finally Prof Suresh Mukherji for the invitation.

Pia C. Sundgren, MD, PhD
Department of Radiology
University of Michigan
Ann Arbor, MI 48104, USA
Diagnostic Centre for Imaging and
Functional Medicine
Malmö University Hospital
University of Lund
SE-205 02 Malmö, Sweden

E-mail address:
sundgren@med.umich.edu

Neuroimag Clin N Am 19 (2009) xiii
doi:10.1016/j.nic.2009.08.013
1052-5149/09/$ – see front matter © 2009 Elsevier Inc. All rights reserved.

Advanced MRI: Translation from Animal to Human in Brain Tumor Research

Bradford A. Moffat, PhD[a],*, Craig J. Galbán, PhD[b],
Alnawaz Rehemtulla, PhD[c,d]

KEYWORDS

- Diffusion MRI • Magnetic resonance spectroscopy (MRS)
- Perfusion MRI • Brain tumor • Imaging biomarkers
- Translational research

Advanced magnetic resonance imaging (MRI) techniques, such as magnetic resonance spectroscopy (MRS), diffusion MRI, and perfusion MRI, allow for a diverse range of multiparametric information regarding brain tumor physiology to be obtained in addition to the traditional anatomic images.[1,2] Although it is well documented that MRI of rodent brain tumor models plays an important role in the basic research and drug discovery process of new brain tumor therapies,[3–6] the role that animal models have played in translating these methodologies is rarely discussed in such articles. Even in consensus reports[7,8] outlining the pathway to validation of these techniques, the use of animal models is given scant regard. This is despite the use of rodent cancer models to test advanced MRI techniques predates[9] and was integral to the development of clinical MRI. It is the aim of this article to highlight just how integral preclinical imaging is to the discovery, development, and validation of advanced MRI techniques for imaging brain neoplasms.

From almost the moment MRI was commercially available, its potential to become an indispensable tool central to the multidisciplinary planning of individualized brain tumor patient management was recognized.[10] The inherent high resolution and exquisite soft tissue contrast of MRI allow radiologists, pathologists, neurosurgeons, neuro-oncologists, and radiation oncologists to gain an understanding of the 3-dimensional morphologic problem they face on a patient-by-patient basis. Paralleling this, many people in the research community (clinical and basic science) have been exploring the role that advanced MRI techniques may play in investigating the structural, functional, and metabolic nature of the brain tumor microenvironment. This exploration has been brought about

Funding support: Dr Moffat would like to acknowledge the funding support of the Australian National Health and Medical Research Council (#454790 and #566992) and the Radiation Oncology Branch of the Department of Health and Aging (Australian Government, #509322). Drs Rehemtulla and Galbán would like to acknowledge the funding support of the National Institutes of Health (P50CA093990, PO1CA085878, and U24CA083099).

[a] Department of Radiology, The Royal Melbourne Hospital, University of Melbourne, Parkville, Victoria 3050, Australia
[b] Department of Radiology, University of Michigan, 109 Zina Pitcher Place BSRB, Room D200, Ann Arbor, MI 48109-2200, USA
[c] Department of Radiation Oncology, University of Michigan, 109 Zina Pitcher Place BSRB, Ann Arbor, MI 48109-2200, USA
[d] Department of Radiology, University of Michigan, 109 Zina Pitcher Place BSRB, Room A528, Ann Arbor, MI 48109-2200, USA
* Corresponding author.
E-mail address: brad.moffat@mh.org.au (B.A. Moffat).

by a desire of the clinical researchers and pharmaceutical companies to have access to early and noninvasive biological information that can predict outcome and/or quantify therapeutic efficacy. The most common and most developed techniques (although there are others) can be classified into 3 main categories:

1. MRS for quantifying cell metabolites.
2. Perfusion MRI for quantifying tissue hemodynamics (blood volume, flow, and vessel permeability).
3. Diffusion MRI for quantifying tissue structure and microenvironment (cell density and white matter tractography).

These technologies are currently being investigated as biomarkers for early diagnosis, for predicting outcome in response to specific therapies, and to monitor therapeutic efficacy. The pathway to clinical and regulatory acceptance of MRI biomarkers is not entirely transparent. A biomarker needs to find a niche role in improving patient outcome and/or reducing costs in a clinical setting. For use in the drug discovery process, a biomarker needs to significantly improve a clinical trial of a new therapy by quantifying efficacy, aiding in patient selection, or helping with "go or no go" decisions. Demonstrating these abilities is not trivial and goes beyond clinical or scientific studies. However, what is necessary is that before a biomarker can be accepted as a surrogate marker, it must go through a process of validation and qualification[11] through numerous scientific and clinical studies. In terms of validating biomarkers as surrogate endpoints in oncology research and drug discovery, it is necessary to establish strong scientific evidence of the biologic mechanism involved, acceptable analytical characteristics (sensitivity, specificity, reproducibility, and accuracy), and clinical feasibility.[12] Just as new therapeutic agents must be shown to improve outcome of patients through regulated clinical trials, ultimately much of this validation must occur in the clinical setting by correlating biomarkers with clinical outcome for acceptance. This process is extremely expensive and time consuming, and it is often not ethical or possible to quantify image biomarker standardization and robustness through repeatability and dose-dependent experiments on only patients.

To this end, preclinical imaging of brain tumor animal models has played and will, for some time, play a vital role in the validation of numerous MRI biomarkers. This article shows by example how and why preclinical imaging is important to the validation of and to the fundamental understanding of each imaging biomarker. Although it is not possible to cover all potential brain tumor imaging biomarkers, it is hoped that by covering diffusion MRI, perfusion MRI, and MRS, it is possible to show the immense impact of preclinical imaging has had on the translation from biomarker concept to a clinically useful surrogate endpoint.

MAGNETIC RESONANCE SPECTROSCOPY

In vivo MRS is an MR technique that allows for the detection of cellular metabolites whose protons have different MR frequencies from that of the surrounding water protons.[13] The MRS data are acquired from either large single voxel localized by traditional MRI images (Fig. 1A, B) or from multiple voxels similar to traditional MR images. The data are usually presented in the form of a spectrum (Fig. 1C). Each peak represents the relative abundance of protons with different resonant frequencies caused by differences in their local magnetic field. The unique chemical structure of various metabolites results in different local magnetic fields experienced by their protons and results in a unique fingerprint-like MRS signature. Because MRS can be acquired from human and rodent tumors, it can be an excellent translational research tool or biomarker for quantification and imaging of tumor metabolism.

Investigation of brain tumor metabolism by MRS is one of the oldest clinical research applications of MR and predates[14–16] the availability of clinical MRI scanners. Initially, phosphorous MRS was the most widely used technique, as it allowed for the quantification of high-energy phosphate metabolism[16] as a biomarker of tumor hypoxia.[14] However, since the introduction of clinical scanners, proton MRS has become the most popular MRS technique, as it allows for assessment of tumor metabolites using standard clinical MRI scanners and radio-frequency coils. Preceding the publication of the first clinical MRS results[17] was an MRS study of the well-characterized C6 rat glioma model by Remy and colleagues.[18] In this study the authors were able to resolve several different MRS resonance peaks, identifying 5 different metabolites: N-acetyl aspartate (NAA), lactate, lipid, choline (cho), and creatine (cr). Although it is now possible to quantify more than 10 important tumor metabolites (see Fig. 1) with modern MRI scanners,[19] these original 5 MRS biomarkers are still the most commonly quantified. In addition to identifying these MRS peaks, this early study showed that the relative lactate, lipid, and cho signals increased, whereas NAA and cr

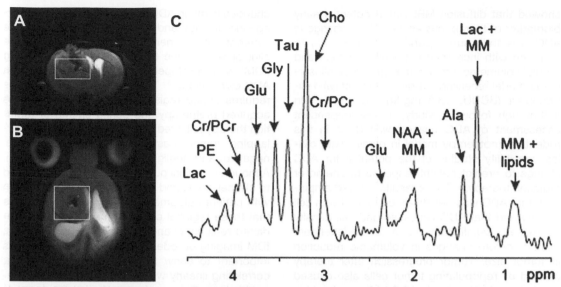

Fig. 1. Proton MRS of a 9L gliosarcoma in the rat brain acquired using a 9.4T MRI scanner. The location of the MRS voxel is shown on the coronal (A) and axial (B) T2-weighted images. (C) The MRS spectrum showing the metabolic signature of this brain tumor model, including lactate (Lac), phosphorylethanolamine (PE), creatine (Cr), phosphocreatine (PCr), glutamate (Glu), glycine (Gly), taurine (Tau), choline (Cho), N-acetyl aspartate (NAA), and macromolecule (MM). (*From* Pfeuffer J, Lin JC, Delabarre L, et al. Detection of intracellular lactate with localized diffusion {1H-13C}-spectroscopy in rat glioma in vivo. J Magn Reson 2005;177(1):134; with permission.)

decreased with increasing tumor burden. This established a link between MRS and tumor biology, showing that MRS had the potential to become an important noninvasive biomarker of tumor malignancy. Early clinical results[17,20] showed that tumors had significantly different metabolic profiles compared with healthy brain tissue when measured by MRS. However, these significant differences between benign and malignant tumors were not universal.[20] This prompted animal studies of various rodent brain tumor models[21–24] to investigate the biologic phenomena that was being quantified by MRS. As a result of these studies, it was identified that MRS measures of tumor metabolism were extremely heterogeneous[21] and brain tumors had overall lower metabolism compared with normal brain tissue contralateral to the tumor.[22] This correlated with decreased tumor metabolism that was independently measured by bioluminescent quantification of tumor adenosine triphosphate, lactate, and glucose distributions.[22] Paralleling the clinical results showed that the MRS tumor metabolic profile was unable to differentiate different types of tumor models[24] or stage of development.[22]

Despite the lack of specificity of MRS to predict tumor grade, these early animal experiments showed that MRS was still a potentially important biomarker because it could quantify tumor metabolic progression and/or therapeutically induced change in tumor metabolism. In a 9L gliosarcoma

model, it was shown that MRS could reproducibly quantify decreased tumor metabolism associated with an efficacious cytotoxic agent.[23]

DIFFUSION MRI

Diffusion MRI is an application of MRI that allows for the quantification and imaging of the random Brownian motion of water molecules within the cellular or tissue microenvironment.[25] At first inspection, this may not seem like an important biophysical property that could help in the assessment of malignant brain tumors. However, it is emerging as an important imaging biomarker of therapeutic efficacy,[26] of tumor invasion,[27–29] and for tracking white matter fiber connectivity.[30] The reason is that the cellular environment causes the restriction of this diffusion by, among other things, cell membranes, and so diffusion MRI can be used as a measure of cellular status and cytoarchitecture.[31]

Although diffusion-weighted MRI is often used clinically, the diffusion process can also be quantified by calculating the apparent diffusion coefficient (ADC), which when determined on a voxel-wise basis can generate a quantitative image. In such representations of the ADC, the membrane dense gray and white matter is hypointense compared with the cerebrospinal fluid. Analogous to MRS, it was the result of ADC measurements[32] of rodent brain tumors that showed that diffusion MRI was a potential early biomarker of therapeutic efficacy. This change in ADC was then subsequently shown (**Fig. 2**) to correlate with increased extracellular space and predict volumetric tumor shrinkage in a 9L gliosarcoma model receiving 1,3-bis(2-chloroethyl)-1-nitrosourea (BCNU, 13.3 mg/kg) treatment.[33] In a thorough follow-up study, a dose-dependent assessment of ADC change was done in this rodent/chemotherapy model in parallel with clinical feasibility studies of the potential for ADC change to predict patient response to chemo or radiation therapy.[34] These results showed empirically that ADC was negatively correlated with cell density and that ADC increased and cell density decreased significantly in a dose-dependent manner before changes in volumetric reduction in tumor size. Tumor progression after therapy caused by repopulating tumor cells also caused a substantial decrease in ADC before volumetric progression was measurable.

Although these initial results did prove promising, there were still several hurdles to overcome to clinically translate diffusion MRI as a biomarker for therapeutic efficacy. The heterogeneity of changes in ADC in human tumors compared with experimental rodent tumors was such that simple

changes in mean ADC were not predictive of therapeutic efficacy and outcome. To overcome the inherent heterogeneity of changes in ADC in the clinical setting, the functional diffusion mapping (fDM) was developed as an alternative to mean ADC calculations.[35] The calculation of fDM maps requires image registration of serial ADC maps acquired pretherapy and during chemo or radiation therapy followed by segmentation of the overlapping tumor mass into regions of positive, negative, and negligible change in ADC (**Fig. 3**). Although the initial publication of fDM was applied to clinical cases and showed excellent correlation with patient outcome, it was impossible to prove that these regional changes in ADC actually predicted regional changes in cellular density. Thus, fDM imaging of rodent brain tumor models[36] was important to show that fDM was reproducible, correlating linearly with survival and chemotherapeutic dose. The use of animal brain tumor models and sophisticated image registration techniques shows that these ADC changes also correlate with regional differences in cell density (**Fig. 4**).[36,37]

The highly ordered cellular environment of white matter causes the ADC to be dependent on the relative angle of the white matter tracts to

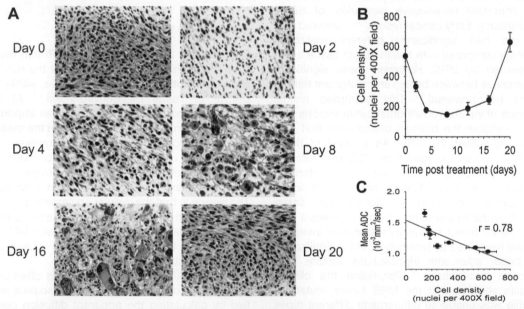

Fig. 2. Correlation of diffusion MRI changes with histopathologic changes in a 9L brain tumor model treated with BCNU (1,3[bis-2-chloroethyl]-1-nitrosourea) chemotherapy. (*A*) Slides showing a decrease in cell density 4 days after chemotherapy (hematoxylin-eosin). As the tumor repopulates, an increase in cell density at day 16 is observed. (*B*) Cell density as a function of time posttherapy. (*C*) Correlation of ADC as a function of tumor cell density. When changes in MR diffusion (mean ADC) are plotted against cell density at each of the time points, a significant correlation is observed, showing that mean ADC is a quantitative surrogate for cell density. (*From* Chenevert TL, Stegman LD, Taylor JM, et al. Diffusion magnetic resonance imaging: an early surrogate marker of therapeutic efficacy in brain tumors. J Natl Cancer Inst 2000;92(24):2032; with permission.)

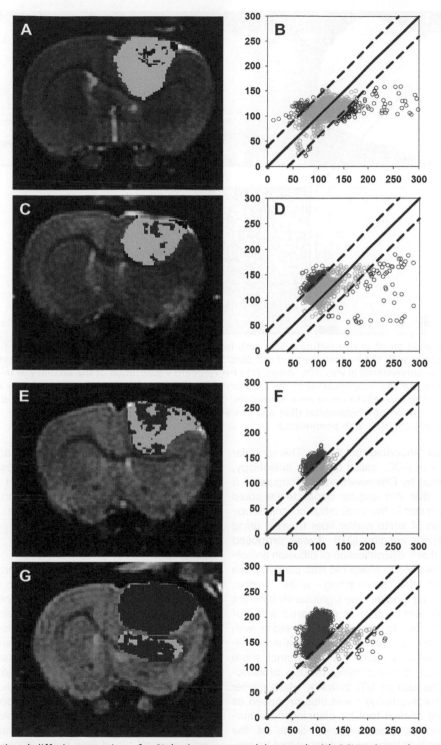

Fig. 3. Functional diffusion mapping of a 9L brain tumor model treated with BCNU chemotherapy. The panel shows examples of fDM maps and corresponding fDM plots following a 0.0 (*A, B*), 0.5 (*C, D*), 1.0 (*D, E*), and 2.0 × LD$_{10}$ (*F, G*) doses of BCNU. These results showed the quantitative nature of diffusion MRI because a dose-dependent increase in tumor cell kill correlated with an increase in the number of voxels that had positive change in diffusion (*red*) compared with pretreatment values (*H*). (*From* Moffat BA, Chenevert TL, Meyer CR, et al. The functional diffusion map: an imaging biomarker for the early prediction of cancer treatment outcome. Neoplasia 2006;8(4):262; with permission.)

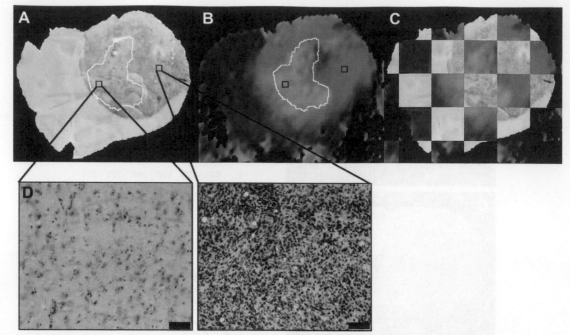

Fig. 4. Coregistration of in vivo diffusion MRI with histology, showing that the heterogeneity of ADC within tumors correlates with the heterogeneity of cell density. (*A*) Hematoxylin-eosin, original magnification ×10 (*B*) Corresponding coregistered in vivo ADC image. (*C*) Checkerboard visualization of the accuracy of the coregistration procedure. (*D*) 40× magnification of the same histology slide showing that the hyper intense ADC regions correspond to the low cellular dense necrotic regions. (*From* Meyer CR, Moffat BA, Kuszpit KK, et al. A methodology for registration of a histological slide and in vivo MRI volume based on optimizing mutual information. Mol Imaging 2006;5(1):22; with permission.)

the diffusion encoding gradients. This angular dependence of ADC, called diffusion anisotropy, was quantified by Chenevert and colleagues.[25] It was shown that this angular dependence could be used to quantify the local diffusion anisotropy and direction of white matter fiber tracts[38] using diffusion tensor imaging (DTI). It was proposed and shown that[39] quantification of diffusion anisotropy could be used to image the infiltration of brain tumors into the surrounding white matter. Although rodent models have significantly different white matter architecture as compared with humans, the ability to correlate DTI metrics with histopathology in these models is essential for validation and determination of which metrics more closely reflect the underlying cellular architecture.[40–42] The use of DTI to track white matter fibers (DTI tractography)[43] was also proposed as an important clinical tool for planning neurosurgical procedures near eloquent areas of the brain.[30] If this is to become a validated tool for presurgical and/or intraoperative planning of tumor resection, then correlation with histopathology and cortical stimulation is imperative. Although cortical stimulation experiments can be performed in clinical studies, rodent imaging is being used to correlate DTI tractography with histopatholgy.[44]

This study by Asunama and colleagues[44] has shown that although tractography does not necessarily provide an accurate neuronal fiber map, tractography does reflect the direction and neural connections around invading gliomas.

PERFUSION MRI

The abnormal vascular microenvironment, which includes a compromised blood-brain barrier, hypervascular proliferation, and tumor cell invasiveness, is a hallmark of malignant brain tumors.[45] Vascular recruitment and neoangiogenesis is thought to be integral to the malignant nature of high-grade primary gliomas and metastatic brain tumors. Strictly speaking, perfusion imaging should be defined as an imaging technique for acquiring spatial maps of tissue blood flow per unit of tissue mass. However, perfusion MRI has become synonymous with quantification of not only cerebral blood flow but also cerebral blood volume (CBV) and blood vessel permeability (K_{trans}). Each of these perfusion parameters was proposed for some time as an important imaging biomarker that may enable noninvasive imaging of tumor malignancy and tumor progression and for quantification of therapeutic efficacy of

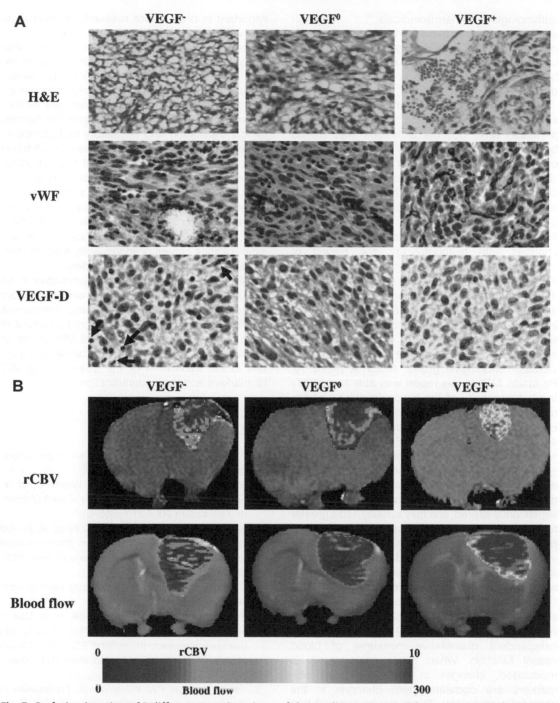

Fig. 5. Perfusion imaging of 3 different genetic variants of the 9L gliosarcoma model. Tumor xenografts of VEGF-A overexpressing (VEGF⁺), underexpressing (VEGF⁻), and wild-type (VEGF⁰) 9L gliosarcoma cells were resected and histologically analyzed. (*A*) Hematoxylin-eosin (H&E), immunohistochemically stained for von Willebrand factor (vWF) and vascular growth factor-D (VEGF-D). (*B*) Tumor-specific perfusion was determined using MRI. Regional CBV (rCBV) and blood flow were calculated and presented as heat maps. Although suppression of VEGF-A production in the VEGF⁻ tumors slowed tumor growth initially, blood flow was higher and blood volume was similar to tumors with wild-type expression of VEGF-A. These studies led to the identification of VEGF-D overexpression in the VEGF⁻ tumors that resulted in restoration of angiogenic activity. (*From* Moffat BA, Chen M, Kariaapper MS, et al. Inhibition of vascular endothelial growth factor (VEGF)-A causes a paradoxical increase in tumor blood flow and up-regulation of VEGF-D. Clin Cancer Res 2006;12(5):1529; with permission.)

antiangiogenic pharmaceuticals.[46,47] Although studies correlating these perfusion metrics with outcome are obviously important for clinical translation,[48] much of the current understanding of the biologic basis of changes in tumor perfusion is derived from rodent studies.

The ability to quantify perfusion using ^{133}Xe single-photon emission tomography predates perfusion MRI, but the technique was limited because of a significantly lower resolution compared with MRI. Steen and colleagues[49] showed that blood flow to tumors became less efficient with increasing tumor size and level of edematous tissue. This work was later replicated using a perfusion MRI technique to quantify blood flow.[50] Apart from the ability to correlate resulting changes with histopathology, the benefit of studying perfusion MRI in rodent brain tumor models is that it is now possible to systematically alter the expression of key vascular growth factors and thereby provide a unique insight into changes in perfusion induced during tumor neoangiogenesis. In a 2006 study,[51] the 9L gliosarcoma model was genetically altered to over- and underexpress vascular endothelial growth factor A (VEGF-A). Perfusion MRI of this model was able to quantify the heterogeneity of the tumor vascular environment, which was histopathologically validated. Histopathologically confirmed perfusion MRI shows that although VEGF-A overexpressing tumors had an expected increase in vascular volume and blood flow, tumors in which VEGF-A expression was inhibited had an initial lag in tumor growth but ultimately their vascular volume was not significantly altered, and they actually had a greater tumor blood flow (Fig. 5). These model systems provided a unique insight into the concept of vascular normalization and led to the identification of alternate vascular growth factors that compensate for the loss of VEGF-A expression.

Perfusion MRI of rodent brain tumor models shows that the different perfusion metrics of blood volume, flow, and permeability provide unique and independent quantitative measures of blood vessel function. When tumor angiogenesis is modulated, changes in these perfusion biomarkers are correlated with changes in the vascular morphology. These results suggest that perfusion MRI may provide important reproducible endpoints for evaluating the effect of antiangiogenic or antivascular therapies on blood vessel function.

SUMMARY

The use of advanced MRI biomarkers such as spectroscopy, diffusion, and perfusion are vitally important in brain tumor research, as they allow for noninvasive, 3-dimensional quantification of important molecular and cellular phenomena without the use of ionizing radiation. The noninvasiveness of these techniques allows for ethical repeat measurements to assess therapeutic response in clinical trials of new therapies without adverse effects on patients. Despite this benefit, clinical translation and regulatory acceptance of these techniques require a process of validation as a surrogate endpoint. Part of this validation process requires scientific evidence of a clear biologic link between the biomarkers and the biologic phenomena that they are supposed to measure. This evidence is almost impossible to obtain clinically, and as such, what is known about these biologic linkages comes predominantly from imaging studies of animal brain tumor models.

Although this article was not exhaustive in its discussion of all MRI biomarkers and the authors cannot fully predict which of these biomarkers will find application in the clinical management of brain tumors, it clearly shows that MRI of animal models is and will for some time be vitally important in the translation of the ever-evolving MRI biomarkers and their quantification.

REFERENCES

1. Young GS. Advanced MRI of adult brain tumors. Neurol Clin 2007;25(4):947–73, viii.
2. Jenkinson MD, Du Plessis DG, Walker C, et al. Advanced MRI in the management of adult gliomas. Br J Neurosurg 2007;21(6):550–61.
3. Rudin M, Beckmann N, Porszasz R, et al. In vivo magnetic resonance methods in pharmaceutical research: current status and perspectives. NMR Biomed 1999;12(2):69–97.
4. Galbraith SM. MR in oncology drug development. NMR Biomed 2006;19(6):681–9.
5. Ross BD, Chenevert TL, Moffat BA, et al. Use of Magnetic Resonance Imaging (MRI) for evaluation treatment response. In: Holland EC, editor. Mouse models of human cancer. Hoboken (NJ): Wiley-Liss; 2004. p. 377–90.
6. Koo V, Hamilton PW, Williamson K. Noninvasive in vivo imaging in small animal research. Cell Oncol 2006;28(4):127–39.
7. Evelhoch J, Garwood M, Vigneron D, et al. Expanding the use of magnetic resonance in the assessment of tumor response to therapy: workshop report. Cancer Res 2005;65(16):7041–4.
8. Padhani AR, Liu G, Koh DM, et al. Diffusion-weighted magnetic resonance imaging as a cancer biomarker: consensus and recommendations. Neoplasia 2009;11(2):102–25.

9. Frey HE, Knispel RR, Kruuv J, et al. Proton spin-lattice relaxation studies of nonmalignant tissues of tumorous mice. J Natl Cancer Inst 1972;49(3):903–6.

10. Hawkes RC, Holland GN, Moore WS, et al. Nuclear magnetic resonance (NMR) tomography of the brain: a preliminary clinical assessment with demonstration of pathology. J Comput Assist Tomogr 1980; 4(5):577–86.

11. Katz R. Biomarkers and surrogate markers: an FDA perspective. NeuroRx 2004;1(2):189–95.

12. Kelloff GJ, Sigman CC. New science-based endpoints to accelerate oncology drug development. Eur J Cancer 2005;41(4):491–501.

13. Aisen AM, Chenevert TL. MR spectroscopy: clinical perspective. Radiology 1989;173(3):593–9.

14. Chapman JD. The detection and measurement of hypoxic cells in solid tumors. Cancer 1984;54(11): 2441–9.

15. Evanochko WT, Ng TC, Glickson JD. Application of in vivo NMR spectroscopy to cancer. Magn Reson Med 1984;1(4):508–34.

16. Koeze TH, Lantos PL, Iles RA, et al. In vivo nuclear magnetic resonance spectroscopy of a transplanted brain tumour. Br J Cancer 1984;49(3):357–61.

17. Bruhn H, Frahm J, Gyngell ML, et al. Noninvasive differentiation of tumors with use of localized H-1 MR spectroscopy in vivo: initial experience in patients with cerebral tumors. Radiology 1989;172(2):541–8.

18. Remy C, Von Kienlin M, Lotito S, et al. In vivo 1H NMR spectroscopy of an intracerebral glioma in the rat. Magn Reson Med 1989;9(3):395–401.

19. Pfeuffer J, Lin JC, Delabarre L, et al. Detection of intracellular lactate with localized diffusion {1H-13C}-spectroscopy in rat glioma in vivo. J Magn Reson 2005;177(1):129–38.

20. Demaerel P, Johannik K, Van Hecke P, et al. Localized 1H NMR spectroscopy in fifty cases of newly diagnosed intracranial tumors. J Comput Assist Tomogr 1991;15(1):67–76.

21. van Vaals JJ, Bergman AH, van den Boogert HJ, et al. Non-invasive in vivo localized 1H spectroscopy of human astrocytoma implanted in rat brain: regional differences followed in time. NMR Biomed 1991;4(3):125–32.

22. Gyngell ML, Hoehn-Berlage M, Kloiber O, et al. Localized proton NMR spectroscopy of experimental gliomas in rat brain in vivo. NMR Biomed 1992;5(6):335–40.

23. Ross BD, Merkle H, Hendrich K, et al. Spatially localized in vivo 1H magnetic resonance spectroscopy of an intracerebral rat glioma. Magn Reson Med 1992; 23(1):96–108.

24. Gyngell ML, Els T, Hoehn-Berlage M, et al. Proton MR spectroscopy of experimental brain tumors in vivo. Acta Neurochir Suppl (Wien) 1994;60:350–2.

25. Chenevert TL, Brunberg JA, Pipe JG. Anisotropic diffusion in human white matter: demonstration with

26. Chenevert TL, Meyer CR, Moffat BA, et al. Diffusion MRI: a new strategy for assessment of cancer therapeutic efficacy. Mol Imaging 2002;1(4):336–43.

27. Price SJ, Burnet NG, Donovan T, et al. Diffusion tensor imaging of brain tumours at 3T: a potential tool for assessing white matter tract invasion? Clin Radiol 2003;58(6):455–62.

28. Lu S, Ahn D, Johnson G, et al. Diffusion-tensor MR imaging of intracranial neoplasia and associated peritumoral edema: introduction of the tumor infiltration index. Radiology 2004;232(1):221–8.

29. Wang W, Steward CE, Desmond PM. Diffusion tensor imaging in glioblastoma multiforme and brain metastases: the role of p, q, L, and fractional anisotropy. AJNR Am J Neuroradiol 2009;30(1):203–8.

30. Holodny AI, Ollenschlager M. Diffusion imaging in brain tumors. Neuroimaging Clin N Am 2002;12(1): 107–24, x.

31. Chenevert TL, Sundgren PC, Ross BD. Diffusion imaging: insight to cell status and cytoarchitecture. Neuroimaging Clin N Am 2006;16(4): 619–32, viii–ix.

32. Ross BD, Chenevert TL, Kim B, et al. Magnetic resonance imaging and spectroscopy: application to experimental neuro-oncology. Quart Magn Reson Biol Med Phys 1994;1:89–106.

33. Chenevert TL, McKeever PE, Ross BD. Monitoring early response of experimental brain tumors to therapy using diffusion magnetic resonance imaging. Clin Cancer Res 1997;3(9):1457–66.

34. Chenevert TL, Stegman LD, Taylor JM, et al. Diffusion magnetic resonance imaging: an early surrogate marker of therapeutic efficacy in brain tumors. J Natl Cancer Inst 2000;92(24):2029–36.

35. Moffat BA, Chenevert TL, Lawrence TS, et al. Functional diffusion map: a noninvasive MRI biomarker for early stratification of clinical brain tumor response. Proc Natl Acad Sci U S A 2005;102(15):5524–9.

36. Moffat BA, Chenevert TL, Meyer CR, et al. The functional diffusion map: an imaging biomarker for the early prediction of cancer treatment outcome. Neoplasia 2006;8(4):259–67.

37. Meyer CR, Moffat BA, Kuszpit KK, et al. A methodology for registration of a histological slide and in vivo MRI volume based on optimizing mutual information. Mol Imaging 2006;5(1):16–23.

38. Basser PJ, Mattiello J, LeBihan D. Estimation of the effective self-diffusion tensor from the NMR spin echo. J Magn Reson B 1994;103(3):247–54.

39. Brunberg JA, Chenevert TL, McKeever PE, et al. In vivo MR determination of water diffusion coefficients and diffusion anisotropy: correlation with structural alteration in gliomas of the cerebral hemispheres. AJNR Am J Neuroradiol 1995;16(2): 361–71.

MR techniques in vivo. Radiology 1990;177(2): 401–5.

40. Inglis BA, Neubauer D, Yang L, et al. Diffusion tensor MR imaging and comparative histology of glioma engrafted in the rat spinal cord. AJNR Am J Neuroradiol 1999;20(4):713–6.

41. Kim S, Pickup S, Hsu O, et al. Diffusion tensor MRI in rat models of invasive and well-demarcated brain tumors. NMR Biomed 2008;21(3):208–16.

42. Lope-Piedrafita S, Garcia-Martin ML, Galons JP, et al. Longitudinal diffusion tensor imaging in a rat brain glioma model. NMR Biomed 2008;21(8): 799–808.

43. Basser PJ, Pajevic S, Pierpaoli C, et al. In vivo fiber tractography using DT-MRI data. Magn Reson Med 2000;44(4):625–32.

44. Asanuma T, Doblas S, Tesiram YA, et al. Diffusion tensor imaging and fiber tractography of C6 rat glioma. J Magn Reson Imaging 2008;28(3):566–73.

45. Vajkoczy P, Menger MD. Vascular microenvironment in gliomas. J Neurooncol 2000;50(1-2):99–108.

46. Barrett T, Brechbiel M, Bernardo M, et al. MRI of tumor angiogenesis. J Magn Reson Imaging 2007; 26(2):235–49.

47. Batchelor TT, Sorensen AG, di Tomaso E, et al. AZD2171, a pan-VEGF receptor tyrosine kinase inhibitor, normalizes tumor vasculature and alleviates edema in glioblastoma patients. Cancer Cell 2007;11(1):83–95.

48. Law M, Young RJ, Babb JS, et al. Gliomas: predicting time to progression or survival with cerebral blood volume measurements at dynamic susceptibility-weighted contrast-enhanced perfusion MR imaging. Radiology 2008;247(2):490–8.

49. Steen RG, Kromhout-Schiro S, Graham MM. Relationship of perfusion to edema in the 9L gliosarcoma. J Neurooncol 1993;16(1):81–7.

50. Moffat BA, Chenevert TL, Hall DE, et al. Continuous arterial spin labeling using a train of adiabatic inversion pulses. J Magn Reson Imaging 2005;21(3):290–6.

51. Moffat BA, Chen M, Kariaapper MS, et al. Inhibition of vascular endothelial growth factor (VEGF)-A causes a paradoxical increase in tumor blood flow and up-regulation of VEGF-D. Clin Cancer Res 2006;12(5):1525–32.

Magnetic Resonance Perfusion and Permeability Imaging in Brain Tumors

Saulo Lacerda, MD[a,b,*], Meng Law, MD[c]

KEYWORDS

- MR perfusion • MR permeability • Brain tumors

PATHOPHYSIOLOGY OF BRAIN TUMOR PERFUSION AND VASCULAR PERMEABILITY

The effects of vascular endothelial growth factor/vascular permeability factor (VEGF/VPF) and other growth factors on vascular perfusion and permeability have been under investigation since Folkman first described the association of tumoral growth with angiogenesis.[1] Recent evidence suggests that vascular permeability and the presence of VEGF/VPF are important mediators of tumor growth in addition to angiogenesis.[2–5] Perfusion and permeability magnetic resonance (MR) imaging can now measure parameters such as cerebral blood volume (CBV) and vascular permeability (K^{trans}), which can be directly correlated with these histopathologic changes as well as molecular markers such as VEGF.[6–9]

There are several reasons for an increase in regional CBV (rCBV) in gliomas. First, gradient-echo sequences exploit the local paramagnetic susceptibility within the vessel lumen, the vessel wall, and surrounding tissues, resulting in intra- and extravascular spins undergoing reduction of T2* signal.[10] Second, pathologic molecular stains such as CD34 demonstrate an increase in the number of tortuous angiogenic vessels, giving the analogy of a "swamp" of numerous, small slow-flowing vessels. This factor is important, as

antiangiogenic therapy has been shown to "normalize" these vessels, increasing the diameter and thereby increasing cerebral blood flow (CBF) and decreasing CBV (due to a decrease in overall vessel density); this is further discussed later in this article. In view of this, it is not surprising that rCBV measurements have been shown to correlate reliably with tumor grade and histologic findings of increased tumor vascularity.[11–24] The degree of vascular proliferation is one of the most critical elements in the histopathologic characterization of tumor biology and determination of prognosis for several reasons. First, the degree of vascular proliferation, or angiogenesis, is one of the most important histologic criteria (along with cellularity, mitosis, pleomorphism, and necrosis) for determination of the degree of malignancy and grade of a glioma. Second, vascular networks are not only the principal route for delivery of oxygen and nutrients to the neoplastic cells but also serve as paths for tumor infiltration along perivascular spaces. Third, the cerebral capillary endothelium (site of the blood-brain barrier, which is composed of a continuous homogeneous basement membrane, numerous astrocytic processes, and tight junctions, and is an important host defense mechanism responsible for the regulation of movement of molecules) is frequently destroyed by malignant tumor cells. Fourth,

[a] Department of Radiology, Mount Sinai Medical Center, One Gustave L Levy Place, Box 1234, 1190 Fifth Avenue, New York, NY 10029, USA
[b] MedImagem-Hospital Beneficencia Portuguesa, Sao Paulo, SP, Brazil
[c] USC Medical Center and LA County Hospitals, Keck School of Medicine, 1500 San Pablo St, Los Angeles, CA 90033, USA
* Corresponding author. Department of Radiology, Mount Sinai Medical Center, One Gustave L Levy Place, Box 1234, 1190 Fifth Avenue, New York, NY 10029.
E-mail address: saulolacerda@hotmail.com (S. Lacerda).

Neuroimag Clin N Am 19 (2009) 527–557
doi:10.1016/j.nic.2009.08.007
1052-5149/09/$ – see front matter © 2009 Elsevier Inc. All rights reserved.

a hyperpermeable blood-brain barrier associated with or without immature angiogenic vessels allows for contrast agent enhancement, extravasation and, hence, measurement of vascular permeability.

These pathophysiologic changes have been shown to provide good correlation between tumor biology and rCBV, CBF, CBV K^{trans}, and V_p measurements. Due to an increase in CBV from microvascular density, as well as many collateral and tortuous vessels (from angiogenesis), it is felt that the mean transit time (MTT) should be prolonged. However, because of the immense heterogeneity of the tumor microvasculature in some regions, MTT may also decrease due to increased CBF, particularly at the tumor margins, where there is rapid shunting of blood flow.[25]

IMAGING TECHNIQUES, PULSE SEQUENCES, PERFUSION MODELS, TECHNICAL PITFALLS, ARTIFACTS, AND LIMITATIONS

The 2 major techniques currently used in both the clinical and research settings are a T1-weighted steady-state dynamic contrast-enhanced MR imaging (DCE MR imaging) method and a T2*-weighted first-pass, dynamic susceptibility contrast-enhanced perfusion MR imaging (DSC MR imaging) method. The advantages and disadvantages of each technique with regard to characterizing tumor biology are discussed here; however, most clinicians and investigators are currently using the DSC MR imaging T2*-weighted technique for brain tumor perfusion MR imaging.

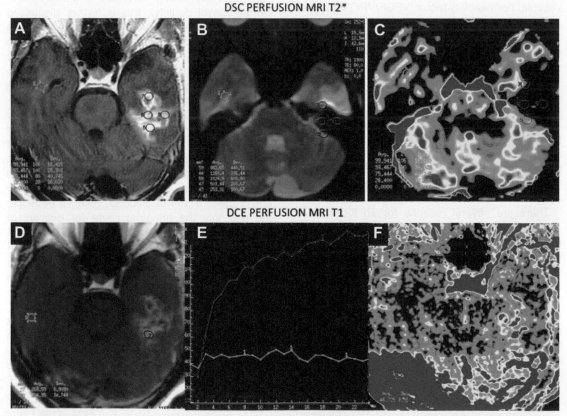

Fig. 1. Heterogeneously enhancing left temporal high-grade glioma (HGG) in a 50-year-old man. (A) Axial T1-weighted image shows an enhancing mass in the left temporal region. (B) Gradient-echo acquisition image shows the proximity of the lesion to the skull base. (C) The DSC MR imaging rCBV color overlay demonstrates apparent no increase in rCBV. (D and E) DCE MR imaging T1 permeability map demonstrates increased vascular permeability, characterized by a very rapid initial increase in the permeability curve. (F) DCE MR imaging T1 steady-state permeability color overlay again demonstrates increased permeability. This case exemplifies a situation whereby spin-echo T1 perfusion can be better than gradient-echo T2* perfusion studies in lesions at the skull base, calvaria, or osseous structures. The fast or turbo spin-echo T1-weighted DCE MR imaging has considerably less susceptibility than the gradient-echo/EPI T2*-weighted DSC MR imaging.

DYNAMIC SUSCEPTIBILITY CONTRAST T2* PERFUSION MR IMAGING

The most common methods for measurement of DSC MR imaging metrics in brain tumors are the indicator dilution methods for nondiffusible tracers[26] and the pharmacokinetic modeling approach developed by Tofts and Kermode.[27–29] In DSC MR imaging, the signal measured is due to the susceptibility T2 or T2* effect induced by the injected contrast agent.

INDICATOR DILUTION THEORY

The theory of nondiffusible tracer kinetics can be used to derive CBV values from the concentration-time curves. On injection of a contrast agent (gadopentetate dimeglumine), a signal intensity versus time curve is obtained. CBV is proportional to the area under the contrast agent concentration, signal intensity-time curve, in the absence of recirculation and contrast leakage. The gadopentetate dimeglumine concentration is proportional to the change in relaxation rate (ie, change in the reciprocal of T2* [$\Delta R2^*$]), which can be calculated from the signal by using the following equation: $\Delta R2^* = [-\ln(SI_t/SI_0)/TE]$, where SI_t is the pixel signal intensity at time t, SI_0 is the precontrast signal intensity, and TE is the echo time.[30] This equation is valid only if T1 enhancement associated with blood-brain barrier disruption has a negligible effect on signal intensity.

SEQUENCE CONSIDERATION: SPIN-ECHO VERSUS GRADIENT-ECHO DSC PERFUSION MR IMAGING

Gradient-echo sequences are much more sensitive in detecting paramagnetic changes in local

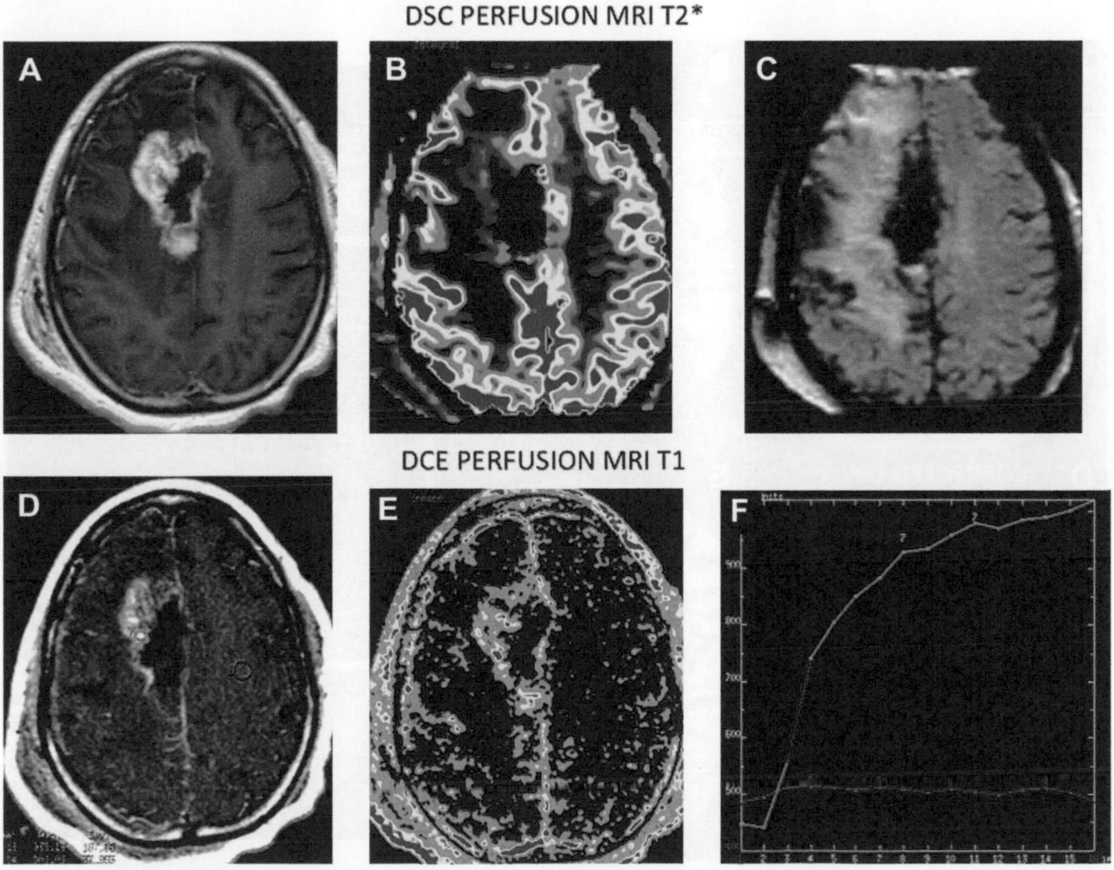

DSC PERFUSION MRI T2*

DCE PERFUSION MRI T1

Fig. 2. Recurrent right frontal GBM. (*A*) Axial T1-weighted postcontrast image shows an enhancing heterogeneous lesion around the surgical cavity in the right frontal lobe. (*B*) DSC MR imaging rCBV color overlay demonstrates no increase in rCBV. (*C*) The DSC MR imaging T2* signal acquisition image demonstrates significant artifact from blood products. (*D–F*) DCE MR imaging T1 permeability color map and permeability intensity curve demonstrate increased vascular permeability. Again this case demonstrates a situation whereby T1 perfusion might be better than T2*-weighted studies. It is well known that the blood products can interfere in the estimation of CBV values as well as the appearance of the rCBV maps.

magnetic susceptibility between vessels and the surrounding tissue, resulting in intra- and extravascular spins undergoing a reduction of T2*. The passage of gadolinium through the microvasculature results in changes in both T2 and T2* so that both spin-echo and gradient-echo sequences will provide reliable and reproducible CBV measurements.

The advantages of using spin-echo sequences include less susceptibility to artifacts, particularly near the skull base or at brain-bone-air interfaces, and the increased sensitivity to spin-echo perfusion to contrast within the capillaries.[11,12] It has been demonstrated that spin-echo sequences are mainly sensitive to smaller vessels (<20 μm) and hence may provide more optimal imaging of tumor capillaries. However, gradient-echo sequences seem to be sensitive to both capillary and larger-vessel perfusion.[14,31] At

most institutions, echo-planar gradient-echo imaging provides excellent signal to noise using a standard dose of contrast (0.1 mmol per kilogram of body weight, typically 20 mL of contrast) for brain tumor perfusion studies. Susceptibility artifact can be reduced by reducing slice thickness.[14,32] The degree of susceptibility effect using 0.1 mmol/kg of gadolinium with gradient-echo sequences is similar in magnitude to using 0.2 mmol/kg with spin-echo sequences.[11] With echo-planar imaging, a new parallel imaging technique, whole brain coverage at 1-second intervals can be achieved using both rapid gradient-echo and spin-echo techniques. Combined spin-echo and gradient-echo techniques can be performed,[33] and this combination can also be used to determine vascular diameter or size, which is important when monitoring antiangiogenic therapy.[34]

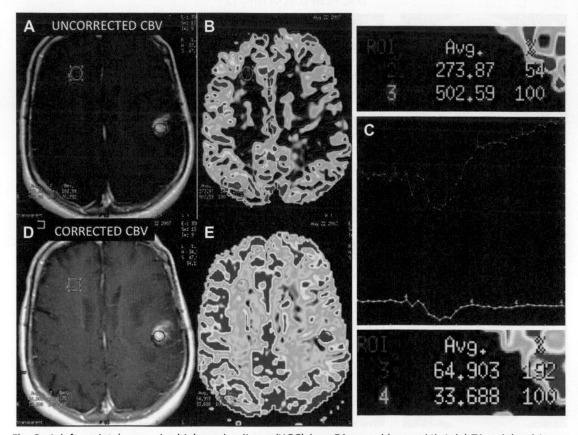

Fig. 3. A left parietal opercular high-grade glioma (HGG) in a 54-year-old man. (A) Axial T1-weighted image shows an enhancing mass in the left parietal opercular region. (B) DSC MR imaging uncorrected rCBV color overlay demonstrating "reduced" rCBV. (C) The DSC MR imaging T2* signal intensity curve demonstrates increased leakiness manifest as an exaggerated T1 effect (signal overshooting the baseline) of gadolinium resulting in underestimation of the rCBV. (D and E) This underestimation can be corrected by preloading with contrast as well as applying baseline correction or gamma variate fit, which will produce corrected rCBV maps providing a more accurate estimation of rCBV.

FIRST-PASS T2* DSC MR IMAGING VERSUS STEADY-STATE T1 DCE MR IMAGING (COMBINED APPROACH)

First-pass pharmacokinetic modeling (FPPM) is used to calculate vascular permeability (K^{trans}) from the same DSC MR imaging data used to calculate rCBV. FPPM uses an exact expression for tissue contrast concentration, assuming that contrast exists in 2 interchanging compartments (plasma and extravascular, extracellular space).[28,29]

Due to the complexity of angiogenesis, the accuracy and reproducibility of different perfusion MR imaging techniques for the measurement of vascular permeability has been under discussion recently. The primary issues are that vascular permeability may be "non–flow limited" or "flow limited"[35] and that the first pass of contrast measures only the permeability in the first pass, which is likely to be different to permeability measured in the steady state, where measurement of bidirectional exchange between 2 interchanging compartments (plasma and extravascular, extracellular space) can be characterized.

Cha and colleagues[36] recently compared vascular permeability measurements, K^{trans} using steady-state T1-weighted (ssT1) with a first-pass T2*-weighted (fpT2*) MR imaging methods in gliomas and meningiomas. The fpT2* K^{trans} was highly correlated with ssT1 K^{trans} in gliomas but not in meningiomas.

Further investigation is likely to demonstrate that there are likely to be 2 types of vascular permeability, very high vascular permeability (which is flow related and can be characterized in the first pass) versus steady-state permeability (which is not necessarily flow limited and more proportional to the surface area product), which may be characterized using steady-state techniques. As a result, some centers, including the authors', are using both ssT1 and fpT2* methods for obtaining perfusion metrics in gliomas.[37] Indeed, there are some inherent advantages to T1 techniques for obtaining perfusion and permeability metrics, such as the ability to estimate fractional blood volume or CBV in the setting of susceptibility from postsurgical blood products or lesions in the temporal lobes or skull base. Three-dimensional T1-weighted dynamic sequences and novel

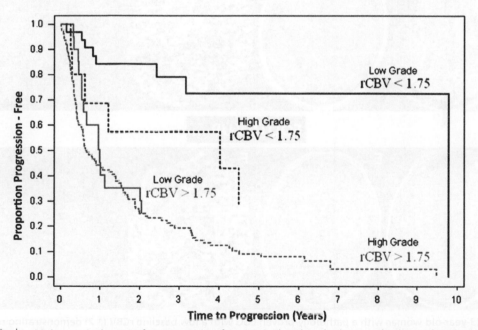

Fig. 4. Kaplan-Meier survival curves for progression-free survival within the low-grade glioma (LGG) group with (rCBV <1.75) and (rCBV >1.75) rCBV groups (*solid lines*) demonstrating a significant difference in time to progression in LGGs stratified by rCBV alone (*P*<.0001). When comparing HGGs (*broken lines*), similarly there was a significant difference in progression in HGGs with high (rCBV >1.75) versus low rCBV (*P*<.0001). Among subjects with low rCBV (rCBV <1.75) there was a significant difference between high- and low-grade tumors with respect to progression-free survival (*P* = .047). However, among subjects with high rCBV (rCBV >1.75), time to progression was not significantly different (*P* = .266) for low- and high-grade tumors. (*From* Law M, Yang S, Babb JS, et al. Comparison of cerebral blood volume and vascular permeability from dynamic susceptibility contrast-enhanced perfusion MR imaging with glioma grade. AJNR Am J Neuroradiol 2004;25(5):746–55; with permission.)

techniques using iterative analysis to estimate permeability and perfusion have been demonstrated.[38,39]

TECHNICAL PITFALLS AND LIMITATIONS

Even though DSC MR imaging is the most commonly used and easily applied technique for studying brain tumor perfusion, there are several important limitations with using a gradient-echo sequence.[40] First, because the technique is weighted to measure susceptibility, it is extremely sensitive to structures of lesions that cause magnetic field inhomogeneity such as blood products, calcium, bone, melanin, metals, or lesions near the brain-bone-air interface, such as the skull base (**Figs. 1** and **2**).

Solutions to reduce the inhomogeneity and susceptibility include decreasing the slice thickness, which also reduces the signal to noise ratio (SNR) and slice coverage. Parallel imaging methods can also reduce both susceptibility and the scan time to allow for more brain coverage and SNR. If there is a larger lesion that requires increased brain coverage, then the interslice gap can be increased while maintaining thinner slices to reduce susceptibility. Second, as discussed earlier, the quantification of perfusion metrics such as CBV and K^{trans} can be inaccurate in lesions where there is a very leaky blood-brain barrier, such as glioblastoma multiforme, choroid plexus tumors, and meningiomas. Therefore, extremely low or high perfusion values must taken with caution. Correction algorithms can be applied to

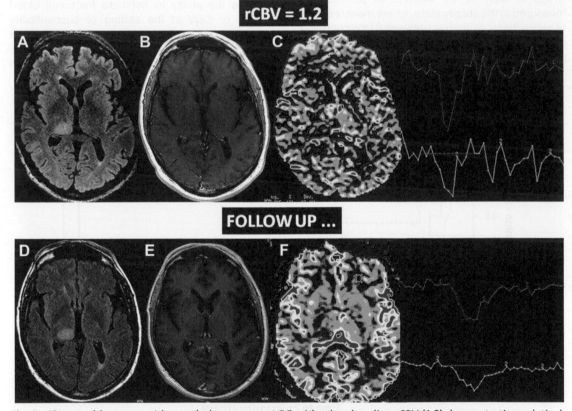

Fig. 5. 43-year-old woman with a pathology-proven LGG with a low baseline rCBV (1.2) demonstrating relatively stable disease. (*Top row*) (*A*) Axial fluid-attenuated inversion recovery (FLAIR) shows increased signal involving the right posterior thalamus/pulvinar, in keeping with an LGG. (*B*) Contrast-enhanced axial T1-weighted image demonstrates no contrast enhancement in the right thalamus. (*C*) DSC MR imaging image with rCBV color overlay map shows a lesion with low initial perfusion with a rCBV of 1.2, in keeping with an LGG. The T2* signal intensity curve (*purple*) confirms the lack of increased perfusion compared with the contralateral white matter (*green curve*). (*Bottom row*) MR imaging at 6 months' follow-up. (*D*) Axial FLAIR image demonstrates no interval change confirming a true LGG. (*E*) Contrast-enhanced axial T1-weighted image demonstrates no contrast enhancement. (*F*) Gradient-echo axial DSC MR imaging image with rCBV color overlay map shows a lesion with low perfusion with an rCBV of 1.2, in keeping with an LGG.

compensate for leakiness.[41] When confined to the intravascular space, paramagnetic contrast agents produce low signal intensity on T2-weighted scans that occur over a dynamic first-pass injection. However, because gadolinium/diethylenetriamine pentaacetic acid (Gd-DTPA) is also an effective T1 relaxation enhancer, the susceptibility contrast signal intensity loss can be masked by signal intensity increase in regions where T1 effects are significant. This situation occurs in enhancing tumors, where Gd-DTPA extravasates into the interstitial space of lesions with significant blood-brain barrier breakdown. In such instances, rCBV will be underestimated, which may affect tumor grade prediction (Fig. 3). Preloading with a small dose of contrast (which can also serve to produce T1 steady-state permeability maps) along with gamma

variate, and linear fitting and baseline correction to correct for this leakage will improve accuracy of rCBV estimations. Extreme tumor leakiness can cause rCBV to be greatly underestimated or overestimated using DSC MR imaging techniques. This divergence will impact on the qualitative appearance of rCBV maps and the estimation of rCBV. Paulson and Schmainda[42] recently demonstrated the importance of preloading with a small dose of gadolinium to reduce the error caused by extremely leaky lesions. As a result, at the authors' institution 2 separate injections are performed. A smaller initial injection of 5 to 7 mL of gadolinium also acquires T1 steady-state DCE MR imaging permeability data; this also serves as a preloading dose for the second injection whereby the DSC MR imaging perfusion data are acquired.

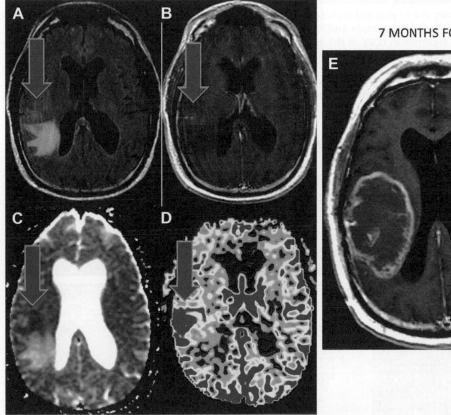

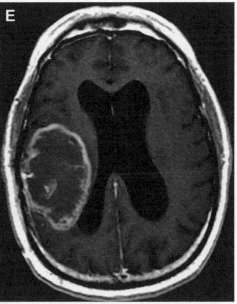

7 MONTHS FOLLOW-UP

Fig. 6. 62-year-old man with pathology-proven low-grade astrocytoma with a high baseline rCBV (3.2). (A) Axial FLAIR image shows increased signal intensity tumor in the right parietal opercular region, surrounded by moderate amount of infiltrating and vasogenic edema. (B) Contrast-enhanced axial T1-weighted image demonstrates no clear region of enhancement within the tumor. (C) Apparent diffusion coefficient (ADC) maps demonstrate diffusion restriction within the lesion, suggesting hypercellularity. (D) Gradient-echo axial DSC MR imaging image with rCBV color overlay map shows a lesion with high initial perfusion with a rCBV of 3.2, more in keeping with an HGG than an LGG. Note the excellent correlation between the ADC values and the hyperperfusing region. (E) MR imaging at 7 months' follow-up. Axial postcontrast T1-weighted image shows a substantial increase in enhancing tumor volume, again in keeping with an HGG and not an LGG. These images indicate that pathology can sometimes underestimate tumor biology.

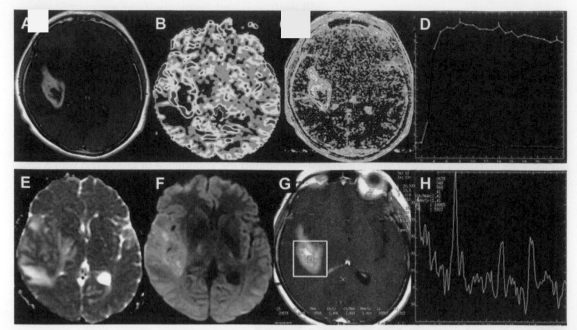

Fig. 7. High-grade tumor in a 67-year-old man. (*A*) Axial postcontrast T1-weighted image shows a predominantly peripheral enhancing lesion in the insula and right temporal region. (*B*) DSC MR imaging T2* perfusion color overlay demonstrates elevation in rCBV in the enhancing component of the lesion. (*C* and *D*) DCE MR imaging T1 steady-state permeability color maps and curve demonstrate a very rapid initial increase in permeability, compatible with a high-grade tumor. (*E* and *F*) ADC maps and axial diffusion-weighted imaging demonstrate diffusion restriction within the lesion, in keeping with very cellular tumors. (*G* and *H*) Spectroscopy of the lesion demonstrates high levels of choline, reduced *N*-acetylaspartate (NAA), and moderate increase in LI/LAC (lipid and lactate) levels.

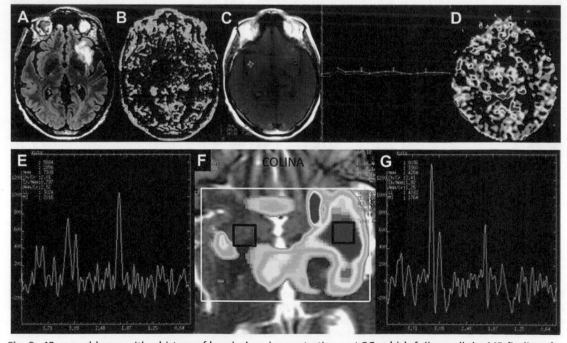

Fig. 8. 48-year-old man with a history of headaches demonstrating an LGG, which follows all the MR findings for an LGG. (*A*) Axial FLAIR image demonstrates a hyperintense left insula tumor. (*B* and *C*) Spin-echo DCE T1 MR imaging shows a decrease in vascular permeability. (*D*) Gradient-echo axial DSC T2* MR imaging with rCBV color overlay demonstrates reduced relative cerebral blood volume within the lesion. (*E–G*) MR spectroscopy demonstrates only mild increase in the choline when the choline is compared with the contralateral normal brain and reduced levels of NAA, in keeping with LGG.

CLINICAL APPLICATIONS OF PERFUSION MR
Primary Gliomas

Histologic grading limitations with neuropathology and World Health Organization classification in measuring tumor angiogenesis with CBV, CBF, and permeability

The existence of multiple approaches to pathologic classification of human glioma implies that there is a lack of consensus among experts as to which is the single best approach.[43-48] These multiple grading systems do, however, agree on the histologic parameters that are important in the determination of glioma biology, namely hypercellularity, pleomorphism, vascular endothelial proliferation, mitotic activity, and necrosis.

There have been numerous publications demonstrating the relatively low reproducibility of this system. Coons and colleagues[49] demonstrated that 4-observer concordance is 52%, 3-observer concordance is 60%, and after 3 common reviews and agreement on pathologic features, the 4-observer concordance improved minimally to 69% and 3-observer concordance to 75%. Furthermore, there are other issues affecting pathologic reproducibility that must also to be considered. (1) Because only a few small samples of tissue are assessed, particularly from stereotactic biopsy, the most malignant portion of a tumor may not be sampled. (2) It may be difficult to obtain a range of samples if the tumor is inaccessible to the surgeon (in eloquent brain). (3) There are numerous classification/grading systems used between different institutions. (4) The dynamic nature of central nervous system (CNS) tumors, with at least 50% dedifferentiating into more malignant grades.[50,51]

Despite these shortcomings, the World Health Organization (WHO) classification scheme remains the standard reference for guiding therapy and predicting prognosis in patients with brain tumors. Law and colleagues[52] recently compared

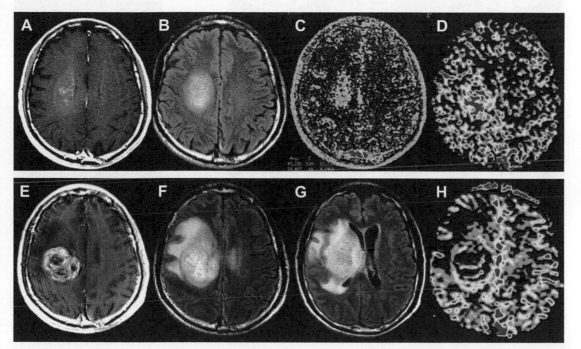

Fig. 9. 53-year-old man with pathology-proven anaplastic oligoastrocytoma with a high baseline rCBV (3.7). (*Top row*) (*A*) Contrast enhanced axial T1-weighted image demonstrates patchy contrast enhancement in the right semi-ovale region. (*B*) Axial FLAIR image shows a hyperintense mass in the right semi-ovale region with mild mass effect. (*C*) Spin-echo DCE MR imaging permeability overlap map demonstrates mild increase in vascular permeability. (*D*) Gradient-echo axial DSC MR imaging image with rCBV color overlay map shows a lesion with high initial perfusion with an rCBV of 3.7, again suggesting a higher-grade glioma. (*Bottom row*) MR imaging at 5 months' follow-up. (*E*) Contrast-enhanced axial T1-weighted image demonstrates markedly increase in enhancing tumor volume. (*F* and *G*) Axial FLAIR image shows a substantial increase in tumor volume and volume of T2 signal abnormality, with significant mass effect and compression of the right lateral ventricle. (*H*) Gradient-echo axial DSC MR imaging image with rCBV color overlay map demonstrates progressively increasing rCBV.

the value of rCBV measurements in predicting tumor biology (**Fig. 4**), using patient outcome as the gold standard. In this study, patients with the histopathologic diagnosis of high-grade gliomas (HGGs) and low-grade gliomas (LGGs) (from stereotactic biopsy and resection) were stratified into 2 groups based on rCBV. The Kaplan-Meier curve demonstrated that progression-free survival within the LGG group with (rCBV <1.75) and (rCBV >1.75) rCBV groups (solid lines in **Fig. 4**) was significantly different (*P*<.0001). When comparing HGGs (broken lines in **Fig. 4**), similarly there was

a significant difference in progression in HGGs with high (rCBV >1.75) versus low rCBV (*P*<.0001). Lesions with low baseline rCBV (<1.75) demonstrated stable tumor volumes when followed over time (**Fig. 5**), and lesions with high baseline rCBV (>1.75) demonstrated progressively increasing tumor volumes over time (**Fig. 6**). These results demonstrate that perhaps rCBV measurements from DSC MR imaging may overcome some of the limitations of the current histologic methods to provide an additional prognostic factor for tumor biology.

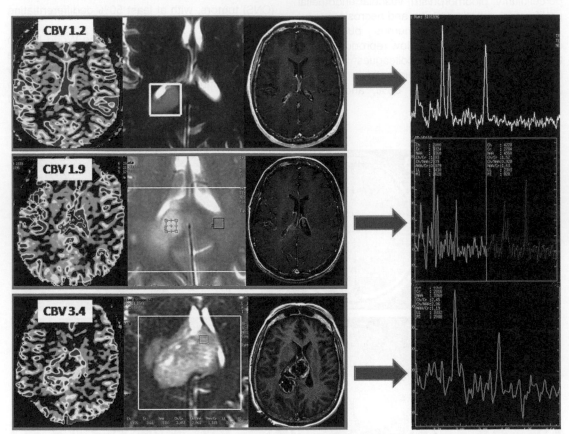

Fig. 10. Tumor progression "the angiogenic switch" demonstrated by DSC MR imaging perfusion maps. (*Top row*) Gradient-echo axial DSC MR imaging image with rCBV color overlay map shows low initial perfusion with a rCBV of 1.2, more in keeping with an LGG than an HGG. Axial FLAIR image shows increased signal within the right splenium of the corpus callosum with some mass effect on the adjacent lateral ventricle. Axial postcontrast T1-weighted image shows no enhancement within the lesion. Spectroscopy of the lesion demonstrates high levels of choline and reduced NAA levels. (*Middle row*) MR imaging at 6 months' follow-up. Gradient-echo axial DSC MR imaging image with rCBV color overlay map shows an increase in rCBV in comparison to the previous examination (1.2–1.9), more in keeping with an HGG than an LGG (*arrow*). However, there is no enhancement, and no change was observed in the spectroscopy. This "angiogenic switch" may herald early malignant transformation. (*Bottom row*) MR imaging at 8 months' follow-up. At this time there is clear tumor progression, characterized by a marked increase in tumor volume and enhancement as well as mass effect. There is now obvious evidence of tumor infiltration across the corpus callosum and extension into the lateral ventricle. DSC MR imaging image with rCBV color overlay shows a further increase in rCBV (3.4), in keeping with tumor progression. It has been demonstrated in the literature that the rCBV increase can precede the contrast enhancement, probably reflecting the angiogenic switch in the tumor biology.

Several studies have demonstrated that rCBV measurements have clinical utility in glioma grading. Comparison of rCBV measurements between LGG and HGG has demonstrated LGG to have maximal rCBV values of between 1.11 and 2.14, and HGG to have maximal rCBV values of between 3.54 and 7.32.[11,17,20,21,53] A larger study (n = 160) demonstrated LGG to have rCBV values of 2.14 and HGG to have rCBV values of 5.18 (Figs. 7 and 8).[17]

DSC MR imaging increases the sensitivity and predictive value in predicting glioma grade compared with conventional contrast-enhanced MR imaging.[17] In clinical practice, 95% to 100% sensitivity has been reported for differentiating HGGs from LGGs using thresholds of 1.75 and 1.5 for rCBV, respectively (Fig. 9).[17,18] In the same studies, 57.5% to 69% specificity can be achieved using the same threshold values. Law and colleagues[17] reviewed 160 glioma patients, of whom 120 were HGGs and 40 were LGGs. The relatively lower specificity is due in part to the high number of false positives. Several LGGs with elevated rCBV can be misclassified as HGGs, giving more false positives.

The role of VEGF, also known as VPF, as a mediator of tumor growth and angiogenesis has also resulted in several investigators demonstrating a good correlation between vascular permeability and glioma grade. It seems clear, however, in part due to the heterogeneity of glioma vasculature, that the regions of increased rCBV are spatially heterogeneous and different to areas of increased permeability.[54,55]

The dynamic nature of CNS tumors, with at least 50% dedifferentiating into more malignant grades, is well known and for some neurosurgeons, if one allows enough time, all low-grade tumors will progress to high-grade tumors. What is still unknown is how, when, and why a dormant (silent) tumor becomes aggressive.[56] A very important concept related to the tumoral progression is the "angiogenic switch."[56,57] This concept refers to the transition of an avascular tumor to an angiogenic one, and represents a distinct step in the malignant transformation of gliomas.[56,58–61] Overexpression of angiogenic factors or hypoxia results in the production of certain growth factors and cytokines that ultimately induce angiogenesis in gliomas.

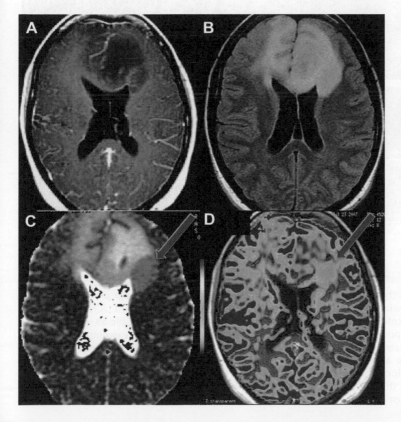

Fig. 11. Minimally enhancing left frontal glioma in a 50-year-old man. (A) Axial T1-weighted image post gadolinium demonstrates minimal if any enhancement within the tumor. (B) Axial FLAIR image shows a hyperintense mass in the left frontal lobe, extending through the corpus callosum to the right frontal lobe, with mass effect in both lateral ventricles. (C) ADC map demonstrates a focal region of diffusion restriction adjacent to the left lateral ventricle, suggesting that this area has higher cellularity when compared with the rest of the tumor. (D) Gradient-echo axial DSC T2* MR imaging with rCBV color overlay demonstrates focal increase in the relative cerebral blood volume within the lesion, in the same area where there is diffusion restriction. This patient had a biopsy directed to that region, resulting in a diagnosis of high-grade tumor (WHO IV). Biopsy of a region with lower rCBV or lower cellularity may have resulted in a lower grade tumor, an effect of sampling error.

Danchaivijitr and colleagues[62] recently demonstrated that in transforming LGG, DSC MR imaging perfusion imaging can demonstrate significant increases in rCBV up to 12 months before contrast enhancement is apparent on T1-weighted MR images. This result indicates that an increase in microvascular density occurs well in advance of blood-brain barrier leakage reflected by pathologic contrast enhancement. rCBV increase is therefore likely to provide an earlier noninvasive indicator of malignant progression, and may likely indicate this "angiogenic switch" (Fig. 10).

Guiding stereotactic biopsy and radiosurgery

The rationale for using perfusion MR imaging to guide stereotactic brain biopsy is again based on the utility of these techniques in defining the most vascular regions of the tumor.[63] Most

biopsies are guided with contrast-enhanced T1-weighted MR or computed tomography images,[64] which only reflect blood-brain barrier disruption and may not indicate the most malignant or vascular region of the tumor. Often the region of highest vascularity and hence malignancy is found within the region of T2 signal abnormality and not necessarily within the region of contrast enhancement (Figs. 11 and 12).

Therapeutic monitoring

- Therapy-induced necrosis and recurrent tumor
- Chemoradiation-induced pseudoprogression
- Antiangiogenesis therapies, surrogate biomarker

The differentiation of therapy-induced necrosis (radiation or chemotherapy) from recurrent or residual tumor is challenging, from

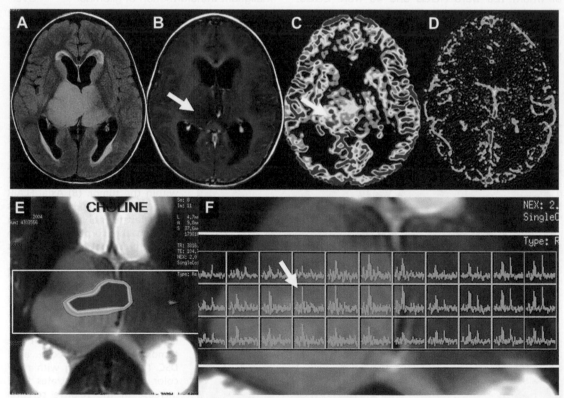

Fig. 12. Nonenhancing low-grade bithalamic tumor in an 8-year-old boy. (A) Axial FLAIR image demonstrates a bithalamic hyperintense tumor. (B) Axial T1-weighted image shows no contrast enhancement. (C) Gradient-echo axial DSC MR imaging with rCBV color overlay demonstrates increased relative cerebral blood volume within the right thalamus (arrow). (D) Spin-echo DCE T1 MR imaging shows a decrease in vascular permeability. (E and F) MR spectroscopy demonstrates higher choline levels in the right lesion, well demonstrated in the choline color map (arrow). Despite all of the advanced methods suggesting a high-grade tumor, the biopsy showed a low-grade tumor. The biopsy was done in the most anterior aspect of the right thalamus, and the most malignant areas of the tumor (high rCBV and high choline), which were located in the posterior thalamus seen best on images C and F were not biopsied again, demonstrating some of the limitations of biopsy and histopathologic sampling error.

a clinical point of view and also from conventional MR imaging. Unfortunately, most of the time in clinical practice and also at histopathology, both of these entities coexist. After all, it is primarily in the setting of residual tumor that the patient is receiving adjuvant radiation or chemotherapy.

Delayed radiation necrosis (DRN) is histopathologically an occlusive vasculopathy that results in "strokelike episodes." Endothelial proliferation can be seen in the early phase of DRN (which may represent "pseudoprogression"—see later discussion); this usually results in obliteration of the vessel lumen in the later phase. The endothelial injury from radiation leads to fibrinoid necrosis of small vessels, endothelial thickening, hyalinization, and vascular thrombosis. Recurrent tumor, on the other hand, demonstrates vascular proliferation and angiogenesis without vascular luminal obliteration.

Hu and colleagues[65] recently published a paper in which they studied 13 patients with new enhancing lesion in the follow-up of HGGs previously treated with multimodality therapy, correlating the CBV values with tissue specimen. Using an in-house Matlab-based MR perfusion technique, they found that in the radionecrosis group the rCBV values ranged from 0.21 to 0.71 and in the tumor group the values ranged from 0.55 to 4.64. In 8.3% of the tumor group, the rCBV values fell within the radionecrosis group range. These investigators concluded that (rCBV >0.71) predicted tumor growth, whereas (rCBV <0.71) predicted radionecrosis, with approximately 95.9% accuracy.[65]

Sugahara and colleagues[66] previously studied 20 patients with new enhancing lesions, and found that all the recurrent tumors presented with CBV values greater than 2.6, whereas the radionecrosis group presented with CBV values less than 0.6.

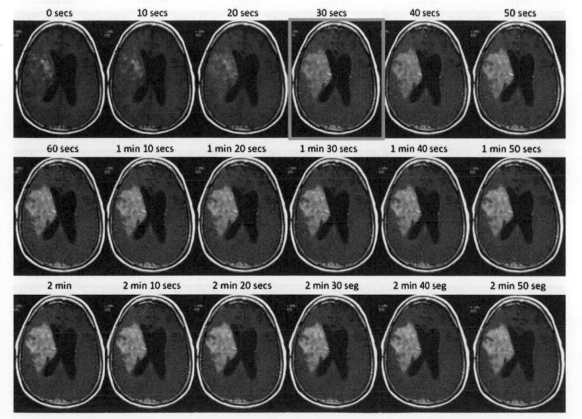

Fig. 13. DCE MR imaging T1 steady-state permeability dynamic acquisition images demonstrates a very rapid increase in signal intensity following the gadolinium injection, compatible with a leaky blood-brain barrier from a very vascular lesion. Within 30 seconds, there is avid contrast enhancement indicating a vascular recurrent tumor in these 10-second snapshots of the steady-state permeability dataset.

These investigators suggested that patients with CBV values between those numbers should undergo a new modality.[66]

Despite the fact that DSC MR imaging is proving to be a sensitive technique in differentiating DRN from recurrent tumor,[14,67–69] to date accurate threshold rCBV values that accurately differentiate radionecrosis from tumor have yet to be published.

The use of a multiparametric approach that incorporates normalized choline/choline ratio (Cho/Cho(n)) and permeability DCE perfusion studies in the follow-up of these patients certainly adds further diagnostic accuracy. Typically in radioinduced necrosis the vascular permeability (K^{trans}) is reduced because even though there may be enhancement, the rate of enhancement is typically very slow; pathologically it appears as an occlusive vasculopathy (**Figs. 13–17**). There will also be a decrease in normalized Cho/Cho(n) compared with the contralateral Cho. On the other hand, in recurrent tumor, the DCE MR imaging T1 steady-state permeability study usually demonstrates a very rapid initial increase in the vascular permeability curve, compatible with a vascular phase then a more steady leakage typical for a highly vascular and highly permeable recurrent tumor (see **Figs. 13–15; Fig. 18**). Also, spectroscopy will show an increase in normalized Cho/Cho(n) compared with the contralateral Cho (**Fig. 19**).

Perfusion (rCBV) and vascular permeability seem to be measuring different pathophysiologic changes in the brain. As a result there are some instances where there are not only spatial differences in the distribution of the rCBV versus permeability, but changes in one metric may be better than the other in differentiating radiation necrosis from recurrent tumor (**Figs. 20 and 21**).

Data recently reported in the randomized EORTC 22981/26981-NCIC CE.3 (European Organization for Research and Treatment of Cancer/National Cancer Institute of Canada) phase 3 trial on newly diagnosed patients with glioblastoma (GBM)

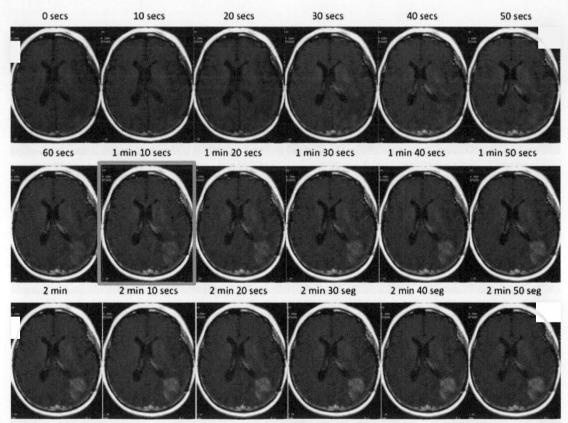

Fig. 14. DCE MR imaging T1 steady-state permeability demonstrates a very slow increase in signal compatible with a leaky blood-brain barrier from radionecrosis but no rapid vascular phase. The lesion enhances but at 30 seconds there is very little enhancement; the lesion does not fully enhance until 2 minutes following the injection. This pattern indicates a leaky blood-brain barrier but not a vascular lesion, and would be compatible with radiation necrosis.

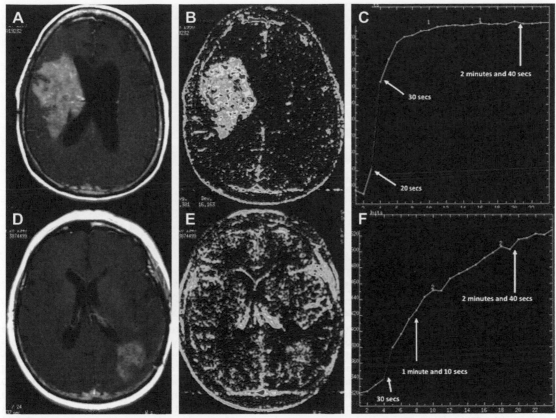

Fig. 15. High-grade tumors treated with surgery and radio-chemotherapy. Each one of these patients presented with a new enhancing lesion. (*A–C*) T1 postcontrast permeability maps and steady-state signal intensity curves generated from the data in **Fig. 13** (*upper*) demonstrate a very rapid increase in signal intensity following the gadolinium injection, compatible with a leaky blood-brain barrier from a very vascular lesion (ie, recurrent tumor). (*D–F*) T1 postcontrast permeability maps and DCE MR imaging T1 steady-state signal intensity curves generated from the data in **Fig. 14** (*lower*). Steady-state permeability demonstrates a very slow increase in signal compatible with a leaky blood-brain barrier from radionecrosis but no vascular phase, rapid initial increase.

patients given temozolomide (TMZ) plus radio-therapy (RT) have provided a new standard of care.[70] Since the introduction of chemo-radio-therapy with temozolomide as the new standard of care for patients with glioblastoma, there has been an increasing awareness of post-therapeutic progressive and enhancing lesions on MR imaging, noted immediately after the end of treatment, which are not related to tumor progression but which are a treatment effect.[71–75] This so-called therapy-induced enhancement/encephalitis or pseudoprogression, which can occur in up to 20% of patients who have been treated with temo-zolomide chemo-radiotherapy, can explain about half of all cases of increasing lesions and enhance-ment after the end of this treatment.[73] These lesions decrease in size or stabilize without addi-tional treatments, and often remain clinically asymptomatic (**Fig. 22**).[73] These findings suggest

that pseudoprogression represents a continuum between the subacute radiation encephalitis/reac-tion and treatment-related necrosis. The mecha-nisms behind these events have not yet been fully elucidated, but the likelihood is that chemo-radio-therapy causes a higher degree of (desired) tumor cell and endothelial cell killing. This increased cell kill might lead to secondary reactions, such as edema and abnormal vessel permeability in the tumor area, mimicking tumor progression, in addi-tion to subsequent early treatment-related necrosis in some patients and milder subacute radiotherapy reactions in others.[73]

Advanced neuroimaging findings in pseudo-progression have not yet been published, but preliminary findings suggest a decrease in CBV values and an increase in vascular permeability (as well as increase in choline levels), keeping with the proposed pathophysiology previous

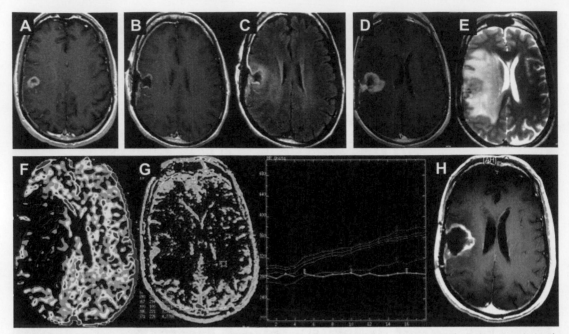

Fig. 16. Patient with a primary, biopsy-proven, high-grade glioma (HGG) presenting with radionecrosis in the follow-up. (*A*) Axial T1-weighted image post gadolinium shows a peripherally enhancing mass in the right frontoparietal region. (*B* and *C*) Axial T1-weighted image post gadolinium and FLAIR weighted image in the first postoperative day demonstrate radical resection of the tumor and small amount of edema surrounding the surgical cavity. Six months following radiotherapy and chemotherapy, the patient presents with left-sided hemiparesis. (*D* and *E*) Axial T1-weighted image post gadolinium shows an enhancing lesion adjacent to the surgical bed and axial FLAIR demonstrates significant amount of "edema" with mass effect. (*F*) Gradient-echo axial DSC MR imaging with rCBV color overlay map demonstrates reduced perfusion throughout the lesion. (*G* and *H*) DCE MR imaging T1 steady-state permeability color overlay and curve demonstrates a considerably slower increase in signal, suggesting radionecrosis. (*H*) Axial T1-weighted image post gadolinium post resection of the lesion, which proved to be radionecrosis.

described (**Fig. 23**). These findings usually appear in the first 3 months of treatment, earlier than the typical time period in which radionecrosis is described, and usually regress 6 to 9 months following the initial commencement of temozolomide and radiation therapy (and possibly other chemo-radiation regimes). Further research is needed to establish reliable imaging parameters that distinguish between true tumor progression and pseudoprogression or treatment-related necrosis. It is certainly critical to determine which parameter better differentiates early pseudoprogression from early progressive lesions, as the management approaches are completely different for each situation.

PERFUSION MR IMAGING AS BIOMARKERS FOR NOVEL ANTIANGIOGENIC AGENTS

Malignant gliomas, particularly recurrent anaplastic gliomas and glioblastoma multiforme (GBM), are highly refractory to therapy. A key feature of malignant gliomas such as GBM is their tendency to infiltrate surrounding tissues. This invasive property often precludes total surgical resection and makes it difficult to treat with radiation without damaging normal brain parenchyma. Because of the difficulty in obtaining total eradication, patients with GBM have a median survival of less than 1 year, despite aggressive treatment. Of the approximately 35,000 Americans diagnosed with primary brain cancer each year, almost half with high-grade (WHO class III–IV) gliomas will succumb to their disease within 2 years if treated and in less than 6 months if untreated. This extremely poor prognosis has not changed despite 30 years of research, technological progress, and clinical trials. Whereas concomitant use of radiation and temozolomide has been recently defined as the standard first-line approach for therapy for newly diagnosed grade 4 gliomas,[70] the conventional treatment of recurrent high-grade glial tumors remains ill defined.

These gliomas are highly vascular and are likely the result of the tumoral upregulation of angiogenic growth factors, such as VEGF. VEGF is secreted by

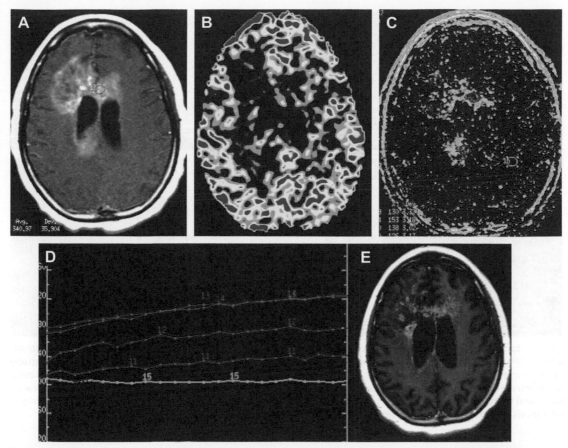

Fig. 17. A large heterogeneously enhancing lesion in a 48-year-old man with a history of high-grade tumor treated with surgery and chemo-radiotherapy. (*A*) Axial postcontrast T1-weighted image demonstrates a large enhancing lesion in the right frontal lobe, extending to the corpus callosum. There is also another enhancing focus posteriorly within the corpus callosum. (*B*) DSC MR imaging T2* perfusion color overlay demonstrates a decrease in rCBV throughout the enhancing lesion. (*C* and *D*) DCE MR imaging T1 steady-state permeability color overlay and curve demonstrates a slower increase in signal compatible with a leaky blood-brain barrier from fibrinoid necrosis, but no vascular phase (rapid increase in signal, as with **Fig. 13**). (*E*) Follow-up study after a small course of steroids shows marked reduction in enhancement.

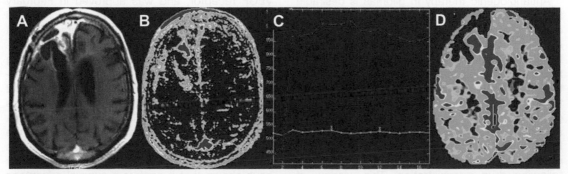

Fig. 18. Recurrent tumor in a 63-year-old woman. (*A*) Axial postcontrast T1-weighted image demonstrating prior right frontal craniotomy with an enhancing lesion adjacent to the surgical cavity. (*B* and *C*) DCE MR imaging T1 steady-state color map and permeability curve demonstrates a very rapid initial increase in permeability compatible with a vascular lesion, typical for a highly vascular and highly permeable recurrent tumor. (*D*) DSC MR imaging T2* perfusion color overlay demonstrates elevation in rCBV in the enhancing component of the lesion.

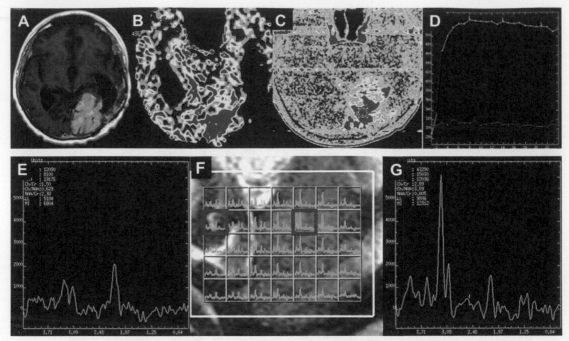

Fig. 19. Imaging of a patient with recurrent tumor. (A) Axial postcontrast T1-weighted image demonstrates a large enhancing mass in the left occipital lobe. (B) DSC MR imaging T2* perfusion color overlay demonstrates increase in rCBV within the lesion. (C and D) DCE MR imaging T1 steady-state color map and permeability curve demonstrates a very rapid initial increase in permeability compatible with a lesion typical with very high vascularity and highly permeable recurrent tumor. (E–G) MR spectrum from the enhancing lesion demonstrates higher Cho levels than the contralateral normal Cho(n) in E, in keeping with recurrent tumor.

tumor cells and acts in a paracrine manner on the VEGF receptors (VEGFRs) on endothelial cells to stimulate endothelial cell proliferation, migration, and survival. The importance of VEGF is highlighted by the fact that the degree of vascularization has been linked to prognosis in gliomas and other solid tumors, and VEGF levels in glioblastomas have been correlated with tumor blood vessel density, invasiveness, and patient prognosis.[76]

Antiangiogenic therapy in gliomas is desirable for multiple reasons, including the prominent role of angiogenesis in glioblastoma growth and proliferation. The accessibility of intravascular VEGFR localized to endothelial cells circumvents the challenge of delivering the drug to the tumor beyond the impermeable blood-brain barrier. In addition to the potential for direct antitumor effects, antiangiogenic therapy has been shown to prune abnormal vessels and "normalize" existing vasculature, which may paradoxically improve drug and oxygen delivery to the tumor for a period of time following drug administration. This window of normalization ideally can lead to a temporary improvement in tumor oxygenation and blood flow, which may enhance the effectiveness of radiation therapy and chemotherapy (Fig. 24). In

addition, anti-VEGF therapy has been shown to reduce cerebral edema through elimination of VEGF, which may reduce the need for steroid use and have a beneficial impact on neurologic function.[76]

One of the few agents currently approved by the Food and Drug Administration (FDA) is Avastin, or bevacizumab. Bevacizumab (Avastin) is a humanized murine monoclonal antibody against the VEGF receptor, and was approved in February 2004 for first-line use against metastatic colorectal cancer when used with 5-fluorouracil based chemotherapy. There are promising data regarding its use in other cancers as well, including renal cell carcinoma, non–small cell lung, pancreatic, and breast cancer.[77] Current phase 2 and phase 3 studies are testing its efficacy in these and other tumor types. However, published data on Avastin's role in primary brain tumors are much more limited. Although bevacizumab seems to have some activity as a single agent, no studies have shown that it confers a survival advantage when used without cytotoxic chemotherapy, suggesting that sequestration of circulating VEGF is not sufficient to produce antitumor activity and that bevacizumab may be able to potentiate the

7 MONTHS POST SURGERY

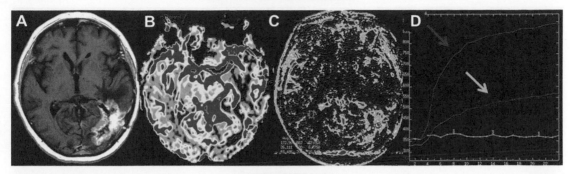

2 MONTHS LATER

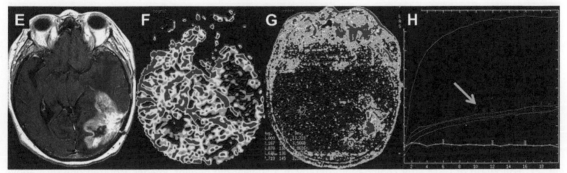

Fig. 20. Follow-up of GBM after chemo-radiotherapy in a 50-year-old patient. (A) Axial T1-weighted postcontrast image shows a heterogeneously enhancing lesion in the left tempoparietal region in the region of the previously resected tumor. (B) Gradient-echo T2* axial DSC MR imaging with rCBV color overlay demonstrates increase relative cerebral blood volume within the lesion. (C) T1 Spin-echo DCE MR imaging shows some foci of high vascular permeability within the lesion. (D) DCE MR imaging T1 steady-state permeability curve demonstrates some foci with a very rapid initial increase compatible with recurrent tumor (*red arrow*) and some foci with slower increase, compatible with radionecrosis (*blue arrow*). (E–H) Volumetric increase in the lesion, with more mass effect. Again, DSC MR imaging with rCBV color overlay demonstrates increased relative cerebral blood volume. There was also volumetric increase in the region with high permeability, but there are still some foci with a slow increase in the permeability curve (*blue arrow*), in keeping with concurrent radionecrosis.

effects of cytotoxic chemotherapy,[76] Fine[78] has recently demonstrated in a phase 2 study that patients with glioblastoma treated with bevacizumab alone had a response rate of 60% and a 6-month progression-free survival rate of 30%. These response and progression-free survival rates are similar to the published data on bevacizumab plus irinotecan, suggesting that most of the radiographic response and clinical benefit may be attributable to bevacizumab and that eliminating irinotecan may improve the therapy's tolerability.

Vredenburgh and colleagues[79,80] published the first phase 2 study of patients treated with bevacizumab and irinotecan, and showed an overall radiographic response rate of 63% based on Mac Donald criteria, against 5% or 6% with the traditional treatments (**Fig. 25**). More importantly, the 6-month progression-free survival was much higher than any in previous series, reaching 30%

in the GBM group treated with bevacizumab and irinotecan, whereas historically it was reported to be around 15%, although it is still unclear whether this new treatment improves overall survival.[80]

One study demonstrated a 50% conventional MR imaging response rate in 14 patients with recurrent HGGs. Of these patients, 4 died (mean survival after treatment: 116 days), 2 of whom had what the investigators described as "mixed progressive disease" and the other 2 with "partial response," suggesting that radiographic improvement does not correlate well with clinical outcome.[81]

There is also evidence that VEGF receptor inhibitors may have activity. In a recent phase 2 study of the pan-VEGF receptor inhibitor AZD2171 in recurrent GBMs, the radiographic response rate was approximately 50%, and 6-month progression-free survival was 27%. It was also demonstrated that in most patients relative tumor vessel size significantly decreased as

7 MONTHS POST SURGERY

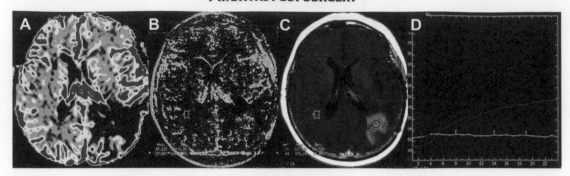

2 MONTHS LATER

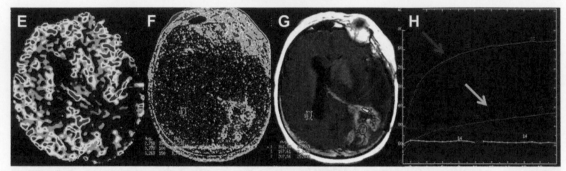

Fig. 21. Follow-up of GBM after chemo-radiotherapy in a 50-year-old patient. Images acquired one slice above the previous images. (*A*) Gradient-echo axial DSC MR imaging with rCBV color overlay demonstrates reduced relative cerebral blood volume within the lesion. (*B–D*) T1 Spin-echo DCE MR imaging shows no foci of high vascular permeability within the lesion, and the permeability curve shows a very slow increase, in keeping with radionecrosis. (*E–H*) MR imaging 2 months later. (*E*) Gradient-echo axial DSC MR imaging with rCBV color overlay demonstrates reduced relative cerebral blood volume within the lesion. (*F–H*) DCE MR imaging T1 steady-state permeability curve now demonstrates some foci with a very rapid initial increase in permeability compatible with recurrent tumor (*red arrow*), whereas other areas demonstrate a slower increase, compatible with radionecrosis (*blue arrow*). This case demonstrates a situation whereby permeability shows recurrent tumor in a lesion with relatively low perfusion, indicating that perfusion (rCBV) and permeability are different metrics correlating with different pathophysiology.

early as 1 day after the onset of AZD2171 treatment, as well as vascular permeability. Reversal of the vascular normalization began by 28 days, being the ideal time for combining with a cycle of concurrent chemotherapy or radiotherapy. It was also shown that the tumor vessels became abnormal following drug withdrawal and "renormalized" after drug resumption.[34] Blood vessel diameter can be measured with MR imaging by comparing spin-echo planar DSC images and gradient-echo DSC images. Gradient-echo planar images are sensitive to vessels of all sizes whereas spin-echo images are sensitive to smaller vessels. The ratio of these 2 sequences provides an estimate of average vessel diameter within the tumor.[34,82] In these patients, the enhancement volume and permeability were smaller before medication was halted, increased substantially

during withdrawal, and then regressed again after the AZD2171 was resumed, giving insight into the plasticity of human tumor vessels.[34]

Although the results suggest benefit from the combination of bevacizumab and irinotecan, there are cases that do not respond. This failure could be due to the heterogeneity in the vascular response to bevacizumab or because of other independent patient characteristics that make them less likely to respond to therapy (**Fig. 26**).[83] These characteristics include differences in the molecular profiles among those with primary and secondary GBM. Also, the tumor escape from anti-VEGF therapy may involve other growth factors important for angiogenesis, including VEGF-C, VEGF-D, placental growth factor, platelet-derived growth factor, and basic fibroblast growth factor.[76]

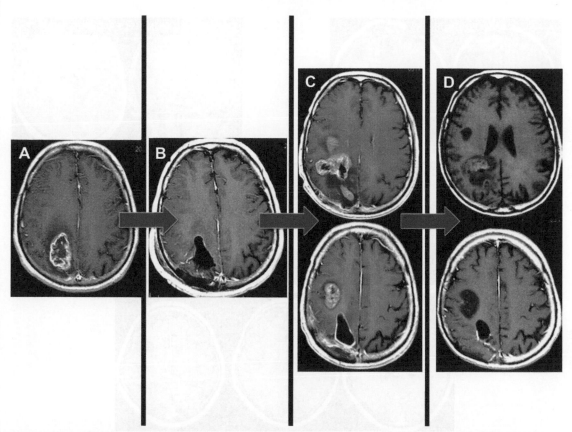

Fig. 22. 52-year-old man with a glioblastoma multiforme in the right parietal lobe. (*A*) Axial T1-weighted image post contrast shows a mass with heterogeneous enhancement located in the right parietal lobe. (*B*) Axial T1-weighted image post contrast in the first day postoperatively demonstrates radical resection of the tumor. (*C*) Axial T1-weighted image post contrast 2 months following the beginning of the radio- and chemotherapy shows the appearance of new enhancing lesions adjacent to the surgical cavity. (*D*) Postcontrast T1-weighted imaging demonstrates a significant decrease in contrast enhancement within the lesions just 1 month following steroid treatment, findings likely related to pseudoprogression.

A critically important issue is the brain tumor community's definition of response, which is still largely based in the MacDonald response criteria. These criteria use standard MR imaging to measure changes in tumor size based on T1-weighted post-gadolinium techniques. Dramatic decreases in contrast enhancement as early as 24 hours following a single dose of anti-VEGF therapy have been demonstrated. This result would qualify as a response, but it is unlikely that there would have been a significant, if any, antitumor effect.[76] These changes are best reclassified as a decrease in vascular permeability or vascular response rather than a true tumor "response" (**Fig. 27**).[76] However, it does not seem that these anti-VEGF agents are acting just as "supersteroids," because many patients have prolonged disease-free survival while receiving bevacizumab alone or in combination with irinotecan, suggesting that in selected patients anti-VEGF therapy has a true antitumor effect.

It seems clear that new response criteria need to be formulated to better define the effect of these treatments on MR imaging scans and to assist with end-point definition for clinical trials that evaluate the efficacy of these antiangiogenic agents. Being essentially antiangiogenic drugs, the question that still needs to be answered is: can the potential antitumor effects of these drugs be separated from their antipermeability effects?

Noninvasive imaging techniques are being used to determine whether changes in vascular permeability are predictive of long-term response. In a recent study by Desjardins and colleagues, changes in the permeability constant (K^{trans}) value were highly correlated with the percentage of

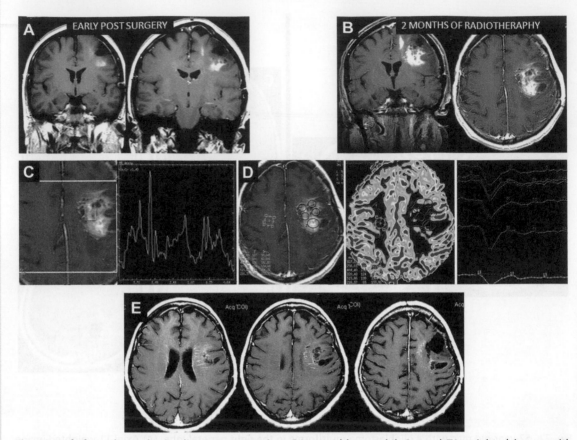

Fig. 23. Left frontal anaplastic oligoastrocytoma in a 34-year-old man. (*A*) Coronal T1-weighted image with contrast demonstrates postoperative surgical cavity with minimal residual tumoral enhancement. (*B*) Coronal T1-weighted image post gadolinium demonstrates increased enhancement within the surgical cavity. (*C*) Spectroscopy of the lesion demonstrates high levels of choline, reduced NAA, and moderate increase in LI/LAC levels. (*D*) DSC MR imaging T2* color overlay imaging demonstrates reduced perfusion. Therapy was continued as the findings were felt to be due to pseudoprogression from chemoradiation therapy. (*E*) Eight months following therapy there was a decrease in contrast enhancement, confirming that this is likely pseudoprogression, which tends to appear in the first 3 months following commencement of therapy, with regression 6 to 9 months after therapy. This situation has been reported in approximately 20% of patients treated with radiation and temozolomide therapy.

decline in tumor volume from baseline to the end of the first cycle of bevacizumab and irinotecan treatment. However, no dynamic contrast-enhanced-MR imaging measures at either 24 hours or 6 weeks from the beginning of treatment were predictive of progression-free survival or overall survival.[76]

This new antiangiogenic drug widens the use of perfusion metrics, because CBV has been the most used hemodynamic parameter in evaluating brain tumors. Besides CBV, CBF seems to have an important role in the evaluation of those patients. These 2 parameters measure different aspects of the tumoral hemodynamic and frequently they are not related to each other. An area of tumor may contain an increased volume of blood because of increased vessel size or number of vessels, but the blood flow through that area may be slow and inefficient because of the underlying abnormal tumor vasculature.[84] Restoration of normal vessel architecture with an antiangiogenic agent can improve the efficiency of tumor blood flow (ie, improve CBF) but decrease CBV, as was shown in a mouse glioma model.[82,84]

Initial studies with antiangiogenic agents such as thalidomide demonstrated that perfusion imaging was able to more accurately predict overall survival and progressive disease than conventional MR imaging.[85] More recently, the authors have used CBV and permeability measurements to follow patients on Avastin. So far, it seems as

CD34 PRE AVASTIN   CD34 POST AVASTIN

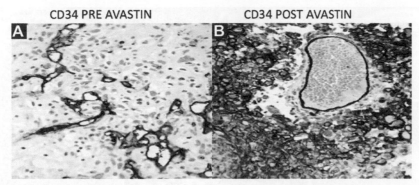

Fig. 24. Histologic findings in a patient before (*A*) and after (*B*) treatment with the angiogenesis inhibitor Avastin (bevacizumab) in combination with irinotecan (CPT-11). CD34 special stains highlight vascular arcades before Avastin and increased tumor cell staining after treatment. Not also the "normalization" of the vessels from the very small tortuous angiogenic vessels to the more "normal" larger caliber vessels. (*Reproduced from* Fischer, et al. Glioma before and after Avastin, Neuro-oncology October 2008; with permission.)

PRE-AVASTIN

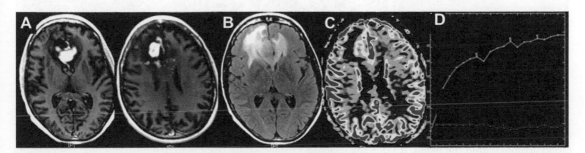

POST-AVASTIN

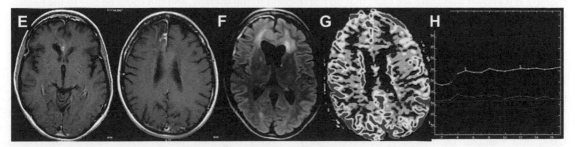

Fig. 25. Pathologically recurrent glioblastoma multiforme (WHO Grade IV). (*A*) Axial T1-weighted post-gadolinium image demonstrates a recurrent enhancing glioma in the right mesial frontal region. (*B*) Axial FLAIR image demonstrates substantial associated T2 signal abnormality with mass effect on the frontal horns of the ventricles. (*C*) Gradient-echo axial T2* DSC MR imaging with rCBV color overlay demonstrates high relative cerebral blood volume within the lesion. (*D*) Spin-echo T1 DCE MR imaging with the signal intensity curve shows increased vascular permeability. (*E* and *F*) Follow-up T1 and FLAIR imaging after Avastin therapy demonstrate a good response. (*G*) Gradient-echo axial T2* MR imaging with rCBV color overlay demonstrates reduced relative cerebral blood volume within the lesion. (*H*) Spin-echo T1 DCE MR imaging with the signal intensity curve shows a decrease in vascular permeability after Avastin therapy.

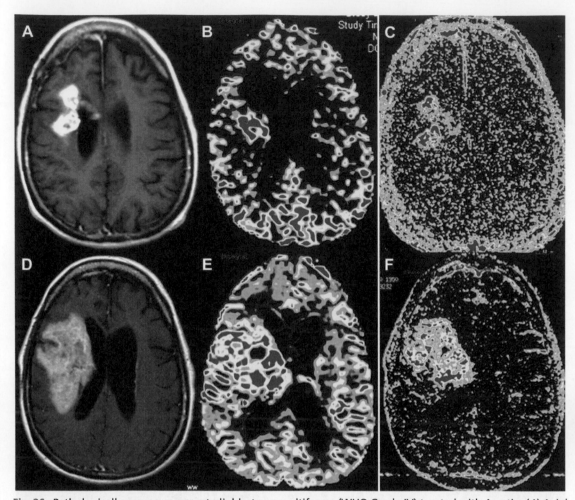

Fig. 26. Pathologically proven recurrent glioblastoma multiforme (WHO Grade IV) treated with Avastin. (*A*) Axial T1-weighted post-gadolinium image demonstrates a new enhancing lesion in the deep right frontal white matter. (*B*) Gradient-echo axial DSC MR imaging with rCBV color overlay demonstrates high relative cerebral blood volume within the lesion. (*C*) DCE MR imaging T1 steady-state color map demonstrates high permeability within the lesion. (*D–F*) Three-month follow-up images demonstrate increase in tumor volume and enhancement as well as mass effect. Again, DSC and DCE perfusion studies show high perfusion and permeability after Avastin therapy. It is known that there are cases that do not respond to the therapy, and this could be due to the heterogeneity in the vascular response to bevacizumab or because of other independent patient characteristics that make them less likely to respond to therapy.

though radiographically on conventional MR imaging, CBV, and permeability measurements, most patients demonstrate a response to treatment with a decrease in the enhancing volume, CBV, and vascular permeability; however, many of these patients do not demonstrate significant improvement in time to progression or overall survival.

Recent evidence has demonstrated that a subset of patients treated with bevacizumab and irinotecan may develop nonenhancing tumor progression without evidence of an increase in tumor vascularity.[76,86] Experimental evidence has shown that glioma tumors treated with the anti-VEGFR-2 antibody DC-101 demonstrated an increase in the number and total area of small satellite tumors.[87] Tumor cells were found to have migrated along blood vessels over long distances to eventually reach the pial surface and spread in the subarachnoid space, a process known as co-option vascular.[87] The results suggest that in a therapeutic situation whereby angiogenesis is inhibited, tumors cells can co-opt preexistent cerebral vessels to provide their blood supply before they induce neovascularization, and this may be demonstrated in the MR

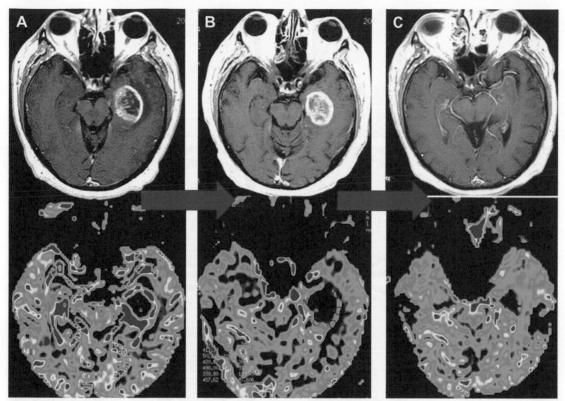

Fig. 27. Pathologically proven recurrent glioblastoma multiforme (WHO Grade IV) treated with an antiangiogenic agent. (*A*) Axial T1-weighted post-gadolinium image shows a peripherally enhancing lesion in the left temporal lobe. Gradient-echo axial DSC MR imaging with rCBV color overlay demonstrates high relative cerebral blood volume within the enhancing component of the lesion. (*B*) Follow-up study 3 months later shows no significant change in the contrast enhancement; however, there is a clear reduction in rCBV values within the lesion. Using the traditional MacDonald criteria this would not have been classified as a response, but the perfusion study demonstrated an excellent response to therapy. (*C*) Follow-up T1-weighted imaging demonstrates marked decrease in the enhancement component of the lesion. Again, DSC MR imaging with rCBV color overlay demonstrates reduced relative cerebral blood volume within the lesion. This case is an example of a good therapeutic response demonstrated earlier by the perfusion study. It is clear now that new response criteria need to be formulated to better define the effect of these new treatments on MR imaging scans.

imaging as an increase in the hyperintense surface area on fluid-attenuated inversion recovery (FLAIR) sequences (**Fig. 28**). Again, there is no standard method to quantify this pattern of progression radiographically. There is normally no increase in the CBV values, even though the spectroscopy can show high choline levels and diffusion-weighted image low levels of apparent diffusion coefficient (ADC) (**Fig. 29**).

At present, the genetic tumor profile is becoming increasingly important when selecting patients for novel new treatment strategies. Until recently, antiangiogenic drugs were chosen and used regardless of the genetic profile of a tumor, which can lead to erroneous conclusions about efficacy.[60] In a phase 1 study by Haas-Kogan and colleagues,[88] 43% of patients with EGFR mutations or low phosphorylation of protein kinase B (PKB)/Akt demonstrated an objective response to erlotinib (an anti-EGFR antibody) compared with 0% in the absence of EGFR mutations or high phosphorylation of PKB/Akt. Thus, it is more than likely that future individualization of a patient's treatment should be based on the patient's molecular signature.

In future it is likely, as with many other disease processes such as human immunodeficiency virus and tuberculous infection, that a combination of drugs that will target different components of glioma biology will be most effective. Regardless of therapy, it is evident that quantitative MR measures of perfusion, diffusion, and other pathophysiologic parameters will become early surrogate biomarkers of therapeutic response.

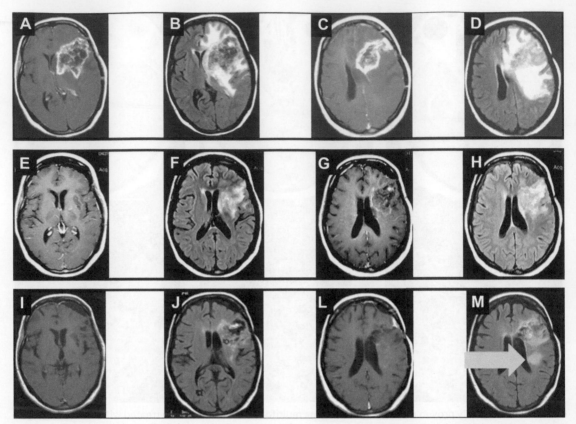

Fig. 28. Recurrent tumor treated with Avastin. (*A–D*) Axial postcontrast T1-weighted image shows a large hetero-geneous enhancing lesion in the left frontal lobe, with mass effect, surrounded by a large amount of vasogenic edema. (*E–H*) MR imaging at 1 month following commencement of therapy. There has been significant reduction in the enhancing areas as well as in the vasogenic edema, suggesting a good response to the therapy. (*I–M*) MR imaging at 3-month follow-up. Again, there has been reduction in contrast enhancement as well as mild decrease in the hyperintense areas around the enhancement lesion. However, there is a new hyperintense area (*red arrow*) adjacent to the left ventricle, probably related to tumor infiltration. The literature suggests that in a therapeutic situation whereby angiogenesis is inhibited, tumors cells can co-opt preexistent cerebral vessels to provide their blood supply before they induce neovascularization, which will be demonstrated in the MR imaging as an increase in the hyperintense area in the FLAIR sequence.

STANDARDIZED METHODS FOR PERFORMING PERFUSION MR IMAGING, AUTOMATED METHODS FOR CLINICAL TRIALS, AND END POINTS

Reliable and reproducible determinations of tumor angiogenesis and neovascularity are important in the clinical management of patients with cerebral gliomas. Such accuracy is also becoming increas-ingly important in the numerous clinical trials investigating the efficacy of antiangiogenic agents in cancer. Reliable, reproducible data may be obtainable by experienced operators in a research setting or in the clinics of large radiology depart-ments. Simple, objective methods with the highest intra- and interinstitutional reproducibility are

necessary to detect subtle changes, especially because perfusion MR imaging is being used to determine the efficacy of antiangiogenic thera-pies.[89] Pharmaceutical companies certainly are motivated by having reproducible methods that governmental agencies such as the FDA can acknowledge as imaging biomarkers in the deter-mination of therapeutic efficacy and safety. Furthermore, agencies that ultimately determine which MR techniques are applicable clinically and can be reimbursed will need to have methods that are easily reproducible in the clinical setting. Determination of perfusion metrics is currently undertaken in the research and clinical settings using software that relies on accurate region-of-interest (ROI) analysis. When using an ROI

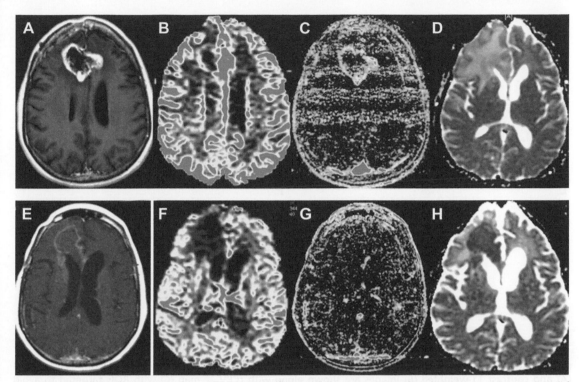

Fig. 29. Pathologically recurrent glioblastoma multiforme, following 2 months of therapy with Avastin. (A) Axial T1-weighted post-gadolinium image demonstrates recurrent tumor in the frontal lobes. (B) Gradient-echo axial DSC MR imaging with rCBV color overlay demonstrates increased relative cerebral blood volume within the lesion. (C) DCE MR imaging T1 permeability color map demonstrates increased vascular permeability. (D) ADC map demonstrates high diffusion within the lesion. 2 months after Avastin therapy. (E) Axial T1-weighted post-gadolinium image demonstrates marked reduction in the enhancement pattern within the lesion. (F) Gradient-echo axial DSC MR imaging depicts a decrease in rCBV and perfusion. (G) DCE MR imaging T1 permeability color map demonstrates reduced vascular permeability. (H) Diffusion-weighted ADC image demonstrates a marked decrease in signal, suggesting possible increase in tumor cellularity and possible increase in invasiveness within the recurrent glioma, which may be a biologic response to the removal of the angiogenic component as well as decrease in edema from the decrease in vascular permeability.

approach, there are several methods that have been shown to increase inter- and intraobserver reproducibility.[90] In terms of rCBV estimations, it is also important when placing the ROIs to avoid large intratumoral and extratumoral vessels.[91] However, any ROI measurement still remains operator dependent and somewhat subjective, with an unavoidable component of interobserver and intraobserver variability.

Histogram analysis is a quantitative technique used in several neuroimaging studies. Histogram analysis of DSC MR imaging data in focal disease such as primary glial neoplasms has not been previously well studied. The authors and other investigators have recently used histogram analysis for quantifying perfusion data in cerebral gliomas. The histogram can be applied to the rCBV color map to display the pixel values from the magnitude image.

Histogram analysis of rCBV data was found to be as effective as $rCBV_{max}$ derived from an ROI analysis in the correlation with glioma grade. Inexperienced operators may obtain perfusion metrics using histogram analysis that are comparable to those obtained by experienced operators using ROI analysis. Representative cases of LGG and HGG are shown in Fig. 30. The authors also examined the reproducibility of histogram-based versus ROI-based techniques, and found that the interobserver and intraobserver reproducibility of rCBV was acceptable using ROI and non-ROI histogram techniques. Further refinement of non-ROI analysis of perfusion MR data may lead to standardized, automated methods for tumor quantification. This refinement will be critical in both single and multi-institutional studies involving quantification of perfusion metrics for predicting glioma biology and also

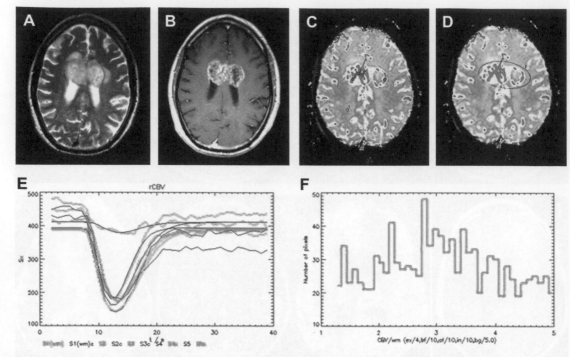

Fig. 30. HGG, glioblastoma multiforme (grade IV/IV) in frontal lobes spanning the corpus callosum. T2-weighted (*A*) and contrast T1-weighted (*B*) images are shown along with rCBV$_{max}$ map (*C*) with ROIs targeted to avoid areas of radiologic necrosis to determine perfusion curves (*E*). rCBV histogram map (*D*) and histogram curve (*F*) are derived from the maximal tumor diameter regardless of heterogeneity. (*From* Law M, et al. AJNR 2007(121).)

for assessing therapeutic response to novel anti-angiogenic agents.

REFERENCES

1. Folkman J. Tumor angiogenesis: therapeutic implications. N Engl J Med 1971;285:1182–6.
2. Vajkoczy P, Menger MD. Vascular microenvironment in gliomas. J Neurooncol 2000;50(1–2):99–108.
3. Vajkoczy P, Menger MD. Vascular microenvironment in gliomas. Cancer Treat Res 2004;117:249–62.
4. Dvorak HF, Brown LF, Detmar M, et al. Vascular permeability factor/vascular endothelial growth factor, microvascular hyperpermeability, and angiogenesis. Am J Pathol 1995;146(5):1029–39.
5. Dvorak HF, Nagy JA, Feng D, et al. Vascular permeability factor/vascular endothelial growth factor and the significance of microvascular hyperpermeability in angiogenesis. Curr Top Microbiol Immunol 1999; 237:97–132.
6. Provenzale JM, Wang GR, Brenner T, et al. Comparison of permeability in high-grade and low-grade brain tumors using dynamic susceptibility contrast MR imaging. AJR Am J Roentgenol 2002;178(3):711–6.
7. Roberts HC, Roberts TPL, Brasch RC, et al. Quantitative measurement of microvascular permeability in human brain tumors achieved using dynamic contrast-enhanced MR imaging: correlation with histologic grade. AJNR Am J Neuroradiol 2000; 21(5):891–9.
8. Roberts HC, Roberts TP, Ley S, et al. Quantitative estimation of microvascular permeability in human brain tumors: correlation of dynamic Gd-DTPA-enhanced MR imaging with histopathologic grading. Acad Radiol 2002;9(Suppl 1):S151–5.
9. Maia ACM Jr, Malheiros SMF, da Rocha AJ, et al. MR cerebral blood volume maps correlated with vascular endothelial growth factor expression and tumor grade in nonenhancing gliomas. AJNR Am J Neuroradiol 2005;26(4):777–83.
10. Sorensen AG, Reimer P. Cerebral MR perfusion imaging: principles and current applications. 152nd edition. New York: Thieme; 2000.
11. Aronen HJ, Gazit IE, Louis DN, et al. Cerebral blood volume maps of gliomas: comparison with tumor grade and histologic findings. Radiology 1994; 191(1):41–51.
12. Aronen HJ, Perkio J. Dynamic susceptibility contrast MRI of gliomas. Neuroimaging Clin N Am 2002;12: 501–23.
13. Bruening R, Kwong KK, Vevea MJ, et al. Echo-planar MR determination of relative cerebral blood

volume in human brain tumors: T1 versus T2 weighting. AJNR Am J Neuroradiol 1996;17(5):831–40.

14. Cha S, Knopp EA, Johnson G, et al. Intracranial mass lesions: dynamic contrast-enhanced susceptibility-weighted echo-planar perfusion MR imaging. Radiology 2002;223(1):11–29.

15. Cha S. Perfusion MR imaging: basic principles and clinical applications. Magn Reson Imaging Clin N Am 2003;11(3):403–13.

16. Cha S, Johnson G, Wadghiri YZ, et al. Dynamic, contrast-enhanced perfusion MRI in mouse gliomas: correlation with histopathology. Magn Reson Med 2003;49(5):848–55.

17. Law M, Yang S, Wang H, et al. Glioma grading: sensitivity, specificity, and predictive values of perfusion MR imaging and proton MR spectroscopic imaging compared with conventional MR imaging. AJNR Am J Neuroradiol 2003;24(10): 1989–98.

18. Lev MH, Rosen BR. Clinical applications of intracranial perfusion MR imaging. Neuroimaging Clin N Am 1999;9(2):309–31.

19. Petrella JR, Provenzale JM. MR perfusion imaging of the brain: techniques and applications. Am J Roentgenol 2000;175(1):207–19.

20. Shin JH, Lee HK, Kwun BD, et al. Using relative cerebral blood flow and volume to evaluate the histopathologic grade of cerebral gliomas: preliminary results. Am J Roentgenol 2002;179(3):783–9.

21. Sugahara T, Korogi Y, Kochi M, et al. Correlation of MR imaging-determined cerebral blood volume maps with histologic and angiographic determination of vascularity of gliomas. AJR Am J Roentgenol 1998;171(6):1479–86.

22. Sugahara T, Korogi Y, Shigematsu Y, et al. Value of dynamic susceptibility contrast magnetic resonance imaging in the evaluation of intracranial tumors. Top Magn Reson Imaging 1999;10(2):114–24.

23. Wong ET, Jackson EF, Hess KR, et al. Correlation between dynamic MRI and outcome in patients with malignant gliomas. Neurology 1998;50(3): 777–81.

24. Wong JC, Provenzale JM, Petrella JR. Perfusion MR imaging of brain neoplasms. Am J Roentgenol 2000; 174(4):1147–57.

25. Law M, Young R, Babb J, et al. Comparing perfusion metrics obtained from a single compartment versus pharmacokinetic modeling methods using dynamic susceptibility contrast-enhanced perfusion MR imaging with glioma grade. AJNR Am J Neuroradiol 2006;27(9):1975–82.

26. Zierler KL. Circulation times and the theory of indicator-dilution methods for determining blood flow and volume. In: Handbook of physiology. Baltimore (MD): Williams & Wilkins; 1962. p. 585–615.

27. Johnson G, Wetzel SG, Cha S, et al. Measuring blood volume and vascular transfer constant from dynamic, T(2)*-weighted contrast-enhanced MRI. Magn Reson Med 2004;51(5):961–8.

28. Tofts PS, Brix G, Buckley DL, et al. Estimating kinetic parameters from dynamic contrast-enhanced T(1)-weighted MRI of a diffusible tracer: standardized quantities and symbols. J Magn Reson Imaging 1999;10(3):223–32.

29. Tofts PS, Kermode AG. Measurement of the blood-brain barrier permeability and leakage space using dynamic MR imaging. 1. Fundamental concepts. Magn Reson Med 1991;17(2):357–67.

30. Rosen BR, Belliveau JW, Vevea JM, et al. Perfusion imaging with NMR contrast agents. Magn Reson Med 1990;14:249–65.

31. Weisskoff R, Belliveau J, Kwong K, et al. Functional MR imaging of capillary hemodynamics. In: Potchen E, editor. Magnetic resonance angiography: concepts and applications. St Louis (MO): Mosby; 1993. p. 473–84.

32. Young IR, Cox IJ, Coutts GA, et al. Some consideration concerning susceptibility, longitudinal relaxation time constants and motion artifact in vivo human spectroscopy. NMR Biomed 1989;2:329–39.

33. Schmainda KM, Rand SD, Joseph AM, et al. Characterization of a first-pass gradient-echo spin-echo method to predict brain tumor grade and angiogenesis. AJNR Am J Neuroradiol 2004;25(9): 1524–32.

34. Batchelor TT, Sorensen AG, di Tomaso E, et al. AZD2171, a pan-VEGF receptor tyrosine kinase inhibitor, normalizes tumor vasculature and alleviates edema in glioblastoma patients. Cancer Cell 2007;11(1):83–95.

35. Padhani AR, Dzik-Jurasz A. Perfusion MR imaging of extracranial tumor angiogenesis. Top Magn Reson Imaging 2004;15(1):41–57.

36. Cha S, Yang L, Johnson G, et al. Comparison of microvascular permeability measurements, Ktrans, determined with conventional steady-state T1-weighted and first-pass T2*-weighted MR imaging methods in gliomas and meningiomas. AJNR Am J Neuroradiol 2006;27(2):409–17.

37. Parks LD, Choma MA, York GE, et al. Correlation of DCE and rCBV values for patients with high grade glial neoplasms. Proceedings of the Radiological Society of North America. Chicago (IL); 2005. p. 346.

38. Li KL, Zhu XP, Waterton J, et al. Improved 3D quantitative mapping of blood volume and endothelial permeability in brain tumors. J Magn Reson Imaging 2000;12(2):347–57.

39. Li KL, Zhu XP, Checkley DR, et al. Simultaneous mapping of blood volume and endothelial permeability surface area product in gliomas using iterative analysis of first-pass dynamic contrast enhanced MRI data. Br J Radiol 2003;76(901): 39–51.

40. Cha S. Update on brain tumor imaging: from anatomy to physiology. AJNR Am J Neuroradiol 2006;27(3):475–87.

41. Boxerman JL, Schmainda KM, Weisskoff RM. Relative cerebral blood volume maps corrected for contrast agent extravasation significantly correlate with glioma tumor grade, whereas uncorrected maps do not. AJNR Am J Neuroradiol 2006;27(4):859–67.

42. Paulson ES, Schmainda KM. Comparison of dynamic susceptibility-weighted contrast-enhanced MR methods: recommendations for measuring relative cerebral blood volume in brain tumors. Radiology 2008;249(2):601–13.

43. Burger PC. Classification, grading, and patterns of spread of malignant gliomas. In: Apuzzo, editor. Neurosurgical topics: malignant cerebral glioma. Park Ridge (IL): America Association of Neurological Surgeons; 1990. p. 3–17.

44. Daumas-Duport C, Beuvon F, Varlet P, et al. [Gliomas: WHO and Sainte-Anne Hospital classifications]. Ann Pathol 2000;20(5):413–28.

45. Kleihues P, Soylemezoglu F, Schauble B, et al. Histopathology, classification, and grading of gliomas. Glia 1995;15(3):211–21.

46. Kleihues P, Ohgaki H. Primary and secondary glioblastomas: from concept to clinical diagnosis. Neuro-oncol 1999;1(1):44–51.

47. Kleihues P, Cavanee P. WHO classification of tumors: pathology and genetic of tumors of the nervous system. Lyon: IARC Press; 2000.

48. Ringertz J. Grading of gliomas. Acta Pathol Microbiol Scand 1950;27:51–64.

49. Coons SW, Johnson PC, Scheithauer BW, et al. Improving diagnostic accuracy and interobserver concordance in the classification and grading of primary gliomas. Cancer 1997;79(7):1381–93.

50. Gilles FH, Brown WD, Leviton A, et al. Limitations of the World Health Organization classification of childhood supratentorial astrocytic tumors. Children Brain Tumor Consortium. Cancer 2000;88(6):1477–83.

51. Jackson RJ, Fuller GN, Abi-Said D, et al. Limitations of stereotactic biopsy in the initial management of gliomas. Neuro-oncol 2001;3(3):193–200.

52. Law M, Young RJ, Babb JS, et al. Gliomas: predicting time to progression or survival with cerebral blood volume measurements at dynamic susceptibility-weighted contrast-enhanced perfusion MR Imaging 10.1148/radiol.2472070898. Radiology 2008;247(2):490–8.

53. Yang D, Korogi Y, Sugahara T, et al. Cerebral gliomas: prospective comparison of multivoxel 2D chemical- shift imaging proton MR spectroscopy, echoplanar perfusion and diffusion-weighted MRI. Neuroradiology 2002;44(8):656–66.

54. Law M, Yang S, Babb JS, et al. Comparison of cerebral blood volume and vascular permeability from dynamic susceptibility contrast-enhanced perfusion MR imaging with glioma grade. AJNR Am J Neuroradiol 2004;25(5):746–55.

55. Lupo JM, Cha S, Chang SM, et al. Dynamic susceptibility-weighted perfusion imaging of high-grade gliomas: characterization of spatial heterogeneity. AJNR Am J Neuroradiol 2005;26(6):1446–54.

56. Verheul HM, Voest EE, Schlingemann RO. Are tumours angiogenesis-dependent? J Pathol 2004;202(1):5–13.

57. Carmeliet P, Jain RK. Angiogenesis in cancer and other diseases. Nature 2000;407(6801):249–57.

58. Kerbel RS. Tumor angiogenesis. N Engl J Med 2008;358(19):2039–49.

59. Bergers G, Benjamin LE. Tumorigenesis and the angiogenic switch. Nat Rev Cancer 2003;3(6):401–10.

60. Jouanneau E. Angiogenesis and gliomas: current issues and development of surrogate markers. Neurosurgery 2008;62(1):31–50 [discussion: 50–2].

61. Jain RK, di Tomaso E, Duda DG, et al. Angiogenesis in brain tumours. Nat Rev Neurosci 2007;8(8):610–22.

62. Danchaivijitr N, Waldman AD, Tozer DJ, et al. Low-grade gliomas: do changes in rCBV measurements at longitudinal perfusion-weighted MR imaging predict malignant transformation? 10.1148/radiol.2471062089. Radiology 2008;247(1):170–8.

63. Martin AJ, Liu H, Hall WA, et al. Preliminary assessment of turbo spectroscopic imaging for targeting in brain biopsy. AJNR Am J Neuroradiol 2001;22(5):959–68.

64. Kelly PJ, Daumas-Duport C, Kispert DB, et al. Imaging-based stereotaxic serial biopsies in untreated intracranial glial neoplasms. J Neurosurg 1987;66(6):865–74.

65. Hu LS, Baxter LC, Smith KA, et al. Relative cerebral blood volume values to differentiate high-grade glioma recurrence from posttreatment radiation effect: direct correlation between image-guided tissue histopathology and localized dynamic susceptibility-weighted contrast-enhanced perfusion MR imaging measurements. AJNR Am J Neuroradiol 2008.

66. Sugahara T, Korogi Y, Tomiguchi S, et al. Posttherapeutic intraaxial brain tumor: the value of perfusion-sensitive contrast-enhanced MR imaging for differentiating tumor recurrence from nonneoplastic contrast-enhancing tissue. AJNR Am J Neuroradiol 2000;21(5):901–9.

67. Essig M, Waschkies M, Wenz F, et al. Assessment of brain metastases with dynamic susceptibility-weighted contrast-enhanced MR Imaging: initial results 10.1148/radiol.2281020298. Radiology 2003;228(1):193–9.

68. Fuss M, Wenz F, Scholdei R, et al. Radiation-induced regional cerebral blood volume (rCBV) changes in normal brain and low-grade astrocytomas: quantification and time and dose-dependent occurrence. Int J Radiat Oncol Biol Phys 2000;48(1):53–8.

69. Wenz F, Rempp K, Hess T, et al. Effect of radiation on blood volume in low-grade astrocytomas and normal brain tissue: quantification with dynamic susceptibility contrast MR imaging. Am J Roentgenol 1996; 166(1):187–93.

70. Stupp R, Mason WP, van den Bent MJ, et al. Radiotherapy plus concomitant and adjuvant temozolomide for glioblastoma. N Engl J Med 2005;352(10): 987–96.

71. Brandes AA, Franceschi E, Tosoni A, et al. MGMT promoter methylation status can predict the incidence and outcome of pseudoprogression after concomitant radiochemotherapy in newly diagnosed glioblastoma patients. J Clin Oncol 2008; 26(13):2192–7.

72. Brandes AA, Tosoni A, Spagnolli F, et al. Disease progression or pseudoprogression after concomitant radiochemotherapy treatment: pitfalls in neurooncology. Neuro-oncol 2008;10(3):361–7.

73. Brandsma D, Stalpers L, Taal W, et al. Clinical features, mechanisms, and management of pseudoprogression in malignant gliomas. Lancet Oncol 2008;9(5):453–61.

74. de Wit MC, de Bruin HG, Eijkenboom W, et al. Immediate post-radiotherapy changes in malignant glioma can mimic tumor progression. Neurology 2004;63(3):535–7.

75. Chamberlain MC, Glantz MJ, Chalmers L, et al. Early necrosis following concurrent Temodar and radiotherapy in patients with glioblastoma. J Neurooncol 2007;82(1):81–3.

76. de Groot JF, Yung WK. Bevacizumab and irinotecan in the treatment of recurrent malignant gliomas. Cancer J 2008;14(5):279–85.

77. de Gramont A, Van Cutsem E. Investigating the potential of bevacizumab in other indications: metastatic renal cell, non-small cell lung, pancreatic and breast cancer. Oncology 2005;69(Suppl 3):46–56.

78. Fine HA. Promising new therapies for malignant gliomas. Cancer J 2007;13(6):349–54.

79. Vrodonburgh JJ, Desjardins A, Herndon JE 2nd, et al. Phase II trial of bevacizumab and irinotecan in recurrent malignant glioma. Clin Cancer Res 2007;13(4):1253–9.

80. Wong ET, Hess KR, Gleason MJ, et al. Outcomes and prognostic factors in recurrent glioma patients enrolled onto phase II clinical trials. J Clin Oncol 1999;17(8):2572–8.

81. Pope WB, Lai A, Nghiemphu P, et al. MRI in patients with high-grade gliomas treated with bevacizumab and chemotherapy 10.1212/01.wnl.0000208958.29600.87. Neurology 2006;66(8):1258–60.

82. Quarles CC, Schmainda KM. Assessment of the morphological and functional effects of the anti-angiogenic agent SU11657 on 9L gliosarcoma vasculature using dynamic susceptibility contrast MRI. Magn Reson Med 2007;57(4):680–7.

83. Buie LW, Valgus J. Bevacizumab: a treatment option for recurrent glioblastoma multiforme. Ann Pharmacother 2008;42(10):1486–90.

84. Gerstner ER, Sorensen AG, Jain RK, et al. Advances in neuroimaging techniques for the evaluation of tumor growth, vascular permeability, and angiogenesis in gliomas. Curr Opin Neurol 2008;21(6): 728–35.

85. Cha S, Knopp EA, Johnson G, et al. Dynamic, contrast-enhanced T2*-weighted MR imaging of recurrent malignant gliomas treated with thalidomide and carboplatin. AJNR Am J Neuroradiol 2000;21(5):881–90.

86. Rubenstein JL, Kim J, Ozawa T, et al. Anti-VEGF antibody treatment of glioblastoma prolongs survival but results in increased vascular cooption. Neoplasia 2000;2(4):306–14.

87. Kunkel P, Ulbricht U, Bohlen P, et al. Inhibition of glioma angiogenesis and growth in vivo by systemic treatment with a monoclonal antibody against vascular endothelial growth factor receptor-2. Cancer Res 2001;61(18):6624–8.

88. Haas-Kogan DA, Prados MD, Tihan T, et al. Epidermal growth factor receptor, protein kinase B/ Akt, and glioma response to erlotinib. J Natl Cancer Inst 2005;97(12):880–7.

89. Akella NS, Twieg DB, Mikkelsen T, et al. Assessment of brain tumor angiogenesis inhibitors using perfusion magnetic resonance imaging: quality and analysis results of a phase I trial. J Magn Reson Imaging 2004;20(6):913–22.

90. Wetzel SG, Cha S, Johnson G, et al. Relative cerebral blood volume measurements in intracranial mass lesions: interobserver and intraobserver reproducibility study. Radiology 2002;224(3): 797–803.

91. Caseiras GB, Thornton JS, Yousry T, et al. Inclusion or exclusion of intratumoral vessels in relative cerebral blood volume characterization in low-grade gliomas: does it make a difference? AJNR Am J Neuroradiol 2008;29(6):1140–1.

Diffusion Imaging for Therapy Response Assessment of Brain Tumor

Thomas L. Chenevert, PhD*, Brian D. Ross, PhD

KEYWORDS

- Diffusion-weighted MRI • Apparent diffusion coefficient
- Diffusion anisotropy • Brain tumor
- Treatment response • Parametric response map

It is estimated there will be over 22,000 newly diagnosed cancers of the brain and central nervous system in the United States in 2009 and that nearly 13,000 individuals will die of cancer of the brain and central nervous system.[1] Despite the emergence of many new treatment strategies and multimodality therapies, successful management of brain tumors in adults and children remains largely unsatisfactory. In particular, glioblastoma multiforme (GBM) presents a major challenge given its moderate response rates to essentially all available standard-of-care therapies leading to a median survival time of only 12.2 to 18.2 months in these patients.[2] This is in contrast to patients with anaplastic astrocytomas, who survive over 40 months on average,[3] and low-grade gliomas, which have a better prognosis, although most of these individuals eventually succumb to their disease.[4] To date, patient age, tumor histology, patient functional status, and the combination of these parameters are considered the most reliable prognostic indicators of overall survival.[5,6] This is an unfortunate fact considering remarkable advances in neuroimaging that have occurred over the last couple decades. Despite major strides in spatial resolution and contrast of anatomic features, along with information-rich functional, metabolic, and physiologic representations of tissues, these undeniable achievements in

neuroimaging have not had a commensurate impact on brain tumor patient survival outcome. The reader is referred to other articles in this issue for reviews of other advanced imaging approaches applied to brain tumor. One must remember that the therapy and not the imaging ultimately treats the tumor, and lack of any major improvement in brain tumor treatment outcome is more of an indictment of these therapies than of imaging. Moreover, although advanced imaging techniques have been available for many years, these methodologies are still evolving rapidly and have not been standardized or applied uniformly in large clinical trials. In most instances imaging is used as a simple indicator of change in tumor size well after therapy administration by way of subjective or objective assessment of lesion dimensions. Unfortunately, early change in size is not a reliable indication of tumor response, particularly for patients receiving combination therapy of temozolomide with radiation. The phenomena of "pseudoprogression" is indistinguishable from true tumor progression by conventional imaging.[7–9] Pseudoprogression is characterized by an increase in size or number of contrast-enhancing lesions soon after treatment with temozolomide plus radiation, which eventually resolves or stabilizes without additional treatment. Pseudoprogression is observed in an estimated 15% to 30% of patients receiving this treatment

Supported in part by Grant Nos. P01CA85878, P01CA59827, P01CA87634, and P50CA93990 from The National Institutes of Health and the National Cancer Institute.
Department of Radiology, University of Michigan Medical Center, 1500 East Medical Center Drive, Ann Arbor, MI 48109, USA
* Corresponding author.
E-mail address: tlchenev@umich.edu (T.L. Chenevert).

Neuroimag Clin N Am 19 (2009) 559–571
doi:10.1016/j.nic.2009.08.009
1052-5149/09/$ – see front matter © 2009 Published by Elsevier Inc.

neuroimaging.theclinics.com

and most of these patients remain clinically stable despite the progression-like appearances.[7-9] It is often unclear whether current therapy should be maintained or second-line therapy initiated.

Although a fully satisfactory method to determine tumor response by imaging has not been developed, solid tumor response based on a simple single linear summation of lesion dimension termed "response evaluation criteria in solid tumors" is still in use today.[10] Use of advanced imaging as an integral intervention to customize delivery of treatment on an individual patient basis remains largely untested. This article summarizes the concepts and use of diffusion MR imaging as a prognostic indicator and a potential biomarker of brain tumor treatment response. The scope briefly refers to basic diffusion principles and preclinical diffusion work, and focuses on clinical investigations in use of diffusion for oncologic applications. To date most of these clinical studies are single institution trials and involve modest patient numbers. Despite these limitations, diffusion imaging has shown promise as a tool for oncologic imaging of treatment response.

DIFFUSION CONCEPTS

The essential element of diffusion-based imaging is thermally driven random motion of water molecules, which are the sole source of desired signal. Although water is the sole signal source, it is all the nonwater constituents that provide the contrast and interest in diffusion imaging of tissue. Indeed, in pure water the only relevant modifier to water mobility is temperature; pure water maintained at body temperature has no contrast. Classic diffusion theory provides a statistical estimate for the average random displacement of water molecules over a given time interval. Assuming body temperature (37°C), water molecules migrate approximately 30 μm over a 50-millisecond interval but only if they are totally free of impediments. The 50-millisecond interval was chosen because it is representative of typical diffusion-weighted imaging (DWI) echo time TE. The fact that the diameter of a mammalian cell is approximately a few micrometers to tens of micrometers and that other subcellular structures (ie, membranes, organelles, and macromolecules) have smaller dimensions, the likelihood that a given water molecule encounters nonwater cellular constituents is extremely high. The water molecule likely has many interactions with large obstructions over the diffusion measurement interval. As a result the reduction of water mobility in tissue is a strong reflection of presence and density of nonwater cellular

constituents, such as cell membranes, organelles, and macromolecules. Given that water moves within and across intracellular and extracellular domains, water also encounters impediments presented by tortuosity in the extracellular interstitium.[11-13]

The reader is referred elsewhere for excellent reviews on technical aspects of how diffusion imaging is performed,[14-17] although for the interest here it is sufficient to summarize a few key concepts. Sensitivity of the MR imaging sequence to water mobility is determined by the strength, duration, and direction of gradient pulses interleaved within the imaging sequence. The single most important parameter selected by the operator for diffusion imaging is the "b-value," which is calculated based on gradient waveform amplitude and duration properties. As the b-value is increased, the signal strength decays because of spin dephasing secondary to random molecular displacements. The resultant DWI exhibits tissues where less mobile water seems hyperintense compared with hypointense tissues where water is more mobile. Keen sensitivity to acute ischemic insult leading to cytotoxic edema manifest as a hyperintensity on DWI is a classic example of this principle.[18,19] Although diffusion-based contrast increases with b-value, there are practical signal-to-noise and hardware limitations such that a reasonable b-value range for each particular application is reasonably well established. For example, most clinical DWI of the human brain is performed in the b-value range 0 to 1000 s/mm^2. Aside from qualitative interpretation of heavily DWI (eg, at b = 1000 s/mm^2), the combination of at least two DWIs allows quantitative calculation of an apparent diffusion coefficient (ADC) given by,

$$ADC = \frac{1}{(b_2 - b_1)}\log_e\left[\frac{S_1}{S_2}\right] \qquad (1)$$

where S_1 and S_2 represent signal intensity of images acquired at low b-value, b_1, and high b-value, b_2, respectively.

The simplicity of Eq(1) implies monoexponential signal decay with increasing b-value; however, water diffusion in tissue is well known to exhibit nonmonoexponential behavior observed at very high b-values (b >3000 s/mm^2).[20-23] The existence of nonmonoexponential behavior is not surprising considering the complex nature of the extracellular and subcellular domains, although which biophysical model and means to interpret multiexponential in vivo data remains the subject of debate.[21,23-25] In addition, signal-to-noise ratio limitations and long scan times to acquire a wide b-value range necessary to demonstrate multiexponential features have hampered clinical use of this phenomenon. **Fig. 1** illustrates signal loss and gain in diffusion-weighted contrast of normal tissues and glioma with increasing b-value. Nonmonoexponential behavior is demonstrated by the graphs of signal versus b-value for regions of interest (ROI) defined on normal brain and glioma. Two functional forms proposed to fit these signal decay features are a bi-exponential model[17,20,25] and the stretched exponential model.[24] Model fit parameter values and their functional form are

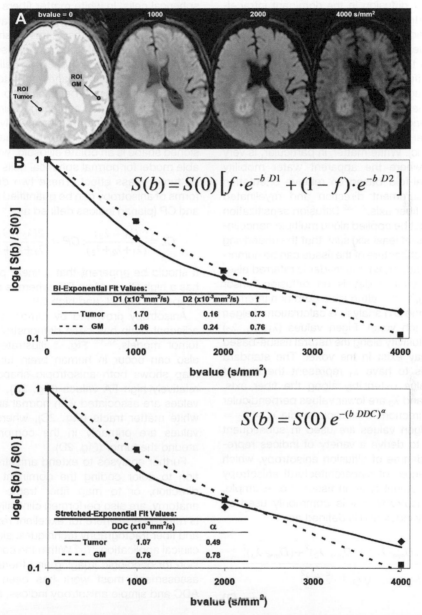

Fig. 1. DWI contrast at high b-value in a 61-year-old patient with a GBM. (A) DWI of the brain typically performed at b-value = 0, 1000 s/mm², although conspicuity of cellular dense central tumor increases at higher b-values. ROI, region of interest. (B) Tissue has multiexponential diffusion decay properties as is evident by curvature in log (*signal*) with b-value, which can be fit by a bi-exponential function to yield fast diffusion D1, slow diffusion D2 coefficients, and relative fraction of fast diffusion component f. (C) The stretched exponential is an alternative functional form to fit multiexponential decay, where DDC is the distributed diffusion coefficient and a lower α value indicates greater heterogeneity of diffusion contributions in the curve. Both the bi-exponential and stretched exponential fits indicate there is a greater spread in diffusion values in tumor relative to normal gray matter for this patient.

illustrated on the graphs for these examples of tumor and normal gray matter. Note the dominant compartment signified by f >0.5 has a higher diffusion coefficient than the minority compartment (ie, D1 > D2). This finding is consistent with other studies and indicates a simple conceptual assignment of lower diffusion in the dominant intracellular compartment and higher diffusion in the smaller extracellular compartment is not valid; more complex models are required.[20,25] The α index from the stretched exponential relates to intravoxel diffusion heterogeneity. A lower α in solid tumor suggests a greater spread in intravoxel diffusion values relative to gray matter.[26]

Another fundamental consideration relates to the fact that water mobility in tissue can be directional (ie, anisotropic). White matter, in particular, is very anisotropic where the apparent water mobility varies several-fold based on relative orientation of the measurement direction and myelinated white matter fiber axis.[27–32] Diffusion sensitization gradients must be applied along multiple noncolinear directions (at least six) such that the underlying directional architecture of the tissue can be numerically estimated. Again, the reader is referred elsewhere for technical details on diffusion tensor imaging (DTI),[16,30,31] although a common intermediate step in the DTI analysis is calculation of eigen values for each voxel. Eigen values (λ_1, λ_2, λ_3) represent diffusivity along the natural tissue-based axes that may exist in the voxel. The standard convention is to have λ_1 represent the highest diffusivity value ostensibly along the fiber axis, whereas λ_2, and λ_3 are lower values perpendicular to the fiber direction. In isotropic media $\lambda_1 \approx \lambda_2 \approx \lambda_3$. These eigen values are used in subsequent calculations to derive a variety of indices representing the degree of diffusion anisotropy, which infers the degree of cytoarchitectural anisotropy and omnidirectonal order in tissue. For example, fractional anisotropy (FA) is commonly used as an anisotropy index and is defined as,

$$FA = \sqrt{3/2} \frac{\sqrt{(D_{ave}-\lambda_1)^2 + (D_{ave}-\lambda_2)^2 + (D_{ave}-\lambda_3)^2}}{\sqrt{\lambda_1^2 + \lambda_2^2 + \lambda_3^2}}$$

(2)

where D_{ave} is the average of the eigen values, which is effectively equivalent to ADC. Mathematically, FA is a dimensionless quantity bound between 0 (nondirectional isotropic) and 1 (highly directional anisotropic), although in actual anisotropic tissue, such as the splenium of the corpus callosum, the maximum FA value is approximately 0.7 to 0.8 and varies with patient age.[31]

FA is just one of several indices available to characterize isotropic and anisotropic elements of tissue.[17,33,34] In addition to the degree of anisotropy there are geometric "shape" indices that may be particularly relevant in tumor that may induce anisotropy by compression of otherwise isotropic spherical cells. In white matter fibers the principle eigen value is significantly greater than the second and third eigen value; the "diffusion shape" is envisioned as an elongated prolate ellipsoid (ie, $\lambda_1 \gg \lambda_2 \approx \lambda_3$). Imagine a spherical cell undergoing compression, however, analogous to a spherical balloon compressed between two planes. For such a shape the first and second eigen value are nearly equivalent and are significantly greater than the third (ie, $\lambda_1 \approx \lambda_2 \gg \lambda_3$). In this situation the envisioned shape is an oblate ellipsoid, which is a suitable model for normal spherical cells compressed by tumor mass effect. These two distinct shape forms of anisotropy can be quantified by CL (linear) and CP (planar) indices defined as,[33,35]

$$CL = \frac{(\lambda_1 - \lambda_2)}{(\lambda_1 + \lambda_2 + \lambda_3)}; CP = \frac{2(\lambda_2 - \lambda_3)}{(\lambda_1 + \lambda_2 + \lambda_3)}$$

(3)

It should be apparent that a linear prolate shape has a high CL and low CP, whereas planar oblate shape has low CL and high CP.

Anisotropy provoked by tumor mass effect in adjacent brain has been demonstrated in animal tumor models.[36,37] **Fig. 2** illustrates this effect also can occur in human brain tumor. The FA map shows both anisotropic shapes can have relatively high FA values (**Fig. 2B**). The high CL values are associated with normal and displaced white matter tracts (**Fig. 2C**), whereas high CP values are primarily in the compression zone around the tumor (**Fig. 2D**).

Further analyses to extend anisotropy information to color coding the dominant eigen value direction, or to map fiber tracts through the anatomy, are also performed clinically. The reader is referred elsewhere for excellent reviews on DTI and fiber tractography techniques, along with their clinical application.[30,38] Within the context of diffusion for oncologic imaging and therapy response assessment, most work has been done using ADC and simple anisotropy indices, such as FA.

DIFFUSION IMAGING IN CHARACTERIZATION OF TUMOR

Water mobility is extremely sensitive to interactions with nonwater constituents in tissues, which provides DWI contrast and diagnostic content. Indeed, DWI is used extensively in clinical practice because of its exquisite sensitivity to cellular status, cytotoxic versus vasogenic edema, cellular

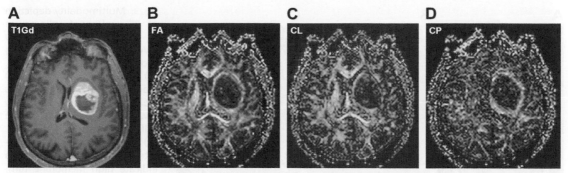

Fig. 2. Diffusion anisotropy is typically associated with normal white matter structures but may be induced by tumor mass-effect compression of adjacent tissues. (*A*) Conventional postcontrast T1-weighted image shows a well-delineated lesion in this 56-year-old GBM patient. (*B*) Fractional anisotropy map shows high anisotropy in normal white matter structures and anisotropy around surrounding the lesion. (*C*) Anisotropy shape analysis of DTI eigen values shows linear-shaped structures on CL map based on high contrast between first and second eigen values. (*D*) Planar-shaped anisotropic zones are apparent on the CP map, which is based on high contrast between second and third eigen values. The conspicuous rim around the lesion is likely caused by compression of cells immediately adjacent to the expanding tumor mass.

density, and directional organization of tissues. In application to tumor, several studies have demonstrated a clear relationship between ADC and tissue-tumor cellularity by histology.[39–42] It is generally noted that low ADC values are associated with cellular-dense zones on histology; ADC and cellular density are inversely related. These studies suggest the lowest ADC values measured in the most solid elements of the tumor may be valuable to characterize and grade tumor in analogy to histologic sampling the most malignant portion of the tumor.[39,41–43] Tumor heterogeneity remains problematic, however, and leads to overlap between groups stratified solely by ADC. A high choline concentration in proton MR spectroscopy is indicative of membrane turnover; choline tends to be high in the viable solid portion of a brain tumor. Combining this with the known relationship between ADC and cellularity, one would expect choline and ADC to be inversely related as was demonstrated in a study of 20 glioma patients.[44] Fig. 3 exemplifies this in a patient with a high-grade glioma where the tumor is highly perfused as seen on the blood flow map, and has high choline with low *N*-acetylaspartate suggesting viable tumor and membrane production. This tumor also has a relatively low ADC, which supports a cellular-dense microenvironment consistent with the MR spectroscopy characterization.

ADC maps have been evaluated in distinguishing solid enhancing tumor, noncontrast enhancing tumor, peritumoral edema, and necrotic or cystic tumor from normal surrounding brain tissue. Some studies indicate ADC values can be helpful to discriminate edema from tumor[45,46] but there are also conflicting studies.[43,47,48] It has been noted that one likely explanation for contradictory

results is the methodologic variability in image acquisition and postprocessing including ROI definition criteria. Some have concluded it is unlikely ADC values alone can reliably differentiate between peritumoral edema and non–contrast-enhancing neoplasm in individual patients,[49] although several studies have shown cystic or necrotic regions consistently have high ADC values relative to contrast-enhancing presumably viable portions of the tumor.[46,50,51]

In terms of the diagnostic value of FA over ADC in distinguishing tumor elements from peritumoral edema, a common observation is that as ADC increases, FA tends to decrease. Although ADC and FA represent fundamentally distinct features of the tissue they are still mathematically linked by their eigen values. Studies have shown a significant increase in mean diffusivity and significant decrease in FA in the peritumoral region of both gliomas and metastatic tumors when compared with those of normal-appearing white matter.[52,53] The peritumoral ADC of metastatic lesions was significantly greater than those of gliomas, however, whereas the FA values showed no discrepancy between tumor and metastasis, suggesting that the FA changes in tissue surrounding gliomas can be attributed to both increased water content and tumor infiltration.[52,53] A clear challenge in measurement of peritumoral FA values is the fact that white matter is the main source of anisotropy; the peritumoral FA value is heavily influenced by the anatomic location of the tumor.

DIFFUSION IMAGING TO GRADE TUMOR

DWI and DTI have been explored as aids to grade tumor in adult and pediatric populations. Several

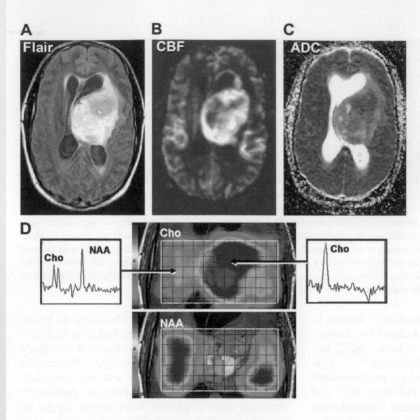

Fig. 3. Multimodality depiction of a malignant glioma in a 29-year-old patient. (A) FLAIR contrast MR imaging shows a large central mass. (B) Cerebral blood flow (CBF) map indicates the tumor is well perfused. (C) Relatively low ADC suggests a high cellular density in the tumor. (D) Choline and N-acetylaspartate maps with extracted spectra indicate high membrane turnover in the tumor. High choline content, high CBF, and low ADC are mutually consistent and support the diagnosis of a cellular dense, viable, malignant tumor. This patient expired within 1 month after this MR imaging examination.

studies have shown that low-grade astrocytoma has higher ADC values relative to lower ADC in high-grade malignant glioma. These studies refer to increased tumor cellularity as the source of reduced ADC in high-grade glioma.[40,41,43] In use of anisotropy, one group showed FA values in grades 1 and 2 gliomas were significantly lower compared with grades 3 and 4 gliomas[54]; they concluded that FA values can distinguish between high- and low-grade gliomas. Consistent with other studies, they also noted ADC was significantly higher in grade 1 than in grades 3 and 4 glioma. There remains controversy in the literature on use of FA values, however, which are generally reduced in tumors suggesting structural disorder may not add much information for tissue classification across tumors.[46] That said, FA may help in the understanding of the effect of brain tumors on nearby white matter fibers, which may be important to assess tumor infiltration and for presurgical planning.[29,55] Again, one must keep in mind the high degree of normal variation in FA depending on location in the brain,[56,57] which must be considered and may help explain disparity across studies. Depending on how fiber tracts are altered, one may expect normal anisotropy from shifted tracts; increased anisotropy caused by compression of tracks[50]; or a reduction of anisotropy caused by edema, infiltration, and

destruction of white matter.[49] Directionally encoded color maps of FA were categorized into four major patterns of tumor-altered white matter tracts: (1) deviated, (2) edematous, (3) infiltrated, and (4) destroyed.[58] Classification by these patterns may aid presurgical planning and thereby potentially avoid damaging an intact tract during surgery. **Fig. 4** illustrates three clinical examples where directionally encoded color FA maps illustrate gradations of white matter anisotropy affected by tumor. In the example on the left the white matter tracts are shifted but otherwise intact, whereas the examples in the middle and right illustrate reduced and obliterated anisotropy, respectively, caused by greater tumor invasion.

DIFFUSION IMAGING FOR PROGNOSIS AND TREATMENT MONITORING

Undoubtedly, many of the challenges in use of diffusion and anisotropy to characterize and grade tumor stem from heterogeneity within and across tumor types. Consider an alternative scenario, however, wherein a given lesion is followed over time during anticancer treatment. In this application, diffusion is used to detect change in the lesion microenvironment presumably caused by a direct therapeutic impact on the lesion. In this regard, there is less concern with pretreatment diffusion

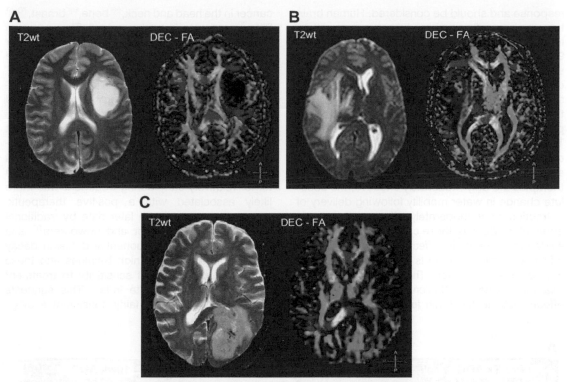

Fig. 4. The effect of tumor on normal white matter structures can be studied by directionally encoded color FA maps. (A) A 26-year-old patient with white matter and normal tissues shifted and somewhat compressed by this anaplastic astrocytoma. (B) This 48-year-old patient has reduced anisotropy and mass effect caused by infiltration of his GBM. (C) This 62-year-old GBM patient has lost all anisotropy because of tumor replacement of white matter in portions of the splenium.

properties of lesion; rather, emphasis is placed on its evolution during and after treatment. Furthermore, if one assumes the therapy is an effective cytotoxic therapy it is reasonable to expect tissue changes by way of cellular necrosis, apoptosis, and membrane lysis should occur before removal of cellular debris and subsequent mass shrinkage. Based on the linkage between water mobility and microscopic cellular features, it has been hypothesized that these positive therapeutic events can be quantified noninvasively by diffusion before traditional measures of therapeutic response (ie, lesion size) reflect the change. Although this section deals with serial change in response to treatment, one group also demonstrated pretreatment ADC may have prognostic value for brain tumor patients.[59] This study showed a low baseline ADC presumably caused by cellular-viable tumor was more responsive to treatment than tumor having a pre-existing high ADC from necrosis.

There are numerous preclinical studies to support the hypothesis that serial change in ADC may be a biomarker of treatment response. Original work on a 9L glioma model treated by single dose of chemotherapy (1,3-bis[2-chloro-ethyl]-1-nitrosourea) demonstrated the increase in tumor diffusion values following treatment was reflective of cellular density changes observed by histology.[36] Furthermore, dose-response experiments involving low chemotherapeutic doses suggest diffusion is sensitive to subtle effects provoked at relatively low cell-kill rates.[60] In this and other tumor models the increase in tumor diffusion occurred before mass shrinkage thereby supporting the argument that ADC may serve as an early biomarker of response.[61–67]

In translating diffusion as a therapy response indicator to the clinic, several inherent features work in its favor. Unlike many other MR imaging quantities, water mobility is not a magnetization property per se, and diffusion measurement is relatively independent of field strength and vendor platform. Moreover, because DWI and DTI are already commonplace sequences in human brain imaging protocols feasibility to acquire the data is well established. There are several key differences between human and animal scenarios, however, that lessen biomarker sensitivity to response and should be considered. Human brain tumors are often more heterogeneous than implanted tumor in animal studies, such as the 9L glioma in rodents. Also, tumor evolution time scales tend to be shorter in animal studies in terms of therapy delivery, tumor growth, and response such that tissue-tumor alteration caused by therapy tends to appear more slowly and less pronounced in humans than in animal studies. The typical situation in treating human brain cancer is that therapies are administered over an extended interval (eg, several weeks). Because therapies are only moderately effective, the absolute change in water mobility following delivery of a fraction of a moderately effective therapy is attenuated. Despite these concerns there is good evidence therapeutic effects are detectable by diffusion, which supports its investigation as a response biomarker. There are other recent examples where diffusion reveals therapeutic effects outside the brain for patients treated for

cancer in the head and neck,[68] bone,[69] breast,[70,71] liver,[72] sarcoma,[73] and cervix.[74] The common trend in these studies is that an increase in tumor ADC values seems to be correlated with positive clinical response.

Original work in human brain tumor demonstrated the feasibility to detect therapy-induced tumor ADC changes relatively early into therapy,[60] and was found to be consistent with subsequent studies involving chemotherapy,[75] chemoradiation,[76] and stereotactic radiotherapy.[77,78] As with extracranial tumor sites, an ADC increase in brain tumor relatively early during treatment was more likely associated with a positive therapeutic response measured at a later date by traditional means. Work by Mardor and coworkers[76] also involved use of multiexponential diffusion decay features measurable at high b-values and these authors found additional sensitivity to treatment response in a composite index. This suggests that although there are fairly consistent findings

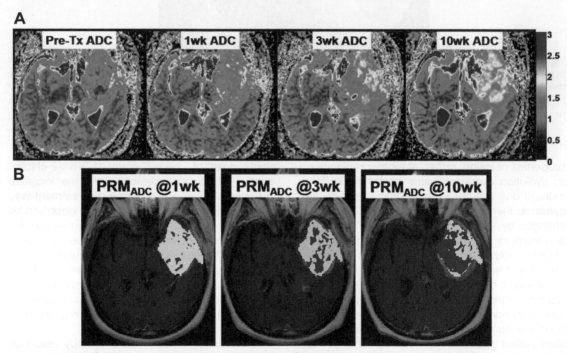

Fig. 5. PRMADC of a 45-year-old GBM patient. (A) Series of coregistered ADC maps 1 week before therapy and 1, 3, and 10 weeks from start of chemoradiotherapy. ADC maps are on a quantitative color scale in units of 10^{-3} mm^2/s. (B) Series of PRMADC maps showing an increase in ADC beyond a $+0.55 \times 10^{-3}$ mm^2/s significance threshold as red voxels; or a decrease in ADC by more than -0.55×10^{-3} mm^2/s as blue voxels and the remainder (nonsignificant change) as green voxels. These voxels are superimposed on the co-registered T1-weighted gadolinium image used to define the tumor volume of interest. PRMADC at 1, 3, and 10 weeks corresponds to ADC changes measured at 1, 3, and 10 weeks from start of therapy relative to pretherapy baseline. This patient had a relatively large fraction of the tumor that exhibited an increase in ADC early into treatment and was considered a "responder" by PRMADC analysis, which was consistent with this patient's 33-month survival. (Adapted from Hamstra DA, Galban CJ, Meyer CR, et al. Functional diffusion map as an early imaging biomarker for high-grade glioma: correlation with conventional radiologic response and overall survival. J Clin Oncol 2008;26:3387–94; with permission.)

across tumor sites and therapies, there remain technical issues in how to best analyze ADC data.

Definition of lesion extent and tumor heterogeneity are recognized challenges to use of image-based biomarkers including diffusion. In general, the studies cited previously used conventional ROI analysis to yield whole-tumor average ADC values. Standard ROI summary statistics of mean or median, however, do not address intralesion spatial heterogeneity or variable spatial response across the lesion. Cellular changes in tumor after therapy may involve a combination of cell swelling caused by loss of cellular water homeostasis, and subsequent cell lysis or apoptotic cell shrinkage. In addition, there may be a redistribution or resorption of excess water from edema and cysts. The balance of these effects can yield transient and spatially focal reduction and increases in diffusion values. The magnitude of these regional changes may be underestimated by ROI-derived whole-tumor averages. An alternative potential remedy to these effects is to deal with changes on a voxel-by-voxel basis. This concept originally applied to diffusion was referred to as "functional diffusion mapping" (fDM).[79] An essential element of fDM is spatial alignment of three-dimensional ADC maps into a common geometric framework. In this way diffusion changes are measurable on a voxel-by-voxel basis by subtraction of pretherapy from midtherapy or pretherapy from posttherapy three-dimensional image sets. In addition, co-registered ADC maps can be spatially aligned with high-quality three-dimensional anatomic data, such as postcontrast T1- and T2-weighted FLAIR images. Typically, multiple contrasts are co-registered using a mutual information algorithm and an affine transformation.[80] A clear advantage of this is that tumor boundaries can be drawn with the aid of the best available tumor contrast and defined over multiple slices

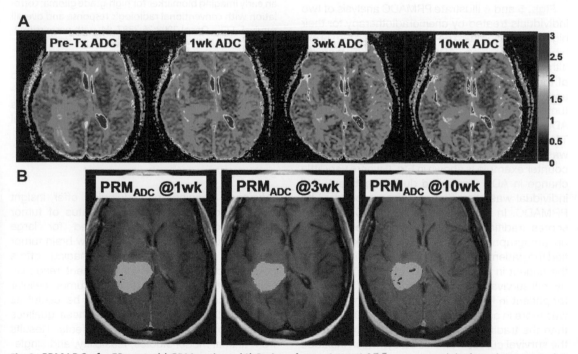

Fig. 6. PRMADC of a 53-year-old GBM patient. (A) Series of coregistered ADC maps 1 week before therapy; and 1, 3, and 10 weeks from start of start of chemoradiotherapy. ADC maps are on a quantitative color scale in units of 10^{-3} mm²/s. (B) Series of PRMADC maps showing an increase in ADC beyond a $+0.55 \times 10^{-3}$ mm²/s significance threshold as red voxels; or a decrease in ADC by more than -0.55×10^{-3} mm²/s as blue voxels and the remainder (nonsignificant change) as green voxels. These voxels are superimposed on the co-registered T1-weighted gadolinium image used to define the tumor volume of interest. PRMADC at 1, 3, and 10 weeks corresponds to ADC changes measured at 1, 3, and 10 weeks from start of therapy relative to pretherapy baseline. This patient had a relatively small fraction of the tumor that exhibited an increase in ADC early into treatment and was considered a "nonresponder" by PRMADC analysis, which was consistent with this patient's 7-month survival. (Adapted from Hamstra DA, Galban CJ, Meyer CR, et al. Functional diffusion map as an early imaging biomarker for high-grade glioma: correlation with conventional radiologic response and overall survival. J Clin Oncol 2008;26:3387–94; with permission.)

(ie, volume of interest). Because all three-dimensional image sets are spatially aligned, the volumes of interest defined on one type of image contrast are directly applicable to another image type or quantitative map. Another important distinction of this type of analysis is that instead of measuring the intensity of ADC change averaged over the volume of interest, one measures the volume (or fractional volume) of the tumor that exhibits a "significant" change. For this one needs to provide the threshold above which change is considered significant, more likely true than random. One method to determine this threshold was proposed in the original fDM article, although alternative approaches can be applied.[81] This concept has been extended to other modalities and is generally referred to as "parametric response mapping" (PRM).[82] For consistency with the generalized approach the original fDM may be referred to as PRMADC. Recently, PRM principles were applied to diffusion anisotropy[83] and to monitor recurrent brain tumor.[84]

Figs. 5 and 6 illustrate PRMADC analysis of two individuals treated by chemoradiotherapy for their high-grade gliomas. The first patient (see Fig. 5) exhibited increasing ADC early during therapy, although there was not much change in the size of the tumor. By week 3 into treatment PRMADC analysis indicated a relatively large fraction of the tumor volume exhibited a significant increase in ADC as coded by red voxels superimposed on T1-weighted gadolinium images in Fig. 5B, and was classified as a "responder" by PRMADC. A counter example is shown in Fig. 6 where very little change in ADC was noted during treatment; this individual was classified as a "nonresponder" by PRMADC. In contrast to the PRMADC response scores, traditional response criteria based primarily on radiographic size of the tumor at week 10 classified the patient in Fig. 5 as progressive disease and the patient in Fig. 6 as stable disease. The actual overall survival of these two individuals (33 months for patient in Fig. 5, 7 months for patient in Fig. 6) was more in agreement with the PRMADC findings than the traditional response score. Fig. 7 shows the survival curves from this study, which included 55 high-grade tumor patients as stratified by PRMADC.[85] A key finding from this study was that PRMADC was at least as prognostic as the traditional response criteria (Macdonald criteria). PRMADC stratification was available 7 to 8 weeks earlier well before therapy was completed, however, and it potentially allows for individualization of treatments.[85] As exemplified in these examples the PRM also provides a visual indication of tumor that appears more responsive to treatment and regions unaltered and possibly resistant to

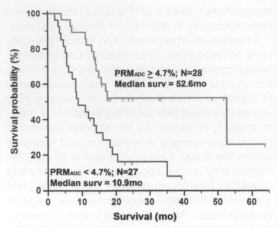

Fig. 7. Overall survival by log-rank test based on PRMADC stratification of 55 high-grade glioma patients at 3 weeks from start of treatment. PRMADC at 3 weeks from start of treatment was found to be at least as predictive of conventional lesion sized-based response criteria measured at 10 weeks. (*Adapted from* Hamstra DA, Galban CJ, Meyer CR, et al. Functional diffusion map as an early imaging biomarker for high-grade glioma: correlation with conventional radiologic response and overall survival. J Clin Oncol 2008;26:3387–94; with permission.)

treatment. This information may be valuable to guide spatially directed therapy, such as radiosurgery, although use of PRM to guide interventions has not yet been tested in large multi-institutional clinical trials.

SUMMARY

Advanced imaging methodologies offer insight into functional and biophysical status of tumor tissue and are being considered for large multi-institutional clinical trials of new brain tumor treatment strategies. Diffusion imaging offers potential as a biomarker of treatment response because it is sensitive to tissue-tumor cellular density and organization and may be useful as a quantitative index of change in these qualities because of positive therapeutic effects. Results from animal model studies, feasibility, and single-institution studies provide supportive evidence for use of diffusion-based quantities as treatment-response biomarkers. A variety of methods to analyze diffusion information have been proposed and range from simple ROI summary of baseline ADC-FA values in the lesion and their change with time, to more elaborate mapping voxel-by-voxel differences. These approaches have shown promise as response indicators, although the voxel-by-voxel response maps have the potential to guide spatially directed therapies.

REFERENCES

1. Horner MJ, Ries LAG, Krapcho M, et al. SEER cancer statistics review, 1975–2006. Bethesda (MD): National Cancer Institute; 2009.

2. Hegi ME, Diserens AC, Gorlia T, et al. MGMT gene silencing and benefit from temozolomide in glioblastoma. N Engl J Med 2005;352(10):997–1003.

3. Keles GE, Chang EF, Lamborn KR, et al. Volumetric extent of resection and residual contrast enhancement on initial surgery as predictors of outcome in adult patients with hemispheric anaplastic astrocytoma. J Neurosurg 2006;105(1):34–40.

4. Sanai N, Berger MS. Glioma extent of resection and its impact on patient outcome. Neurosurgery 2008; 62(4):753–64 [discussion: 264–6].

5. Gaspar LE, Scott C, Murray K, et al. Validation of the RTOG recursive partitioning analysis (RPA) classification for brain metastases. Int J Radiat Oncol Biol Phys 2000;47(4):1001–6.

6. Scott CB, Scarantino C, Urtasun R, et al. Validation and predictive power of Radiation Therapy Oncology Group (RTOG) recursive partitioning analysis classes for malignant glioma patients: a report using RTOG 90-06. Int J Radiat Oncol Biol Phys 1998;40(1):51–5.

7. Brandes AA, Franceschi E, Tosoni A, et al. MGMT promoter methylation status can predict the incidence and outcome of pseudoprogression after concomitant radiochemotherapy in newly diagnosed glioblastoma patients. J Clin Oncol 2008;26(13):2192–7.

8. Brandsma D, Stalpers L, Taal W, et al. Clinical features, mechanisms, and management of pseudoprogression in malignant gliomas. Lancet Oncol 2008;9(5):453–61.

9. Taal W, Brandsma D, de Bruin HG, et al. Incidence of early pseudo-progression in a cohort of malignant glioma patients treated with chemoirradiation with temozolomide. Cancer 2008;113(2):405–10.

10. Therasse P, Arbuck SG, Eisenhauer EA, et al. New guidelines to evaluate the response to treatment in solid tumors. European Organization for Research and Treatment of Cancer, National Cancer Institute of the United States, National Cancer Institute of Canada. J Natl Cancer Inst 2000;92(3):205–16.

11. Kauppinen RA. Monitoring cytotoxic tumour treatment response by diffusion magnetic resonance imaging and proton spectroscopy. NMR Biomed 2002;15(1):6–17.

12. Norris DG. The effects of microscopic tissue parameters on the diffusion weighted magnetic resonance imaging experiment. NMR Biomed 2001;14(2):77–93.

13. Szafer A, Zhong J, Gore JC. Theoretical model for water diffusion in tissues. Magn Reson Med 1995; 33(5):697–712.

14. Haacke EM, Brown RW, Thompson MR, et al. Magnetic resonance imaging: physical principles and sequence design. New York: John Wiley & Sons, Inc; 1999.

15. Hagmann P, Jonasson L, Maeder P, et al. Understanding diffusion MR imaging techniques: from scalar diffusion-weighted imaging to diffusion tensor imaging and beyond. Radiographics 2006; 26(Suppl 1):S205–23.

16. Le Bihan D, Mangin JF, Poupon C, et al. Diffusion tensor imaging: concepts and applications. J Magn Reson Imaging 2001;13(4):534–46.

17. Basser PJ, Jones DK. Diffusion-tensor MRI: theory, experimental design and data analysis. A technical review. NMR Biomed 2002;15(7–8):456–67.

18. Sorensen AG, Buonanno FS, Gonzalez RG, et al. Hyperacute stroke: evaluation with combined multi-section diffusion-weighted and hemodynamically weighted echo-planar MR imaging. Radiology 1996;199(2):391–401.

19. Warach S, Gaa J, Siewert B, et al. Acute human stroke studied by whole brain echo planar diffusion-weighted magnetic resonance imaging. Ann Neurol 1995;37(2):231–41.

20. Clark CA, Le Bihan D. Water diffusion compartmentation and anisotropy at high b values in the human brain. Magn Reson Med 2000;44(6):852–9.

21. Le Bihan D. The wet mind: water and functional neuroimaging. Phys Med Biol 2007;52(7):R57–90.

22. Mulkern RV, Gudbjartsson H, Westin CF, et al. Multicomponent apparent diffusion coefficients in human brain. NMR Biomed 1999;12(1):51–62.

23. Mulkern RV, Haker SJ, Maier SE. On high b diffusion imaging in the human brain: ruminations and experimental insights. Magn Reson Imaging 2009;27(8):1151–62.

24. Bennett KM, Schmainda KM, Bennett RT, et al. Characterization of continuously distributed cortical water diffusion rates with a stretched-exponential model. Magn Reson Med 2003;50(4):727–34.

25. Lee JH, Springer CS Jr. Effects of equilibrium exchange on diffusion-weighted NMR signals: the diffusigraphic shutter-speed. Magn Reson Med 2003; 49(3):450–8.

26. Kwee TC, Galbán CJ, Tsien C, et al. Intravoxel water diffusion heterogeneity imaging of human high-grade gliomas. NMR Biomed 2009, in press.

27. Beaulieu C. The basis of anisotropic water diffusion in the nervous system: a technical review. NMR Biomed 2002;15(7–8):435–55.

28. Chenevert TL, Brunberg JA, Pipe JG. Anisotropic diffusion in human white matter: demonstration with MR techniques in vivo. Radiology 1990;177(2):401–5.

29. Mori S, Frederiksen K, van Zijl PC, et al. Brain white matter anatomy of tumor patients evaluated with diffusion tensor imaging. Ann Neurol 2002;51(3):377–80.

30. Mori S, van Zijl PC. Fiber tracking: principles and strategies: a technical review. NMR Biomed 2002; 15(7–8):468–80.

31. Moseley M. Diffusion tensor imaging and aging: a review. NMR Biomed 2002;15(7–8):553–60.

32. Moseley ME, Kucharczyk J, Asgari HS, et al. Anisotropy in diffusion-weighted MRI. Magn Reson Med 1991;19(2):321–6.

33. Alexander AL, Hasan K, Kindlmann G, et al. A geometric analysis of diffusion tensor measurements of the human brain. Magn Reson Med 2000; 44(2):283–91.

34. Papadakis NG, Xing D, Houston GC, et al. A study of rotationally invariant and symmetric indices of diffusion anisotropy. Magn Reson Imaging 1999;17(6):881–92.

35. Westin CF, Maier SE, Mamata H, et al. Processing and visualization for diffusion tensor MRI. Med Image Anal 2002;6(2):93–108.

36. Chenevert TL, McKeever PE, Ross BD. Monitoring early response of experimental brain tumors to therapy using diffusion magnetic resonance imaging. Clin Cancer Res 1997;3(9):1457–66.

37. Lope-Piedrafita S, Garcia-Martin ML, Galons JP, et al. Longitudinal diffusion tensor imaging in a rat brain glioma model. NMR Biomed 2008;21(8):799–808.

38. Melhem ER, Mori S, Mukundan G, et al. Diffusion tensor MR imaging of the brain and white matter tractography. AJR Am J Roentgenol 2002;178(1):3–16.

39. Gauvain KM, McKinstry RC, Mukherjee P, et al. Evaluating pediatric brain tumor cellularity with diffusion-tensor imaging. AJR Am J Roentgenol 2001;177(2): 449–54.

40. Guo AC, Cummings TJ, Dash RC, et al. Lymphomas and high-grade astrocytomas: comparison of water diffusibility and histologic characteristics. Radiology 2002;224(1):177–83.

41. Kono K, Inoue Y, Nakayama K, et al. The role of diffusion-weighted imaging in patients with brain tumors. AJNR Am J Neuroradiol 2001;22(6):1081–8.

42. Sugahara T, Karogi Y, Kochi M, et al. Usefulness of diffusion-weighted MRI with echo-planar technique in the evaluation of cellularity in gliomas. J Magn Reson Imaging 1999;9(1):53–60.

43. Castillo M, Smith JK, Kwock L, et al. Apparent diffusion coefficients in the evaluation of high-grade cerebral gliomas. AJNR Am J Neuroradiol 2001;22(1):60–4.

44. Gupta RK, Sinha U, Cloughesy TF, et al. Inverse correlation between choline magnetic resonance spectroscopy signal intensity and the apparent diffusion coefficient in human glioma. Magn Reson Med 1999;41(1):2–7.

45. Bastin ME, Sinha S, Whittle IR, et al. Measurements of water diffusion and T1 values in peritumoural oedematous brain. Neuroreport 2002;13(10):1335–40.

46. Sinha S, Bastin ME, Whittle IR, et al. Diffusion tensor MR imaging of high-grade cerebral gliomas. AJNR Am J Neuroradiol 2002;23(4):520–7.

47. Provenzale JM, McGraw P, Mhatre P, et al. Peritumoral brain regions in gliomas and meningiomas: investigation with isotropic diffusion-weighted MR imaging and diffusion-tensor MR imaging. Radiology 2004;232(2):451–60.

48. Stadnik TW, Chaskis C, Michotte A, et al. Diffusion-weighted MR imaging of intracerebral masses: comparison with conventional MR imaging and histologic findings. AJNR Am J Neuroradiol 2001; 22(5):969–76.

49. Field AS, Alexander AL. Diffusion tensor imaging in cerebral tumor diagnosis and therapy. Top Magn Reson Imaging 2004;15(5):315–24.

50. Brunberg JA, Chenevert TL, McKeever PE, et al. In vivo MR determination of water diffusion coefficients and diffusion anisotropy: correlation with structural alteration in gliomas of the cerebral hemispheres. AJNR Am J Neuroradiol 1995;16(2):361–71.

51. Krabbe K, Gideon P, Wagn P, et al. MR diffusion imaging of human intracranial tumours. Neuroradiology 1997;39(7):483–9.

52. Lu S, Ahn D, Johnson G, et al. Peritumoral diffusion tensor imaging of high-grade gliomas and metastatic brain tumors. AJNR Am J Neuroradiol 2003; 24(5):937–41.

53. Lu S, Ahn D, Johnson G, et al. Diffusion-tensor MR imaging of intracranial neoplasia and associated peritumoral edema: introduction of the tumor infiltration index. Radiology 2004;232(1):221–8.

54. Inoue T, Ogasawara K, Beppu T, et al. Diffusion tensor imaging for preoperative evaluation of tumor grade in gliomas. Clin Neurol Neurosurg 2005;107(3):174–80.

55. Wieshmann UC, Symms MR, Parker GJ, et al. Diffusion tensor imaging demonstrates deviation of fibres in normal appearing white matter adjacent to a brain tumour. J Neurol Neurosurg Psychiatr 2000;68(4): 501–3.

56. Pierpaoli C, Jezzard P, Basser PJ, et al. Diffusion tensor MR imaging of the human brain. Radiology 1996;201(3):637–48.

57. Shimony JS, McKinstry RC, Akbudak E, et al. Quantitative diffusion-tensor anisotropy brain MR imaging: normative human data and anatomic analysis. Radiology 1999;212(3):770–84.

58. Field AS, Alexander AL, Wu YC, et al. Diffusion tensor eigenvector directional color imaging patterns in the evaluation of cerebral white matter tracts altered by tumor. J Magn Reson Imaging 2004;20(4):555–62.

59. Mardor Y, Roth Y, Ochershvilli A, et al. Pretreatment prediction of brain tumors' response to radiation therapy using high b-value diffusion-weighted MRI. Neoplasia 2004;6(2):136–42.

60. Chenevert TL, Stegman LD, Taylor JM, et al. Diffusion magnetic resonance imaging: an early surrogate marker of therapeutic efficacy in brain tumors. J Natl Cancer Inst 2000;92(24):2029–36.

61. Hall DE, Moffat BA, Stojanovska J, et al. Therapeutic efficacy of DTI-015 using diffusion magnetic resonance imaging as an early surrogate marker. Clin Cancer Res 2004;10(23):7852–9.

62. Henning EC, Azuma C, Sotak CH, et al. Multispectral tissue characterization in a RIF-1 tumor model:

monitoring the ADC and T2 responses to single-dose radiotherapy (part II). Magn Reson Med 2007;57(3):513–9.

63. Kim H, Morgan DE, Buchsbaum DJ, et al. Early therapy evaluation of combined anti-death receptor 5 antibody and gemcitabine in orthotopic pancreatic tumor xenografts by diffusion-weighted magnetic resonance imaging. Cancer Res 2008;68(20):8369–76.

64. McConville P, Hambardzumyan D, Moody JB, et al. Magnetic resonance imaging determination of tumor grade and early response to temozolomide in a genetically engineered mouse model of glioma. Clin Cancer Res 2007;13(10):2897–904.

65. Stegman LD, Rehemtulla A, Hamstra DA, et al. Diffusion MRI detects early events in the response of a glioma model to the yeast cytosine deaminase gene therapy strategy. Gene Ther 2000;7(12):1005–10.

66. Galons JP, Altbach MI, Paine-Murrieta GD, et al. Early increases in breast tumor xenograft water mobility in response to paclitaxel therapy detected by non-invasive diffusion magnetic resonance imaging. Neoplasia 1999;1(2):113–7.

67. Jennings D, Hatton BN, Guo J, et al. Early response of prostate carcinoma xenografts to docetaxel chemotherapy monitored with diffusion MRI. Neoplasia 2002;4(3):255–62.

68. Kim S, Loevner L, Quon H, et al. Diffusion-weighted magnetic resonance imaging for predicting and detecting early response to chemoradiation therapy of squamous cell carcinomas of the head and neck. Clin Cancer Res 2009;15(3):986–94.

69. Lee KC, Bradley DA, Hussain M, et al. A feasibility study evaluating the functional diffusion map as a predictive imaging biomarker for detection of treatment response in a patient with metastatic prostate cancer to the bone. Neoplasia 2007;9(12):1003–11.

70. Pickles MD, Gibbs P, Lowry M, et al. Diffusion changes precede size reduction in neoadjuvant treatment of breast cancer. Magn Reson Imaging 2006;24(7):843–7.

71. Yankeelov TE, Lepage M, Chakravarthy A, et al. Integration of quantitative DCE-MRI and ADC mapping to monitor treatment response in human breast cancer: initial results. Magn Reson Imaging 2007; 25(1):1–13.

72. Kamel IR, Liapi E, Reyes DK, et al. Unresectable hepatocellular carcinoma: serial early vascular and cellular changes after transarterial chemoembolization as detected with MR imaging. Radiology 2009; 250(2):466–73.

73. Dudeck O, Zeile M, Pink D, et al. Diffusion-weighted magnetic resonance imaging allows monitoring of anticancer treatment effects in patients with soft-tissue sarcomas. J Magn Reson Imaging 2008; 27(5):1109–13.

74. Harry VN, Semple SI, Gilbert FJ, et al. Diffusion-weighted magnetic resonance imaging in the early detection of response to chemoradiation in cervical cancer. Gynecol Oncol 2008;111(2):213–20.

75. Schubert MI, Wilke M, Muller-Weihrich S, et al. Diffusion-weighted magnetic resonance imaging of treatment-associated changes in recurrent and residual medulloblastoma: preliminary observations in three children. Acta Radiol 2006;47(10):1100–4.

76. Mardor Y, Pfeffer R, Spiegelmann R, et al. Early detection of response to radiation therapy in patients with brain malignancies using conventional and high b-value diffusion-weighted magnetic resonance imaging. J Clin Oncol 2003;21(6):1094–100.

77. Tomura N, Narita K, Izumi J, et al. Diffusion changes in a tumor and peritumoral tissue after stereotactic irradiation for brain tumors: possible prediction of treatment response. J Comput Assist Tomogr 2006; 30(3):496–500.

78. Huang CF, Chou HH, Tu HT, et al. Diffusion magnetic resonance imaging as an evaluation of the response of brain metastases treated by stereotactic radiosurgery. Surg Neurol 2008;69(1):62–8 [discussion: 68].

79. Moffat BA, Chenevert TL, Lawrence TS, et al. Functional diffusion map: a noninvasive MRI biomarker for early stratification of clinical brain tumor response. Proc Natl Acad Sci U S A 2005;102(15):5524–9.

80. Meyer CR, Boes JL, Kim B, et al. Demonstration of accuracy and clinical versatility of mutual information for automatic multimodality image fusion using affine and thin-plate spline warped geometric deformations. Med Image Anal 1997;1(3):195–206.

81. Meyer C, Chenevert T, Galban C, et al. Parametric response mapping: a voxel-based analysis of quantitative diffusion MRI changes for individualized assessment of primary breast cancer response to therapy. Proceedings 17th Scientific Meeting, International Society for Magnetic Resonance in Medicine. April 18–24, 2009. p. 2223.

82. Galbán CJ, Chenevert TL, Meyer CR, et al. The parametric response map: an imaging biomarker for early cancer treatment outcome. Nature Medicine 2009;15(5):572–6.

83. Wai Y, Chu J, Wang C, et al. An integrated diffusion map for the analysis of diffusion properties: a feasibility study in patients with acoustic neuroma. Acad Radiol 2009;16(4):428–34.

84. Ellingson B, Malkin M, Rand S, et al. Functional diffusion maps applied to FLAIR abnormal areas are valuable for the clinical monitoring of recurrent brain tumors. Proceedings 17th Scientific Meeting, International Society for Magnetic Resonance in Medicine. April 18–24, 2009. p. 285.

85. Hamstra DA, Galban CJ, Meyer CR, et al. Functional diffusion map as an early imaging biomarker for high-grade glioma: correlation with conventional radiologic response and overall survival. J Clin Oncol 2008;26(20):3387–94.

Presurgical Mapping of Verbal Language in Brain Tumors with Functional MR Imaging and MR Tractography

Alberto Bizzi, MD

KEYWORDS

- Presurgical planning • Intraoperative electrical stimulation
- Functional MR imaging • DTI-MR tractography
- Language • Arcuate fasciculus • Brain tumor • Plasticity

Cortical mapping with direct electrical stimulation mapping (ESM) during surgical craniotomy in awake and cooperative patients was introduced at the beginning of the twentieth century. In the early 1990s the refinement of intraoperative neurophysiologic monitoring, as well as the development of imaging-guided neuronavigational devices and of new functional and anatomic magnetic resonance (MR)-based mapping techniques set the stage for a renaissance of intraoperative ESM. Improvements in lesion localization, and in presurgical and intraoperative assessment of functional brain activity have increased the surgical accessibility of focal brain lesions seated in eloquent areas.

Modern neuroimaging methods provide morphologic, metabolic, and functional measurements that have the potential of guiding and refining surgical treatment. In particular, functional MR (fMR) imaging and diffusion MR tractography have the potential to map nodes and connections of several functional networks. If validated, modern imaging methods may determine hemispheric dominance, establish the relationship of a lesion to adjacent critical gray and white matter structures, and predict postoperative outcome. Neurosurgeons appreciate the value of having functional imaging maps available at their desk when planning a surgical procedure.

MAPPING BRAIN FUNCTIONS
Historical Perspective

The aim of understanding the functional organization of the human brain has motivated philosophers and scientists for centuries. The observation that a focal brain lesion may cause a behavioral or motor deficit was alluded to in an Egyptian papyrus that has been dated to roughly 2500 BC. It is possible that Imhotep, a military surgeon at the time of the pyramids, was the author of this detailed clinical report on 27 cases with head injury.[1] It was at the time of the Alexandria Medical School in the third century BC that Erofilo from Calcedonia (Turkey), an early anatomist, suggested that the brain harbors motor, sensory, and cognitive functions.

It was only in the sixteenth century that Costanzo Varolio (1543–1575) suggested that higher cognitive functions might take place in the brain parenchyma. In the seventeenth century Thomas Willis (1621–1675), the English anatomist and surgeon, localized memory to the cortical gray matter, imagination in the white matter,

Neuroradiology Unit, Fondazione IRCCS Istituto Neurologico Carlo Besta, Via Celoria, 11, 201133 Milan, Italy
E-mail address: alberto_bizzi@fastwebnet.it

Neuroimag Clin N Am 19 (2009) 573–596
doi:10.1016/j.nic.2009.08.010
1052-5149/09/$ – see front matter © 2009 Published by Elsevier Inc.

perception and movement in the striatum, and involuntary actions to the cerebellum and brainstem. It was Giovanni Galvani (1737–1798), an Italian from Bologna, who demonstrated that nervous system activity is an electrophysiological, as opposed to hydrodynamic, phenomenon.

In the nineteenth century, the progress of Neurology was tremendous, due to multiple technical innovations and the application of the anatomoclinical correlation methods introduced by Giovan Battista Morgagni (1682–1771). It was Paul Broca (1824–1880) who declared "Nous parlon avec l'hemisphere gauche" in 1865. Sir Victor Horsley (1857–1916) was the first neurosurgeon to perform direct ESM of the cortex during resection of a deep lesion. Horsley identified an area of motor representation around the central sulcus.

Notwithstanding these innovations, the holistic theory developed by Flourens remained the dominant theory in the academic world throughout the first half of the 1900s. Studies of anatomy and neurophysiology provided more evidence for localization of brain functions during the first 2 decades of the twentieth century. In 1929 Hans Berger, an Austrian neuropsychiatrist, made the first report of the electroencephalogram (EEG) recorded from the scalp. In 1935 Otfrid Foerster (1873–1941) and H. Altenburger acquired the first electrocorticography, and identified the supplementary motor area (SMA). Wilder Penfield (1891–1976), the Neurosurgeon-in-Chief at the Montreal Neurologic Institute, was Foerster's student. Penfield devised direct intraoperative ESM as we know it today. He performed ESM in 1132 epileptic patients, and found that not only motor and somatosensory areas but also language and memory sensations of "deja-vu" can be mapped on the brain surface.

George Ojemann, of the University of Washington in Seattle, provided a more recent historical contribution. He introduced the concept that language localization is highly variable among individuals.[2,3] Ojemann suggested that the classic nineteenth century model of language localization was inaccurate for establishing the risk of aphasia in patients with a focal lesion in the dominant perisylvian cortex. Rather, the risk of developing neurologic deficits could be better assessed in each individual patient using cortical stimulation mapping techniques.[3] Ojemann also performed the first controlled study of language-related activity in the human temporal lobe, using microelectrode recordings.[4]

In the last 20 years modern noninvasive functional imaging techniques, including fMR imaging and positron emission tomography (PET), have been developed and quickly they have become the most popular methods to map the organization of the working human brain. These techniques measure local changes in brain blood flow and blood oxygenation associated with mental activity. The idea of inferring neuronal activity in the brain from a measurement of changes in local blood flow dates back to the observations made by Angelo Mosso, a nineteenth century Italian physiologist from Turin (Italy), in patients with skull defects following neurosurgical procedures.[5,6] Mosso noted that pulsations of the human cortex change during mental activity and "blood very likely may rush to each region of the cortex according as it is most active." He supposed that a very small adjustment in local blood flow follows the needs of the cerebral activity. The idea of using blood flow to map brain activity definitely preceded the ability to do such measurements.[7]

There are at least 3 MR-based techniques that can measure brain function: T2*-weighted susceptibility contrast, perfusion with arterial spin labeling, and in-flow MR angiography. All 3 fMR imaging techniques take advantage of the coupling of cerebral blood flow with oxygen consumption and neural activity. The most robust method with whole brain coverage and higher spatial resolution is susceptibility contrast fMR imaging, based on the discovery made by Ogawa and colleagues[8] in 1990. Deoxyhemoglobin is paramagnetic, and changes in its concentration will affect the MR signal of blood. An increase in deoxyhemoglobin will determine an attenuation of the MR signal that is known as a blood oxygenation level dependent (BOLD) effect. Increments in oxygen content occur at the site of activation. fMR imaging with BOLD contrast provides indirect measurements of neuronal activity by monitoring local hemodynamic changes during performance of a task.

Functional Magnetic Resonance Imaging of Verbal Language

It is important to emphasize that patients with a focal brain lesion should be able to perform the task well to obtain a reliable presurgical mapping of the language network. Even though these patients are usually cooperative and motivated, they may be more anxious than healthy subjects, especially if the fMR imaging study is performed a few days before brain surgery. Because the aforementioned factors may interfere with the subject's performance and the fMR imaging results, a careful preparation and evaluation of these patients is important.

The extension of the cortex activated during the fMR imaging experiment depends on the condition that is experimentally chosen to isolate the function of interest. The essence of language is the capacity to retain, retrieve, and combine arbitrary symbols of a native language into an infinite number of potential expressions. The sensory (input) and motor (output) processes as well as the attention-related functions that are associated with verbal language should be considered distinct from it. The choice of the resting (control) condition is also important, because the brain processes occurring will be inevitably subtracted from the tested condition. The resting condition will have to include all brain processes that are associated with the function of interest but are distinct from it.

Silent language tasks are usually preferred because motion artifacts are reduced.[9] Stimulus input may be visual or acoustic. The former is preferable for evaluating specific language-processing components activating the temporal lobes, because language-related BOLD responses will not be confused with responses in primary auditory areas.

A variety of language paradigms have been developed: verbal fluency with word generation, verb generation, sentence comprehension, and passive listening. All these tasks are easy to implement, perform, and analyze. It has been shown that the use of multiple language paradigms increases the sensitivity and specificity of presurgical fMR imaging.[10,11] Thus it would be preferable to use more than one language paradigm.

Verb generation (VGEN) is the most commonly used and probably the most reliable test in the clinical arena. Instructions are simple: given a word think of the associated verb. Most patients understand it well and are compliant once inside the magnet. Even patients with mild to moderate language deficits can perform it without great difficulty. The VGEN can be administered with a visual or auditory input. At the author's institution the visual input is preferred. Performance of this task includes both language components: comprehension and production. The 3 main linguistic processes are involved: semantics, phonology, and syntax. These linguistic processes evoke a robust BOLD response both in the laterofrontal and temporoparietal language cortex. It has been shown that the VGEN is reliable in assessing language dominance.[12,13]

Two additional tasks that nicely complement the VGEN are the verbal fluency and the sentence comprehension (SC) tasks.[14] Word generation (WGEN) can be used as a verbal phonological fluency task: given a letter the subjects must generate a series of consecutive words starting with the letter shown. The SC task is designed to elicit a stronger response in the posterior language areas: given a one-line sentence to read, the subject has to recognize whichever one of two scenes best illustrates the sentence.

A controversial topic is whether a clear-cut functional parcellation of Broca area can be demonstrated with fMR imaging using different types of verbal fluency tasks: phonological, semantic, and syntactic. Intraoperative ESM studies have shown high specificity of the stimulated cortical areas. The fMR imaging literature suggests that semantic and phonological fluency tasks selectively activate left Brodmann areas (BA) 44 (pars opercularis) and 45 (pars triangularis) in the Broca area, respectively. However, this view has been challenged by a recent fMR imaging study that has shown all different types of verbal fluency tasks to evoke a strong BOLD response in BA 44 and 45.[15] A single paradigm with low linguistic specificity but evoking BOLD response in all language cortical areas may not be so exciting for a cognitive neuroscientist; however, it would indeed be valuable in presurgical fMR imaging. To date, the VGEN language paradigm has been considered the most robust and the most widely used.[10,14,16,17]

Interpretation of fMR imaging studies requires a high degree of experience. The statistical maps must be checked for quality and artifacts. The location of clusters of BOLD response in cortical areas that are putative nodes of the language network must be accurately identified. The spatial extension of the BOLD response in each location must be evaluated at different statistical thresholds to choose the optimal value. Spatial extent of the BOLD response can be highly variable among subjects, because it depends on the quality and quantity of signal acquired rather than on intrinsic boundaries of brain function.[18]

There are several limitations inherent to the fMR imaging technique. There are important differences in the time course of electrophysiological and hemodynamic responses. This uncertainty of neurovascular coupling is a big challenge and a potential source of error in interpreting clinical fMR imaging studies. The BOLD response often localizes in the adjacent sulcus, and it can be a few millimeters away from the electrophysiologically functioning cortex. Colocalization of an important part of the BOLD signal with the draining vasculature is well known and studied.[19] Not least, it should be kept in mind that activation of an area detected by fMR imaging and PET predominantly reflects the input to the area and the corresponding changes in information processing rather than output (ie, neuronal firing) from that area.[20]

Diffusion Tensor Imaging

Diffusion tensor imaging (DTI)[21] measures the effects of tissue microstructure on the random walks (Brownian motion) of water molecules in the brain. In tissues with an orderly oriented microstructure, such as the cerebral white matter, the measured diffusivity of water varies with the tissue's orientation (anisotropic diffusion). Water diffuses fastest along the principal direction of the fibers and slowest along the cross-sectional plane. The DTI model provides the required information to construct a diffusion ellipsoid in each voxel of an imaging volume. DTI measures the diffusivities of water molecules along the 3 orthogonal axes of the ellipsoid (eigenvalues) and their average (mean diffusivity). Fractional anisotropy is a measure of eccentricity of the displacement of water molecules. In the healthy human brain, probably the most relevant factor affecting fractional anisotropy is the intravoxel orientation coherence of white matter fibers.[22]

There are 3 main imaging output of DTI MR imaging: quantitative parametric maps displayed in gray scale (ie, fractional anisotropy maps), color maps showing the principal orientation of diffusion for each voxel, and 3-dimensional maps showing virtual dissection of tracts with streamline tracking methods. The aim of fiber tracking or MR tractography is to infer the 3-dimensional trajectories of white matter bundles by piecing together discrete estimates of the underlying continuous fiber orientation field measured noninvasively with DTI data.[23,24]

Fiber tracking algorithms can be broadly classified into 2 types: deterministic and probabilistic. A DTI tractography atlas for virtual in vivo dissection of the principal human white matter tracts using a deterministic approach has been recently published.[25] Few limitations of fiber tracking performed with the deterministic approach motivated the development of probabilistic tracking algorithms.[26] It is important to understand well the inherent limitations of all methods of DTI-based virtual dissections and measurements. One important limitation is that in each voxel the eigenvector is the average of the orientation of all bundles included in the voxel. In volumes of white matter with many crossing bundles, as in the frontal and parietal paraventricular white matter, fractional anisotropy is low and the degree of uncertainty in the estimation of bundle orientation increases. The limitation of crossing fibers has been addressed with the development of more sophisticated imaging acquisition schemes using high angular resolution diffusion imaging (HARDI).[27]

FUNCTIONAL ANATOMY OF VERBAL LANGUAGE
Topology

The *classic model* of language was developed in the nineteenth century from retrospective studies that correlated neuropathology lesions with different types of aphasic syndromes. The model consists of a frontal expressive area (Broca), a posterior receptive area (Wernicke), and a connecting bundle (arcuate fasciculus, AF).

Topology is the study of places. The word derives from the Greek *topos*, meaning "place." A functional cerebral network is made of specialized cortical areas (places or nodes) and their interconnecting white matter bundles (connections or pathways). Anterior frontal language cortical areas include the posterior part of the inferior frontal gyrus (IFG) that is known as the Broca area, the dorsolateral prefrontal cortex (DLPFC) in the middle frontal gyrus (MFG), and the ventrolateral prefrontal cortex (VLPFC), part of the premotor cortex. Posterior temporal language cortical areas include the superior temporal gyrus (pSTG), middle temporal gyrus (pMTG), and the cortex within the superior temporal sulcus (pSTS). Parietal language cortical areas include the supramarginal gyrus (SMG) and the angular gyrus (AG) in the inferior parietal lobule (Fig. 1).

The robust fMR imaging language tasks that are used in clinical practice and are described herein identify well most of the areas included in the classic model. The tasks are robust also because they evoke simultaneously multiple linguistic processes.

The WGEN task gives a robust BOLD response in the Broca area in the dominant IFG, VLPFC, DLPFC, and STS, but it often gives a less consistent response in the inferior parietal lobule and in the posterior temporal cortex. The SC task gives a robust BOLD response in the dominant VLPFC, DLPFC, AG, and STS, but it gives a less consistent response in the Broca area. The VGEN task gives a robust and consistent BOLD response in all the aforementioned areas.[14]

Modern neuroimaging studies of language processing with PET and fMR imaging suggested that the classic model might be oversimplistic and outdated, although still widely used. The new model represents multiple linguistic processes in the brain. According to the *cognitive model* verbal language is organized in parallel linguistic processes that include orthography, phonology, syntax, and lexical semantics. Functional imaging studies of individual linguistic processes have shown parcellation of activation in the classic language areas.[28,29] Speech and

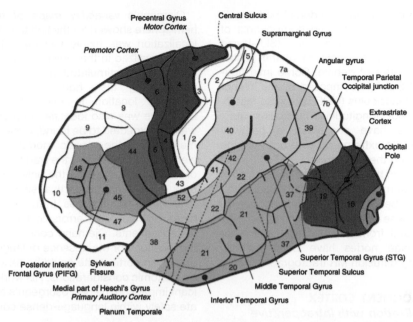

Fig. 1. The lateral surface of the left hemisphere showing the main anatomic structures involved in verbal language. The numbers refer to Brodmann areas (BA). Anterior language areas are located in the inferior frontal gyrus (44–46) and in the dorsolateroprefrontal cortex (6). Language areas in the inferior parietal lobule are located in the supramarginal (40) and angular (39) gyri. Posterior language areas are located in the superior (22) and middle temporal (37) gyri. (*Reproduced from* Démonet JF, Thiérry G, Cardebat D. Renewal of the neurophysiology of language: functional neuroimaging. Physiol Rev 2005;85:49–95; with permission.)

language deficits are now classified according to the selective involvement of each linguistic process. Selection of the appropriate linguistic therapy in aphasic patients is also made according to the cognitive model.

Hodology

Hodology is the study of pathways. The word derives from the Greek *hodos*, meaning "path." In the nineteenth century the anatomy of white matter connections was studied with the fiber dissecting technique at autopsy. In the second part of the twentieth century brain connections were studied with microscopic staining sections, and in vivo in the monkey with tracing autoradiographic techniques. With emerging of diffusion MR tractography it has now become possible to virtually dissect the main white matter pathways in vivo in humans. A new interest on the anatomy and function of the white matter pathways has emerged. In particular for presurgical mapping and speech rehabilitation, MR tractography has the potential to answer 2 very relevant questions: (1) Which bundles are involved in verbal language? (2) Will severing of a specific bundle during surgery lead to permanent language deficits? MR tractography in combination with new advanced neuropathology studies has the potential to test multiple

hypotheses about the role that each pathway may play in several language processes. With diffusion MR tractography the hodological approach can be tested in clinicoanatomic correlation studies.[30–32]

Current theories on brain organization suggest that cognitive functions such as verbal language are organized in widespread, segregated, and overlapping networks.[33] Hickok and Poeppel recently proposed a dual-stream model for auditory language processing.[34–36] From the pSTG, which is engaged in early cortical stages of speech perception, the system diverges into 2 processing streams. The *dorsal stream* projects dorsally toward the inferior parietal lobule and the posterior frontal lobe (DLPFC), and is involved in auditory-motor integration by mapping acoustic speech sounds to articulator representations. The prototype task targeting this dorsal stream is repetition of speech.[34,35] The *ventral stream* projects ventrolaterally to the middle and inferior temporal cortices, and the VLPFC serves as a sound-to-meaning interface by mapping sound-based representations of speech to widely distributed conceptual representations. The prototype task targeting this ventral stream is listening to meaningful speech.[34,35]

In brief, the dorsal pathway mediates sublexical repetition of speech, whereas the ventral pathway mediates comprehension. The dorsal pathway is likely composed of the AF and components of the superior longitudinal fasciculus (SLF-I and SLF-II), whereas the composition of the ventral pathway is a matter of debate. Some investigators[31] suggest that it is composed by the inferior fronto-occipital fasciculus (IFOF), uncinate fasciculus, and inferior longitudinal fasciculus (ILF), whereas others have suggested a pathway coursing along the extreme capsule between the insular cortex and the claustrum.[37]

The relevance of the several bundles involved in language in determination of hemispheric dominance has also been raised. Hemispheric asymmetries of these pathways connecting the inferoventrolateral frontal, temporal, and inferior parietal language nodes have been recently described using diffusion MR tractography.

MAPPING ELOQUENT CORTEX
Cortical Localization with Intraoperative Direct Electrical Stimulation Mapping

Intraoperative direct ESM is a safe, precise, and reliable electrophysiological technique that is currently used to identify eloquent cortical areas and subcortical white matter connections. Devised by Penfield and Roberts,[38] ESM is based on the observation that applying a direct current to an area on the cortical surface may block a specific function, although no local sensation is reported by the awake patient. Intraoperative ESM historically has been used to identify eloquent cortex during resection of epileptic foci, and only more recently for resection of brain neoplasm.

ESM results provide a different perspective from lesion-deficit correlations in patients with chronic stroke, multiple sclerosis or neurodegenerative diseases. The brief duration of the stimulation makes it unlikely that any functional reorganization occurs during the time the current is being applied. Until George Ojemann published his landmark study about "Cortical language localization in the left dominant hemisphere: an ESM investigation in 117 patients" with epilepsy,[39] knowledge of language localization was based on "the lesion method" and clinical-neuropathological correlations.[40] Ojemann was the first to systematically evaluate data from intraoperative ESM of human cortex.[41] Intraoperative ESM studies found that verbal language areas are highly localized in patients and form several mosaics of 1 or less square centimeters.[3,39,42,43] The area of individual mosaics and the total area related to language are usually much smaller than the classic Broca and Wernicke areas.

Ojemann's *variability maps* of the dominant hemisphere showed for the first time that language localization was highly variable. Although often highly localized in the individual patient, essential sites directly stimulated during performance of the naming task had exceedingly different anatomic location in the patient population. Language was also identified in areas in which it was not expected to be found, based on the lesion method and the classic model. Eloquent sites were found far beyond the traditional boundaries of the Broca area. With the only exception of the pars opercularis, no cortical site exceeded 50% of eloquent naming sites. In the temporal-parietal lobes ESM evoked errors in less than 36% of tested patients. Ojemann concluded that neither the location nor the absence of language function at a given cortical site could be reliably predicted by anatomic considerations. His work had a significant impact on the neurosurgeon's ability to operate safely within language-dense cortex.

Variability of Language Localization with Functional Magnetic Resonance Imaging

With the aim to measure interindividual variability of language cortical sites in healthy subjects, Cerliani and colleagues[14] have produced *surface variability maps*. The investigators generated variability maps for the dominant and nondominant hemispheres for each of 3 language tasks (VGEN, WGEN, and SC) in right- and left-handers. The fMR imaging variability maps are color maps that illustrate, for each vertex of the standardized folded cortical mesh, how many subjects show a significant experimental effect. The images are powerful in displaying the variability of the location and extent of the cognitive processes involved during the task. The maps also show that all 3 tasks reliably determine hemisphere dominance. In comparison with the ESM variability maps they offer 2 main advantages: they are semi-automatically generated and both cerebral hemispheres are displayed.

The variability maps may be clinically useful in evaluating the probability that a focal lesion may determine a language deficit in a specific cortical area. The maps also may suggest the language task of choice to study the relationship of an infiltrating mass with the adjacent functioning cortex. For instance, the WGEN and VGEN are better indicated to study a glioma infiltrating the left IFG and the VGEN to study the AG, whereas the VGEN and SC should be used to study lesions in the posterior temporal cortex (**Fig. 2**).

The variability maps may inform the neurosurgeon about the probability to find a positive ESM focus in a particular location. In the presurgical

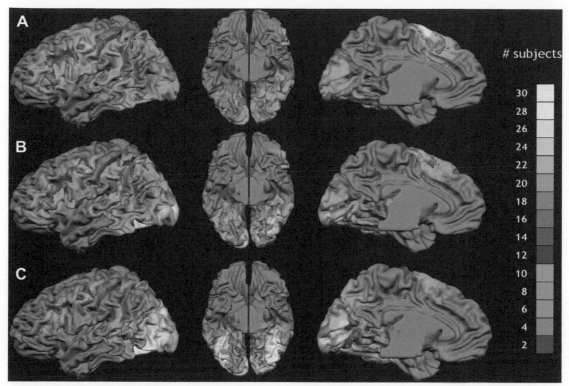

Fig. 2. fMR imaging variability maps from 30 right-handed healthy subjects overlaid over the lateral, inferior, and medial surface of the left hemisphere. The maps were acquired with 3 verbal language tasks: word generation (*A*), verb generation (*B*), and sentence comprehension (*C*). For each vertex of the brain surface the color scale indicates how many subjects showed a BOLD response at the threshold of FDR <0.01. Note the higher number of subjects activating language cortical areas in the inferior frontal gyrus (IFG), dorsolateroprefrontal cortex (DLPFC), AG, and posterior superior temporal sulcus (pSTS) in the lateral surface, and in the supplementary motor area (SMA) in the medial surface. There are differences in percentage and distribution among the 3 tasks. These maps show that language localization is highly variable in healthy subjects: the vertex with the highest percentage is about 65% (*areas in orange*). The high percentage of fMRI activation in the occipital lobes is due to incomplete subtraction of the visual stimuli in the rest condition.

evaluation of patients with a focal mass the fMR imaging variability maps may be useful to answer the following question: "Is the BOLD response in the patient any different from the BOLD response in the normal population?"

In a brain tumor patient the atypical distribution of the BOLD response may be considered evidence of brain reorganization. Of note, plasticity mechanisms may act differently in glioma than in epileptic patients. More extensive reorganization may occur in low grade glioma patients than in epileptic patients, because language function is more frequently preserved in the latter group of patients.

VALIDATION OF FUNCTIONAL MAGNETIC RESONANCE IMAGING RESULTS WITH INTRAOPERATIVE ELECTRICAL STIMULATION MAPPING

Several investigators have focused on presurgical fMR imaging feasibility, the choice of the most

appropriate language task, and the spatial relationship between the lesion and the fMR imaging-activated tissue.[44] In patients with a tumor around the central sulcus, investigators have reported a good correspondence between presurgical fMR imaging and intraoperative ESM results.[45] Validation studies of presurgical language fMR imaging with ESM have involved small samples[10,17,46,47] and the methods used for comparing eloquent foci have often been qualitative and subjective,[10,46–48] with a few exceptions.[16,17]

It must be emphasized that the physiologic measurements made with fMR imaging are different from those of intraoperative direct ESM. ESM is a disruption-based method that identifies nodes and connections essential to language processing. On the contrary, fMR imaging is an activation-based method that potentially identifies all nodes of the network with activity-related changes (essential and supplementary cortical areas).

The diagnostic accuracy of fMR imaging of language was measured by using intraoperative ESM as the reference standard in few studies.[10,16,17,46] In only 3 studies was a site-by-site correlation with a relatively large number of ESM tags performed.[10,16,17]

FitzGerald and colleagues[10] evaluated 140 sites in 11 patients with 5 language tasks, and found a sensitivity of 81% and a specificity of 53%. Sensitivity was higher for results from all tasks combined than for results from a single task. VGEN was the language task with highest sensitivity. Roux and colleagues[17] evaluated 426 tags in 14 patients. Using the VGEN and naming tasks combined and a high statistical threshold ($P < .005$), they measured a sensitivity of 59% and a specificity of 97%, respectively. Decreasing the analysis threshold the sensitivity increased to 66% and the specificity decreased to 91%.

Bizzi and colleagues[16] evaluated 141 tags in 17 patients with a focal mass in the perisylvian cortex (Fig. 3). The location of all stimulated ESM tags was recorded on the fMR imaging dataset (Fig. 3D). This procedure is important in the determination of true and false results, and it may also reduce operator-dependent bias. An overall sensitivity of 80% and specificity of 78% for mapping language with the VGEN task was reported in this study. In addition, the investigators showed that sensitivity and specificity might vary according to lesion type and glioma grade. Sensitivity and specificity were 100% in cavernous angioma. Sensitivity was higher in glioma World Health Organization (WHO) grade II and III (93%) than in glioblastoma multiforme (GBM) (65%). On the contrary, specificity was higher in GBM (93%) than in glioma grade II (79%) and III (76%).[15] There are 2 possible explanations for the higher rate of false-negative fMR imaging results found in GBM. Angiogenesis may lead to abnormal vasculature formation with loss of neurovascular coupling and absence of the BOLD response, despite the presence of neural activity. An alternative explanation is that the larger brain shift occurring in GBM, as the dura is exposed, may diminish the accuracy of the coregistration of preoperative imaging data with the brain tissue on the neuronavigation device.

The sensitivity reported by Roux and colleagues is lower than that reported by the FitzGerald and Bizzi groups. Differences in sensitivity and specificity results among the 3 studies may be explained in part by differences in patient population (tumor type, location, and craniotomy size), fMR imaging paradigms, and methods of analysis used. Bizzi and colleagues[16] reported that sensitivity was higher in anterior than in posterior language areas. A higher percentage of ESM-positive sites for speech arrest in the anterior frontal cortex was reported by Ojemann and colleagues.[39] This finding is relevant for presurgical evaluation, because verbal fluency and verbal memory are 2 functions that are critical to preserve, especially in patients who have built their professional career on those skills. The 2 linguistic processes are most likely segregated in the anterior frontal cortex.

Patient outcome for permanent deficits was 11% in the Bizzi series of 34 patients: 1 patient had severe morbidity due to surgical complications independent of functional localization techniques and 3 patients had moderate or mild permanent postoperative deficits. Other investigators have shown a low rate of postoperative deficits in patients who had eloquent tissue within the tumor when the mass was near the surface and could be evaluated with ESM. Roux and colleagues[17] found fMR imaging intratumoral activated foci in 6 patients.

The ideal mapping technique should be both sensitive and specific. A method with a low rate of false-negative foci will have high sensitivity and will rarely miss functioning tissue. A method with a low rate of false positivity will have high specificity. The investigators of the studies reported here have shown that sensitivity of presurgical fMR imaging of language is consistently high, whereas its specificity may be lower than desired.

Notwithstanding these encouraging results, if fMR imaging is to be used as a reliable and accurate tool for planning and performing function-preserving radical tumor exeresis, its results will also have to be validated with postoperative clinical outcome.

AIMS OF PRESURGICAL PLANNING WITH FUNCTIONAL MAGNETIC RESONANCE IMAGING

The importance of functional localization has been only recently emphasized and, as discussed earlier, is only in part predictable by anatomic landmarks.[49] fMR imaging and diffusion MR tractography are adding pieces of information once unthought-of of, and they may be useful for guiding surgical planning and intraoperative mapping.

Patient Selection Criteria for Awake Craniotomy

The localization of language eloquent cortex is the most critical factor in planning a cortical trajectory and resection of a tumor. Selection of patients for awake craniotomy has been historically based on

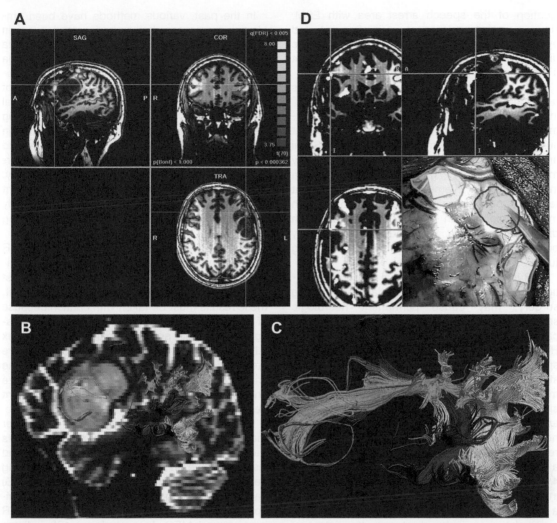

Fig. 3. (A) Presurgical fMR imaging of language (word generation task) in a 43-year-old man. The patient was diagnosed with GBM (WHO-IV) infiltrating the left dorsolateroprefrontal cortex. Sagittal (SAG), coronal (COR), and axial (TRA) fMR imaging maps (threshold FDR <0.005) show a strong BOLD response in the left IFG anterior to the mass, in the precentral cortex (M1) superior to the mass, and in the left superior temporal sulcus. The BOLD response in the IFG is bilateral and lateralized more on the left. (B) Virtual dissection of the 3 segments of the left arcuate fasciculus (AF) with DTI MR tractography. The 3 segments of the AF are color coded: direct (in red), anterior (in green), and posterior (in yellow). In the sagittal view (C), note that the projections of the AF overlap with the fMR imaging clusters (A) in the anterior frontal and posterior temporal lobes. The mass slightly dislocated medially the AF that appears virtually intact. The patient had very mild verbal language deficits including repetition, which were unchanged after surgical resection of the mass. (D) Validation of fMR imaging with intraoperative direct cortical electrical stimulation mapping (ESM). Intraoperative ESM interrupted language production during word generation in the left dorsolateroprefrontal cortex, as illustrated in the intraoperative optic microscopic view (bottom right). With the aid of neuronavigational device, the position of each ESM tag on coronal (top left), sagittal (top right), and axial (bottom left) views of presurgical fMR imaging data set was determined. In this 43-year-old man 1 true positive (red) and 2 true negative (green) fMR imaging BOLD responses were found using ESM as reference index.

clinical presentation and proximity of the tumor to putative functional cortex on conventional MR imaging. It is important to understand functional anatomy of verbal language. Prompt identification of sulcal anatomy on 3-dimensional morphologic MR images is the key.

Unfortunately, the reliability of anatomic landmarks is low in healthy subjects and even lower in patients with a focal mass. Quiñones-Hinojosa and colleagues[49] have addressed this issue and retrospectively found a strict correlation between anatomic variant types of sulcal anatomy and location of the speech arrest area with ESM. However, normal sulcal anatomy is often distorted by glioma infiltration, and eloquent cortex may be displaced by the mass or even reorganized at a distance.

High variability of language localization has been demonstrated by Cerliani and colleagues[14] in healthy subjects with fMR imaging, and by Ojemann and colleagues[39] in patients who underwent surgery for epilepsy with intraoperative ESM. Sanai and colleagues[43] have shown that variability may be even higher in patients with a brain glioma infiltrating Broca, Wernicke, or even the dominant temporal pole. Localization of speech is even more problematic in patients who are fluent in different languages.[50,51] Eloquent tissue may occasionally be found even within the infiltrating tumor.[52]

fMR imaging has the potential to identify functional cortical tissue that, if damaged during surgery, may cause permanent neurologic sequelae. In the last decade the use of presurgical fMR imaging has increased tremendously. However, it is consistently applied only in highly specialized medical centers. It has been demonstrated that presurgical fMR imaging with DTI may reduce the risks and favor a more aggressive resection of the tumor. According to Ulmer and colleagues[53] the risk of developing permanent postoperative deficits is low when the resection margin is at least 5 mm away from a functional site. These investigators reported 4% of unplanned surgically induced motor deficit in a series of 24 patients with the tumor near a motor eloquent area. In certain patients surgical time may be shortened, the extent of resection increased, and craniotomy size decreased.[54]

Can Functional Magnetic Resonance Imaging Replace the Wada Test?

Functional hemispheric language lateralization has been correlated with handedness: approximately 90% of right-handers and 70% of left-handers show left-sided hemispheric language dominance, whereas 15% of left-handers show right-sided lateralization and the remaining 15% a bilateral representation. Of note, approximately 10% of the population is a true left-hander, and left-handedness is less common in women than in men. However, the influence of gender on hemisphere dominance remains a controversial issue. These data imply that roughly 92.5% of the population is left-hemisphere dominant and that only approximately 4% is right-hemisphere language dominant.[55]

In the past, various methods have been employed to assess hemispheric dominance in epileptic patients. For the last 50 years the Wada test has been the standard of care.[56] The Wada test is an invasive procedure with selective catheterization of both carotid arteries, and injection of amobarbital in the anterior and middle cerebral arteries of one hemisphere at a time. The drug causes temporary anesthetization of the brain tissue. Cerebral dominance for language and memory is determined on the patient's performance during the period of functional disability. The Wada is a procedure associated with patient discomfort, high cost, and morbidity that greatly exceed those of noninvasive functional imaging methods.

Several investigators have shown that fMR imaging and the Wada test agreed on determination of language lateralization in most patients.[12,57,58] Despite the overall agreement, these results must be taken with caution because of several important technical issues. Most investigators compute an fMR imaging laterality index (LI) using a region-of-interest (ROI) method. There are many experimental choices that can affect the final laterality result: the language task, the size and location of the selected ROI in the left and right hemispheres, and the statistical threshold.

Notwithstanding, fMR imaging has taken over the role of the Wada test in most medical centers because it is noninvasive, more accessible, and less expensive. In few highly specialized imaging centers with magnetoencephalography (MEG) capabilities, determination of the dominant hemisphere is relied on using the combination of fMR imaging and MEG. In a study on 172 patients with brain tumor abutting language areas, it was shown that measurement by fMR imaging and MEG combined increased the reliability of language localization.[48]

Can Functional Magnetic Resonance Imaging Replace Intraoperative Electrical Stimulation Mapping?

At present, ESM is the reference standard for intraoperative decisions because it has been used extensively and it has been validated by clinical outcome.[39,42,43] If eloquent sites identified by ESM are respected, the risk of developing permanent postoperative sequelae is low. Duffau and colleagues[59] have compared 2 series of patients with supratentorial low-grade glioma operated by the same team: those operated with intraoperative ESM (n = 122) versus those operated without (n = 100). The study found that the use of intraoperative direct ESM lead to increasing percentage of surgery in eloquent areas (63% vs 35%) with decreasing severe permanent deficits (3% vs 17%). The quality of tumor resection was improved, with a favorable impact on survival. In a prospective longitudinally study designed to evaluate verbal language postoperative outcome in 149 patients with tumor in close proximity to or within language areas, Ilmberger and colleagues[60] reported new language impairment at 7 days after awake craniotomy in 41 of 128 patients, without preoperative aphasic deficits. At 7 months after surgery, 14 patients continued to show mild language impairment. In this group of patients aphasic disturbance were mostly mild.

For fMR imaging to be mature to replace intraoperative direct ESM, it should be accurate in identifying brain tissue that can be safely removed. False-negative findings could possibly lead to postoperative language deficits. Type I errors occur infrequently in low-grade glioma and cavernous angiomas, as discussed in the validation subsection earlier. False-positive results are also undesirable, because they may discourage radical resection of the tumor. These additional nonessential areas identified by fMR imaging may be part of the network but if damaged will unlikely cause a permanent deficit.

The accuracy of fMR imaging in identifying the tissue that the neurosurgeon may take out must be also confirmed with outcome studies. Few similar studies have been performed thus far.[61,62] Future larger fMR imaging studies will have to show that the long-term postoperative outcome is favorable. At the current state of the art, fMR imaging mapping is a useful guide in presurgical and intraoperative planning but does not replace the need for intraoperative testing in any patient with a functional language site less than 10 mm away from the tumor's resection margin.[16,17]

PRESURGICAL PLANNING WITH DIFFUSION MAGNETIC RESONANCE IMAGING

The integration of functional data acquired with fMR imaging and MEG into the navigational data sets has improved quick identification of eloquent cortex with intraoperative ESM in the operating room. To avoid postoperative neurologic deficits, however, it is also necessary to preserve the white matter tracts connecting eloquent cortex.

Diffusion MR tractography has recently emerged as a potentially valuable clinical tool for presurgical planning[63–65] and intraoperative imaging-guided navigation in the operating room.[66] Diffusion MR tractography can provide the neurosurgeon with additional information about brain anatomy, pathology, and architecture that conventional MR imaging methods cannot.

Diffusion Tensor Imaging Color Maps

Directionally encoded color maps, with hues reflecting tensor orientation and intensity weighted by fractional anisotropy (FA), provide an aesthetic and informative synthesis of tissue microstructure and architecture. The color maps are a promising tool for delineation of tumor extent and infiltration (Fig. 4). DTI color maps indicate whether a mass is displacing, infiltrating, or destroying the main white matter tracts.[67] MR tractography can be used to virtually dissect functionally critical white matter tracts, such as the corticospinal tract and the AF, enabling the neurosurgeon to identify and preserve the tract during resection.[68]

It has been shown that acquisition of DTI color maps is feasible also in the operating room with intraoperative 1.5-Tesla MR scanners. Intraoperative DTI can depict shifting of major white matter tracts that may occur during surgical removal of the mass. It has been shown that shifting of brain structures may be unpredictable; therefore, intraoperative updating of the navigation system is strongly recommended.[66]

Diffusion Magnetic Resonance Tractography

Three-dimensional objects of preoperative virtually dissected tracts can be reliably integrated into a standard neuronavigation system, allowing for intraoperative visualization and localization of the main tracts.[69] MR tractography may show the relationship of the mass to the virtually dissected AF. Virtual dissection of the 3 segments of the AF may show whether the mass has partially interrupted or only displaced the tracts (see Fig. 4). Display of MR tractography results may also be useful in the operating room when the neurosurgeon is approaching an important bundle, and wishes to reinforce his or her anatomic orientation in the operating field and consider whether to use subcortical ESM to test the functional relevance of a specific tract.[70]

Modern cognitive models of language have shown that there is a lot of redundancy in the language network. It is of paramount importance to identify those bundles that if severed may cause permanent language deficits. Definition of which bundles are functionally eloquent and have to be absolutely spared during resection remains an important issue.

There is a long list of important limitations. Few are inherent to the DTI and the MR tractography technology, and they must be well understood before the results of presurgical MR tractography

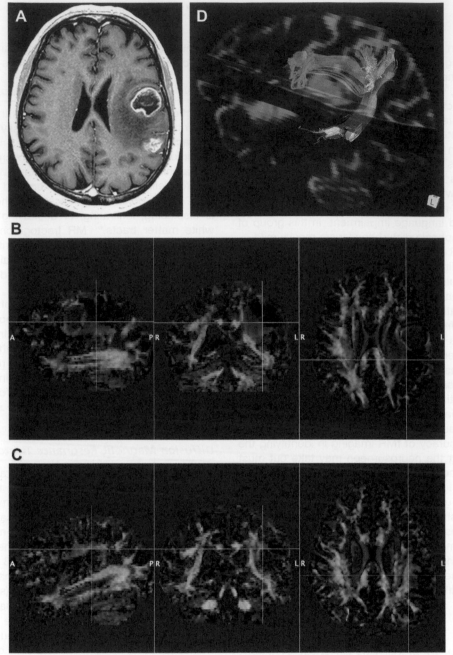

Fig. 4. (A) Axial spin-echo T1-weighted MR image after intravenous injection of gadolinium shows 2 ring-enhancing masses in the dorsolateroprefrontal cortex and supramarginal gyrus in a 62-year-old man. The patient was later diagnosed with GBM (WHO-IV). Before surgery the Aachener Aphasie Test showed discrete language deficits of phonemic and semantic fluency that had completely disappeared 3 months after surgery. (B, C) DTI color maps in the sagittal, coronal, and axial planes before (B) and after (C) surgery. Voxels with the eigenvector oriented along the anterior-posterior direction are displayed in green, those along the right-left direction in red, and those along the craniocaudal direction in blue. In the presurgical DTI color maps, the cursor indicates an area of decreased fractional anisotropy (FA) along the AF (in green). The anterior mass has displaced the AF slightly caudally and medially. It was not possible to reconstruct the 3 segments of the left AF because FA was lower than threshold (0.15) due to the presence of vasogenic edema. Three months after surgery and removal of the prefrontal mass, the vasogenic edema had diminished significantly and FA had increased accordingly along the AF, which is the structure in green indicated by the cursor. At 3 months after surgery it was possible to reconstruct the 3 segments of the AF (direct in red, anterior in green, posterior in yellow) that appeared intact in the image displayed over a T2-weighted axial MR image (D). This case study shows that DTI color maps are useful to identify microscopic changes occurring in white matter tracts. Virtual reconstruction of specific tracts with MR tractography is also very useful, but it may have limitations especially when FA is decreased due to vasogenic edema or infiltration by the tumor.

dissections can be safely exported to the operating room. It is not yet established whether resection of fibers apparently infiltrated by the tumor that on diffusion MR tractography appear to be interrupted or destroyed will result in permanent postoperative neurologic deficits (Fig. 5). On the contrary, it is not yet established whether resection of fibers that appear to be anatomically intact

within the tumor will cause permanent postoperative deficits. There is evidence, however, that severing the pyramidal tract will cause hemiplegia. Whether severing one of the many language connections will cause aphasia is currently a controversial issue.[71]

In conclusion, virtual dissection of the major white matter tracts with the deterministic method should

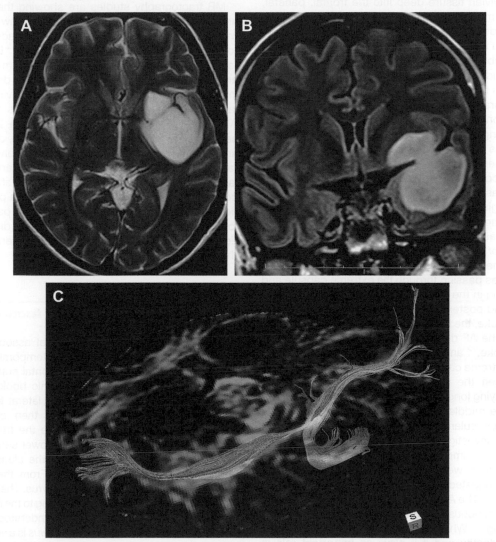

Fig. 5. Axial spin-echo T2-weighted (*A*) and coronal FLAIR (*B*) MR images show a mass infiltrating the temporal stem connecting the basal portion of the left frontal lobe with the anterior part of the temporal lobe in a 42-year-old woman. The patient was later diagnosed with astrocytoma (WHO-II). Before surgery the Aachener Aphasie Test showed no language deficits of phonemic and semantic fluency. Three months after surgery with removal of the mass in the left temporal lobe she had worsening of semantic fluency, with no changes in the phonemic fluency. Virtual reconstruction with DTI MR tractography (*C*) shows the uncinate fasciculus (*in turquoise*) and the inferior fronto-occipital fasciculus (*in orange*) in the right hemisphere, displayed over an FA axial map. Note the mass with very low FA in the left temporal lobe. Reconstruction of the same 2 fascicles was not successful in the left hemisphere. There are 2 possible explanations. The mass infiltrating the temporal stem and capsula extrema may have destroyed the white matter tracts. An alternative hypothesis is that the mass had decreased FA below the threshold (0.15); the white matter tracts cannot be reconstructed even though they may be still functional. The patient's worsening semantic fluency after surgery may support this second hypothesis.

be used as a road map for presurgical planning and as guidance for intraoperative subcortical ESM.

MAPPING CONNECTIONS IN THE LANGUAGE NETWORK

In 1812 Johann Christian Reil identified for the first time a prominent group of fibers arching around the Sylvian fissure deep into the frontal, parietal, and temporal white matter.[31] Ten years later Burdach described in detail the same pathway and named it *arcuate fasciculus*, for the arching shape of its fibers. In his blunt dissection studies Dejerine concluded in 1895 that the "arcuate fasciculus" carries fibers from the caudal superior and middle temporal gyri to the IFG. However, Dejerine was not convinced that the AF contained long fibers coursing along its entire length connecting remote regions of 2 lobes. He had been unable to follow degenerated fibers any further than the immediate neighborhood of the primary focus of the lesion.[72]

It was Karl Wernicke who postulated that a lesion damaging the pathway connecting the frontal and posterior language areas would cause a new type of aphasic syndrome. In the classic form of *conduction aphasia* the patient makes errors in repeating what he hears. Wernicke thought that white matter bundles passing through the extreme capsule and relaying in the anterior insula connected the anterior and posterior language cortices. According to Wernicke, the trajectory of this bundle was distinct from the AF described by Dejerine and Dejerine-Klumpke,[72] and Petrides and Pandya[73] described the extreme capsule as a compact bundle situated between the claustrum and the insular cortex, conveying long association fiber bundles connecting the middle superior temporal region with the pars opercularis (BA 44) of the IFG and the VLPFC. These investigators concluded that the extreme capsule is important for language. Dejerine and colleagues went further beyond this statement and suggested that the AF may not be a "language bundle." The AF may be important for spatial attributes of acoustic stimuli and auditory-related processing.[74] Whether the extreme capsule has its own identity and if it plays an important role in language remains a hot topic and matter of controversy among neuroanatomists and neurosurgeons (Mitch Berger, personal communication).

The Dorsal Pathway

Arcuate fasciculus
In humans the AF and the superior longitudinal fasciculus (SLF) have long been considered synonymous, and the names have been used interchangeably. Recent DTI-MR tractography studies have contributed to this confusion in terminology. In the monkey, however, the SLF comprises 3 subcomponents (SLF-I, -II, and -III) connecting the parietal-occipital lobes with the prefrontal areas. The AF in the monkey is a distinct fiber system, separate from the SLF-II in terms of both its location and trajectory. The AF connects the posterior superior and middle temporal gyri with the DLPFC but not with the IFG.[73]

MR tractography studies are showing that the anatomy of the perisylvian dorsal pathway is more complex than previously thought. In addition to the direct medial segment connecting "Broca territory" with "Wernicke territory," there may be an indirect lateral subcortical pathway divided into 2 segments. Catani and colleagues[75] virtually (and very elegantly) dissected 3 segments of the AF using DTI-MR tractography with the 2-ROI seeding deterministic approach: (1) a long, direct, and medial segment connecting the lateroprefrontal cortex with the temporal lobe; (2) an anterior lateral segment connecting the lateroprefrontal cortex with the inferior parietal lobule; (3) a posterior lateral segment connecting the inferior parietal lobule with the temporal lobe. Postmortem dissections in humans have confirmed the existence of the 3 segments of the AF.[76]

The Ventral Pathway

Uncinate, inferior fronto-occipital fasciculus, and inferior longitudinal fasciculus
The *uncinate fasciculus* is a ventral associative bundle that connects the anterior temporal lobe with the medial and lateral orbitofrontal cortex.[77] Dejerine described it in his anatomic book.[72] In the temporal pole the uncinatus is lateral to the amygdala and hippocampus and then curves upward, passing behind and above the trunk of the middle cerebral artery into the lower segment of the extreme capsule, lateral to the claustrum and medial to the insular cortex. From there, it continues into the posterior orbital gyrus. The uncinate fasciculus is considered to belong to the limbic system but its functions are poorly understood.

The *inferior fronto-occipital fasciculus* is a ventral associative bundle that connects the ventral occipital lobe and the orbitofrontal cortex. In the temporal stem and extreme capsule, the IFOF runs posterior to the uncinatus. In its occipital course the IFOF runs parallel to the ILF.[77] Its functions may be related to reading, attention, and visual processing.

The *inferior longitudinal fasciculus* is a ventral associative bundle with long and short fibers connecting the occipital and temporal lobes. The long fibers connect the amygdala and hippocampus to the visual areas.[77] The ILF is involved in face recognition, visual perception, reading, visual memory, and other functions related to language.

The uncinate and IFOF cross the temporal stem, a narrow structure immediately inferior to the extreme capsule. Although language lateralization has been well established, its anatomic basis is not fully understood as yet. In particular, the role of the uncinate fasciculus, the IFOF, and the ILF in maintaining the integrity and functionality of the language network has been elusive. Intraoperative cortical and subcortical ESM data seem to support the hypothesis that the IFOF in the dominant hemisphere is likely implicated in language specialization.[71,78] Of note, in another intraoperative study subcortical ESM of the left ILF never elicited any language disturbances.[79] In addition, all patients recovered following a transient postoperative language deficit, despite the resection of at least one part of the ILF. This study suggested that the ILF is not essential for language.

LANGUAGE-RELATED HEMISPHERIC ASYMMETRIES AND BRAIN PLASTICITY

Broca and Wernicke first recognized lateralization of function as a key feature of the language network. The left hemisphere is the dominant hemisphere in over 90% of right-handed subjects. Bilateral or right-hemisphere dominance is seen in about 30% of left-handed subjects and in patients with early-onset left-sided lesions.[80] Hemispheric specialization reduces duplication of function between the hemispheres. However, marked asymmetric specialization of anatomy and function might ultimately be a disadvantageous condition for recovery when a disease hits a highly specialized functional network.

Anatomic Asymmetries

Paul Broca discovered that damage to a definite circumscribed area of the brain in the left hemisphere is associated to language loss and motor speech disorders. Broca's discovery went far beyond the description of aphasia. His most important contribution was that the 2 cerebral hemispheres are asymmetric in function and that in most human beings the left hemisphere contains "the language center." The concept of localization of function has been repeatedly demonstrated by clinical and research studies since Broca first articulated it in 1861. Any medical intern or resident is aware that damage caused to the left perisylvian cortex impairs the ability to retrieve object names, at least in the acute stage. Anomie and other dysphasic symptoms are only rarely observed following damage to the right cerebral hemisphere. Despite this clinical robustness, evidence of anatomic asymmetry has been scarce and elusive.

A left-greater-than-right asymmetry of BA 44, the pars opercularis of the IFG, has been reported.[81] The posterior part of the Broca area is a critical area for speech production. A left-dominant asymmetry has been also reported in the planum temporale within the STG.[82] This area is part of the primary auditory cortex and is particularly sensitive to fast-evolving cues and voice-onset time for speech perception.[83]

A larger surface area of BA 44 as well as a leftward white matter volumetric asymmetry of the perisylvian frontal region has also been measured in MR imaging studies of great ape species.[84,85] In monkeys, the mirror-neurons in BA 44 may have been specialized initially for gestural and later for vocal communication.[86] Thus, in great apes BA 44 asymmetry may be associated with the production of gestures accompanied by vocalization. In the scene "The dawn of man" of the inspiring and enthralling movie *2001: A Space Odyssey* Stanley Kubrick magnificently illustrated the combination of gestures and vocalization in our prehistoric ancestors.

Great apes show a humanlike left-dominant asymmetry also in the planum temporale.[87] These findings suggest that the neuroanatomical substrates for left-hemisphere dominance in speech production were present at least 5 million years ago, that they are not unique to hominid evolution, and should be interpreted in evolutionary terms.

Karl Wernicke proposed a "classic model of language" that emphasized the importance of cortical language centers associated with multiple language modalities, but he also stressed the importance of association fiber tracts connecting those centers. He understood that the connections in the brain were just as important as the nodes of the network. In the last few years demonstration of hemispheric asymmetry of the association pathways connecting language-related areas has become the target of extensive research with MR imaging and DTI.[88] An increase in the diameter and myelination of axons may play a role in cognitive development during childhood and adolescence. Paus and colleagues[89] have reported greater maturation of the dominant left AF with 3-dimensional T1-weighted MR imaging in 111 children and adolescents. Hemispheric asymmetry of the AF has been also demonstrated by microscopic examination of postmortem specimens.[90]

Several investigators have demonstrated a significant leftward asymmetry of the AF with

MR tractography analysis. Some investigators used deterministic algorithms with a priori delineation of 1 or 2 anatomic seeding ROIs,[91–96] whereas others used probabilistic methods[97,98] or other more sophisticated models such as spherical deconvolution, every-ball, or diffusion spectrum imaging (DSI).[99]

Powell and colleagues[98] combined probabilistic DTI-MR tractography with 3 fMR imaging language tasks, and demonstrated greater connectivity in the left than in the right hemisphere. Volume of tracts initiated from one seeding functionally defined volume of interest was significantly greater on the left than on the right across all different probabilistic thresholds. A significant correlation between the degree of lateralization of mean FA and lateralization of fMR imaging activation was observed. No significant correlation between tract volumes and functional activation was found.

Catani and colleagues[100] used deterministic DTI-MR tractography to assess the degree of lateralization of the AF direct long segment (as measured by an indirect index of tract volume). Extreme leftward lateralization was found in 62% of right-handed healthy subjects. Mild leftward lateralization was found in 20% and a symmetric direct segment in the remaining 18%. The study also found that extreme left lateralization was higher in males (85%) than in females (40%). A significant association between those subjects with a symmetric AF direct segment and higher performance in learning words by semantic association on the California Verbal Learning Test was found.

Cao and colleagues[101] have shown that leftward asymmetries may be present also in the pathways within the extreme capsule. A leftward asymmetry in right-handers has been shown also in the uncinate fasciculus and IFOF by some investigators,[102] but it has not been confirmed by others.

Functional Asymmetries

The Wada is an excellent test to determine hemispheric dominance for language during a brief period of functional reversible disability. In the majority of patients the Wada test is concordant with fMR imaging production tasks on determination of language lateralization. It is well documented that VGEN and WGEN evoke left-greater-than-right BOLD response in prefrontal language areas. Nevertheless, bilateral activation with a weak left-dominant or without asymmetry has been reported in a substantial number of fMR imaging studies performed in healthy right-handed subjects.[103] In the interpretation of

presurgical fMR imaging of verbal language, it is important to be aware that prevalent bilateral activation is associated with auditory rather than visual input, comprehension rather than production tasks, and figurative rather than symbolic types of stimuli. In healthy subjects detection of BOLD response in the homologous areas of the right hemisphere during a verbal language task may reflect residual and automatic activity that has been competitively diminished by the dominant language network in the left hemisphere. Right-sided regions may be activated, but are neither sufficient nor necessary to perform the task.

In the majority of patients with a recently discovered brain tumor in the left perisylvian areas, the BOLD response is still lateralized to the left dominant hemisphere. On the contrary, enhanced BOLD response in the right-sided language homologous areas has been observed during recovery in aphasic patients after a left-sided stroke, and has been explained as a mechanism of compensation.[104]

The classic left-greater-than-right asymmetry in language processing that is a cornerstone of the "lesion model" still awaits further validation with modern neuroimaging studies. Kimura proposed that the right-sided bias for hand preference could relate to the particular efficient spatial and temporal motor programming skills of the left premotor cortex.[105,106] According to the "temporal hypothesis" the left hemisphere is specifically able to process rapidly changing acoustic signals. Suck skill is obviously also critical for speech comprehension. The larger surface area in the left planum temporale and left BA 44 may be the result of specialization for perceiving and processing rapid acoustic transitions. The "category hypothesis," another complementary hypothesis, proposes that the left hemispheric structures store long-term representations of phonemes. Categorical perception thus reduces acoustic variability by sorting inputs into discrete classes defined by stored prototypes. Predominant BOLD response in the left pSTG and left SMG for categorical perception of syllables and tones have been observed with fMR imaging.[107]

Plasticity in Stroke Patients

Plasticity, or brain reorganization, is defined as a change at the synaptic level that increases communication efficiency in neural networks. Change of the strength of synapses is regulated through molecular and cellular transformation. It is important to distinguish *functional plasticity* from *structural plasticity*. The former changes synaptic strength without changing the anatomic connectivity between neurons, whereas the latter comprises changes in synapse numbers, axonal fiber densities, axonal and dendritic branching patterns, synaptic connectivity patterns, and even neuronal cell numbers. Synaptic rewiring is the retraction of a pre- or postsynaptic element from its target and the subsequent turnover of a different target in reach; it is considered a form of structural plasticity. Synaptic rewiring is probably the most important feature of structural plasticity as it adds a further degree of freedom for changing synaptic connectivity.[108]

Reactive plasticity occurs in the adult brain following a lesion. Recovery may involve unmasking of preexisting, but latent, interhemispheric connections and modulation of synaptic efficacy by long-term potentiation (LTP) or long-term depression (LTD).[109] Reactive plasticity is not restricted to the perilesional cortex but includes also the homologous contralateral cortex. Bilateral rewiring is caused by interhemispheric disinhibition and unmasking of preexisting callosal connections.[110]

Spontaneous recovery is usually observed in patients with aphasia following an acute stroke. The involvement of the right hemisphere during recovery was hypothesized as early as the late nineteenth century by Gowers in his *Lectures on the Diagnosis of the Brain*.[111] In dysphasic patients partially recovered from a left frontal stroke, Blasi and colleagues[112] showed that learning to retrieve words can downregulate activities in the right frontal and right occipital cortex, strongly supporting the compensatory role of the right hemisphere. This fMR imaging study showed a direct relationship between performances and enhanced BOLD response in the right hemisphere. Controversial results have been found with transcranial magnetic stimulation (TMS). Inhibition of right Broca-homologous cortex with TMS induced dysphasia in patients recovering from a left-sided stroke, as evidence that TMS may affect the compensatory functions of the right hemisphere.[113] On the contrary, other investigators have reported improvement of naming abilities during inhibition of the right ventral prefrontal cortex in chronic aphasic patients.[114] These results suggested that increased activity in the contralateral hemisphere might be dysfunctional.

In a longitudinal study in 14 highly selected aphasic stroke patients, Weiller and colleagues[104] showed the dynamics of reorganization of function and related fMR imaging activation patterns in language recovery. All patients recovered clinically. These investigators suggested a model with 3 stages of language recovery, which might be transferable to the motor system and other functional networks as a general concept of reorganization of function after focal brain damage. In the acute stage, patients' group analysis showed minimal activation of noninfarcted left-hemispheric language structures. In the subacute stage, a large increase of BOLD response in both hemispheres with peak activation (upregulation) in the right Broca-homologue and SMA was observed. In the third chronic stage, at 1 year a re-shift of peak activation to the left perilesional cortex was observed, especially in those patients who showed further language improvement.

Plasticity in Brain Tumor Patients

Intraoperative ESM has shown that a functional network is organized into highly specialized functional mosaics. If functional cortex is damaged during surgery, experimental evidence suggests that permanent deficits will follow. However, little is known about spontaneous mechanisms of reorganization of the network that may occur in patients with slow-growing gliomas. Reorganization of the language network probably occurs while the tumor is invading eloquent tissue: this phenomenon may explain the relatively mild clinical symptoms observed in the early stage of this slowly invasive disease, despite the extension and proximity of the mass to eloquent structures.

In 1989 Damasio and Damasio[115] wrote that brain tumors are not a material of choice for clinical-anatomic studies. They wrote: "Even when we look at a region where an abnormal signal definitely exists, this does not mean necessarily that the brain parenchyma is destroyed, or that area is functionally inoperative." Finally today, with the advent of the most modern imaging methods, it has become possible to gather information about residual functional tissue viability in areas infiltrated by the tumors as well as about mechanisms of language reorganization. This information will become valuable to the neurosurgeon who is planning a radical surgery in a patient with minimal preoperative language deficits.

Cortical language activity may increase locally at the lesion periphery, or it may shift to more distant sites in the ipsilateral and contralateral frontal and temporal lobes.[116] Differences in speech organization between patients with and without preoperative speech deficits have been investigated in patients with epilepsy or other lesions associated with seizures. Lucas and colleagues[117] found that focal damage altered the distribution of speech sites in the frontal lobe but not in the temporal lobe. Frontal speech representation expanded into the superior border of the inferior and middle frontal gyri after injury to eloquent speech areas. Damage to an essential language node would result in a shift of the functional load of speech processing to portions of the network already involved, but previously not essential for speech.[117]

Recruitment of distant cortical areas in the ipsilateral and contralateral hemispheres seems to be a more efficient mechanism in slow-growing than in hyperacute occurring lesions. Patients with low-grade glioma may undergo extensive tumor resections without clinically evident dysfunctional consequences.[118] Robles and colleagues[119] used fMR imaging and intraoperative ESM in 2 patients before and during surgery to demonstrate that such plasticity occurs in low-grade glioma infiltrating critical areas. In the interim between 2 consecutive surgical operations to remove a tumor in the left DLPFC, fMR imaging of verbal language showed increased BOLD response in the right nondominant IFG and MFG, left IFG, and bilateral pre-SMA. The investigators interpreted the fMR imaging data as evidence of brain reorganization, and proposed that a multistage surgical approach in conjunction with functional reorganization has the potential to improve the benefit-to-risk balance.

Temporal lobe epilepsy is often associated with atypical, bilateral, or right-sided language dominance.[120] A declining performance in naming is the most common language deficit (30%–40% of patients) after anterior temporal lobe resection (see **Fig. 5**). FMR imaging laterality indices were found to be predictive of outcome measured as severity of naming deficits. A stronger left-lateralized language BOLD response on a fMR imaging semantic decision-making task was found to correlate with a more severe postoperative naming decline.[121] Laterality indices measured in the temporal lobe white matter with probabilistic DTI-MR tractography were correlated with postoperative naming decline. A stronger lateralization of tracts to the dominant hemisphere was associated with more severe decline in naming function.[122] Therefore, presurgical mapping with fMR imaging and MR tractography has the potential to predict the extent of language decline following anterior temporal lobe resection.

However, a word of caution must be said about the accuracy of the fMR imaging and MR tractography methods used to measure the LI. The fMR imaging BOLD response is often measured in eloquent as well as accessory cortical areas. In the same subject the track counts measured with MR tractography may vary according to several factors: the MR diffusion acquisition scheme, the

tractography algorithm, and the choice of the seeding ROI. For instance, Powell and colleagues[122] used a state of the art acquisition scheme and reconstruction algorithm; however, their results were highly dependable on the extension of the selected ROI in the white matter of the temporal lobe. It is important to emphasize that not all temporal white matter bundles are part of the functional and critical connections of the language network. Further prospective studies in larger patient populations with more precise selection of eloquent structures are necessary to confirm that fMR imaging, MR tractography, or both can be used to predict postoperative language deficits.

Can Individual Asymmetries be used as Predictors of Clinical Outcome?

The white matter tracts asymmetries described here may suggest that a strong leftward lateralization of language-related tracts may be a poor prognostic sign of postoperative outcome. On the contrary, patients with symmetric distribution of the AF or IFOF and a focal lesion in the proximity of language eloquent structures may have a more favorable functional outcome after surgery (**Fig. 6**).

However, interpretation of the structure-function relationship between AF asymmetry and language lateralization needs to be considered with some caution. In a recent study performed in left- and right-handed healthy subjects, a predominant leftward asymmetry of the AF was found regardless of functional hemispheric language lateralization.[96]

Another critical and poorly understood issue is the effect of a focal brain lesion on the structure-function relationship. In patients with temporal lobe epilepsy, Rodrigo and colleagues[123] found a correlation between leftward asymmetry of the AF measured by FA with DTI and the leftward asymmetry in functional activation measured by fMR imaging. Patients with higher anisotropy in the left AF showed higher fMR imaging LI (ie, leftward lateralized). However, this correlation was no longer observed in patients with left temporal lobe epilepsy. Atypical language representation is observed more frequently in temporal lobe epilepsy patients with a left-sided epileptic focus, suggesting that the side of the epileptogenic process plays a role in language lateralization.

Together, these data suggest that careful consideration should be given to the AF during surgery of the left hemisphere, irrespective of the side of functional language dominance.[96] Thus, it is important to design studies that investigate whether diffusion MR tractography (and fMR

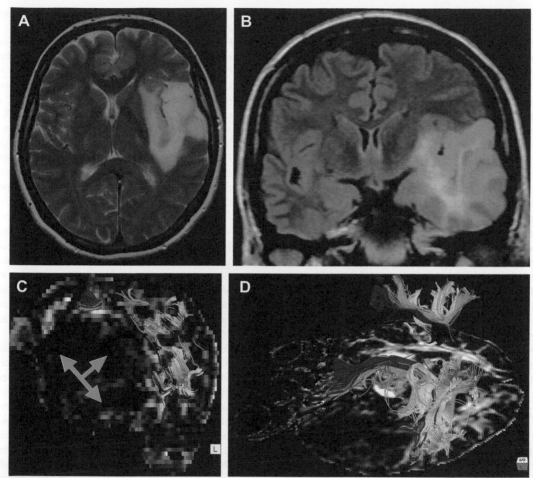

Fig. 6. Axial T2-weighted MR image (*A*) and coronal FLAIR (*B*) show a mass infiltrating the left temporal lobe and insula in a 41 year-old woman later diagnosed with oligoastrocytoma (WHO-II). The patient had very mild verbal language deficits in comprehension and repetition, which were unchanged after surgical resection of the mass. (*C*) Virtual dissection with DTI MR tractography shows the intact left AF that is dislocated cranially and posteriorly by the mass (*triple arrow*) in this sagittal view projected over an FA map. (*D*) Virtual dissection of the 3 segments of the AF in both hemispheres projected over an axial FA map shows symmetry of the direct segments. The 3 segments of the AF are color coded: direct (*in red*), anterior (*in green*), and posterior (*in yellow*).

imaging) results can be valuable as anatomic predictors of clinical outcome in patients with a focal brain lesion. Whether bilateral representation of the language network is an accurate predictor of a more favorable outcome will have to be determined by postoperative outcome.

SUMMARY

fMR imaging and diffusion MR tractography have emerged as valuable tools in the evaluation of language both in healthy individuals and in patients with a focal brain lesion. In healthy subjects, modern neuroimaging methods are contributing toward refining current cognitive and anatomic models. Not only have they confirmed

several theories about language processing but they have also raised unexpected important questions. In patients with brain tumors they have obtained recognition as valuable presurgical clinical tools in the determination of hemispheric dominance and in the selection of candidates who may benefit from awake craniotomy.

In the recent past a patient with a brain tumor near eloquent verbal language structures was not considered a "surgical candidate." The localization of language eloquent cortex is the most critical factor in planning the cortical trajectory and resection of the mass. Whereas mapping of motor and sensory functions are relatively straightforward, mapping of verbal language is far more complex. The developments of fMR imaging and more recently of DTI-MR tractography have changed the way neurosurgeons look at patients with a mass in the dominant hemisphere. The aims of presurgical mapping are fourfold: (1) to determine hemispheric dominance; (2) to select candidates for awake craniotomy; (3) to guide the intraoperative surgical procedure; and (4) to assess the risk of postoperative neurologic deficits by measuring the distance between the margin of the lesion resection and critical functional structures.

Several investigators have shown that fMR imaging and the Wada test agreed on determination of hemispheric language dominance in most patients. Few validation studies have been performed, and these showed that fMR imaging sensitivity is relatively high in slow-growing lesions, whereas specificity is relatively low due to inherent technical limitations. Outcome studies and randomized trials showing the benefits of using fMR imaging and MR tractography in the presurgical evaluation of brain tumor patients are needed.

In the near future fMR imaging and diffusion MR tractography may contribute toward elucidating mechanisms of brain plasticity, and may provide predictors of favorable postoperative clinical outcome.

ACKNOWLEDGMENTS

I am especially grateful to Sylvie Piacentini and Francesca Ferrè for neuropsychological evaluation; to Giovanni Broggi, Paolo Ferroli, Carlo Marras, Carlo Solero, and Francesco Di Meco for professional surgery performed in the patients presented in **Figs. 3–6**. Trackvis (www.trackvis.org) version 0.4.2 was used to generate virtual dissections of the white matter tracts displayed on **Figs. 3–6**.

REFERENCES

1. Breasted JH. The Edwin Smith surgical papyrus. Chicago: The University of Chicago Press; 1930.

2. Calvin WH, Ojemann GA. Conversations with Neil's brain: the neural nature of thought and language. Reading (MA): Perseus Publishing; 1995.

3. Ojemann GA. Individual variability in cortical localization of language. J Neurosurg 1979;50(2):164–9.

4. Ojemann GA, Creutzfeldt OD, Lettich E, et al. Neuronal activity in human lateral temporal cortex related to short-term verbal memory, naming and reading. Brain 1988;111:1383–403.

5. Mosso A. Ueber den Kreislauf des Blutes im Menschlichen Gehirn. Leipzig: von Veit; 1881. [in German].

6. Zago S, Ferrucci R, Marceglia S, et al. The mosso method for recording brain pulsation: the forerunner of functional neuroimaging. Neuroimage 2009;48(4):652–6.

7. Raichle ME. Behind the scenes of functional brain imaging: a historical and physiological perspective. Proc Natl Acad Sci U S A 1998;95(3):765–72.

8. Ogawa S, Lee TM, Kay AR, et al. Brain magnetic resonance imaging with contrast dependent on blood oxygenation. Proc Natl Acad Sci U S A 1990;87(24):9868–72.

9. Smits M, Visch-Brink E, Schraa-Tam CK, et al. Functional MR imaging of language processing: an overview of easy-to-implement paradigms for patient care and clinical research. Radiographics 2006;26(Suppl 1):S145–58. Review.

10. FitzGerald DB, Cosgrove GR, Ronner S, et al. Location of language in the cortex: a comparison between functional MR imaging and electrocortical stimulation. AJNR Am J Neuroradiol 1997;18(8):1529–39.

11. Roux FE, Boulanouar K, Ibarrola D, et al. Functional MRI and intraoperative brain mapping to evaluate brain plasticity in patients with brain tumours and hemiparesis. J Neurol Neurosurg Psychiatr 2000; 69(4):453–63.

12. Binder JR, Swanson SJ, Hammeke TA, et al. Determination of language dominance using functional MRI: a comparison with the Wada test. Neurology 1996;46(4):978–84.

13. Lurito JT, Kareken DA, Lowe MJ, et al. Comparison of rhyming and word generation with FMRI. Hum Brain Mapp 2000;10(3):99–106.

14. Cerliani L, Mandelli M.L, Aquino D, et al, editors. Preoperative mapping of language with fMRI: frequency maps and comparison of three tasks in healthy subjects. ISMRM Annual Meeting Proceedings. Berlin, May 19–25, 2007.

15. Heim S, Eickhoff SB, Amunts K. Specialisation in Broca's region for semantic, phonological, and syntactic fluency? Neuroimage 2008;40(3):1362–8.

16. Bizzi A, Blasi V, Falini A, et al. Presurgical functional MR imaging of language and motor functions: validation with intraoperative electrocortical mapping. Radiology 2008;248(2):579–89.

17. Roux FE, Boulanouar K, Lotterie JA, et al. Language functional magnetic resonance imaging in preoperative assessment of language areas: correlation with direct cortical stimulation. Neurosurgery 2003;52(6):1335–45 [discussion: 45–7].

18. Bandettini PA, Wong EC, Hinks RS, et al. Time course EPI of human brain function during task activation. Magn Reson Med 1992;25(2):390–7.

19. Turner R. How much cortex can a vein drain? Downstream dilution of activation-related cerebral blood oxygenation changes. Neuroimage 2002; 16(4):1062–7.

20. Logothetis NK, Pauls J, Augath M, et al. Neurophysiological investigation of the basis of the fMRI signal. Nature 2001;412(6843):150–7.

21. Basser PJ, Mattiello J, LeBihan D. MR diffusion tensor spectroscopy and imaging. Biophys J 1994;66(1):259–67.

22. Pierpaoli C, Jezzard P, Basser PJ, et al. Diffusion tensor MR imaging of the human brain. Radiology 1996;201(3):637–48.

23. Conturo TE, Lori NF, Cull TS, et al. Tracking neuronal fiber pathways in the living human brain. Proc Natl Acad Sci U S A 1999;96(18):10422–7.

24. Mori S, Crain BJ, Chacko VP, et al. Three-dimensional tracking of axonal projections in the brain by magnetic resonance imaging. Ann Neurol 1999;45(2):265–9.

25. Catani M, Thiebaut de Schotten M. A diffusion tensor imaging tractography atlas for virtual in vivo dissections. Cortex 2008;44(8):1105–32.

26. Jones DK. Studying connections in the living human brain with diffusion MRI. Cortex 2008; 44(8):936–52.

27. Seunarine KK, Alexander DC. Multiple fibers: beyond the diffusion tensor. In: Johansen-Berg H, Behrens TE, editors. Diffusion MRI: from quantitative measurement to in vivo neuroanatomy. Oxford, U.K: Elsevier; 2009. p. 55–72.

28. Gitelman DR, Nobre AC, Sonty S, et al. Language network specializations: an analysis with parallel task designs and functional magnetic resonance imaging. Neuroimage 2005;26(4):975–85.

29. Naidich TP, Hof PR, Gannon PJ, et al. Anatomic substrates of language: emphasizing speech. Neuroimaging Clin N Am 2001;11(2):305–41.

30. Catani M. From hodology to function. Brain 2007; 130(Pt 3):602–5.

31. Catani M, Mesulam M. The arcuate fasciculus and the disconnection theme in language and aphasia: history and current state. Cortex 2008;44(8): 953–61.

32. Catani M, Mesulam M. What is a disconnection syndrome? Cortex 2008;44(8):911–3.

33. Mesulam MM. Large-scale neurocognitive networks and distributed processing for attention, language, and memory. Ann Neurol 1990;28(5):597–613.

34. Hickok G, Poeppel D. The cortical organization of speech processing. Nat Rev Neurosci 2007;8(5): 393–402.

35. Hickok G, Poeppel D. Dorsal and ventral streams: a framework for understanding aspects of the functional anatomy of language. Cognition 2004; 92(1–2):67–99.

36. Poeppel D, Hickok G. Towards a new functional anatomy of language. Cognition 2004;92(1–2):1–12.

37. Saur D, Kreher BW, Schnell S, et al. Ventral and dorsal pathways for language. Proc Natl Acad Sci U S A 2008;105(46):18035–40.

38. Penfield W, Roberts L. Speech and brain mechanisms. Princeton, NJ: Princeton University Press; 1959.

39. Ojemann G, Ojemann J, Lettich E, et al. Cortical language localization in left, dominant hemisphere. An electrical stimulation mapping investigation in 117 patients. J Neurosurg 1989;71(3):316–26.

40. Damasio A, Damasio AR. The lesion method in humans. New York: Oxford University Press; 1989.

41. Berger MS. Introduction: language localization in the dominant hemisphere. J Neurosurg 2008;108:410.

42. Ojemann JG, Ojemann GA, Lettich E. Cortical stimulation mapping of language cortex by using a verb generation task: effects of learning and comparison to mapping based on object naming. J Neurosurg 2002;97(1):33–8.

43. Sanai N, Mirzadeh Z, Berger MS. Functional outcome after language mapping for glioma resection. N Engl J Med 2008;358:18–27.

44. Stippich C, Rapps N, Dreyhaupt J, et al. Localizing and lateralizing language in patients with brain tumors: feasibility of routine preoperative functional MR imaging in 81 consecutive patients. Radiology 2007;243(3):828–36.

45. Fandino J, Kollias SS, Wieser HG, et al. Intraoperative validation of functional magnetic resonance imaging and cortical reorganization patterns in patients with brain tumors involving the primary motor cortex. J Neurosurg 1999; 91(2):238–50.

46. Lurito JT, Lowe MJ, Sartorius C, et al. Comparison of fMRI and intraoperative direct cortical stimulation in localization of receptive language areas. J Comput Assist Tomogr 2000;24(1):99–105.

47. Pouratian N, Bookheimer SY, Rex DE, et al. Utility of preoperative functional magnetic resonance imaging for identifying language cortices in patients with vascular malformations. J Neurosurg 2002;97(1):21–32.

48. Grummich P, Nimsky C, Pauli E, et al. Combining fMRI and MEG increases the reliability of presurgical language localization: a clinical study on the difference between and congruence of both modalities. Neuroimage 2006;32(4):1793–803.

49. Quiñones-Hinojosa A, Ojemann SG, Sanai N, et al. Preoperative correlation of intraoperative cortical mapping with magnetic resonance imaging landmarks to predict localization of the Broca area. J Neurosurg 2003;99(2):311–8.

50. Bello L, Acerbi F, Giussani C, et al. Intraoperative language localization in multilingual patients with gliomas. Neurosurgery 2006;59(1):115–25 [discussion: 25].

51. Roux FE, Trémoulet M. Organization of language areas in bilingual patients: a cortical stimulation study. J Neurosurg 2002;97(4):857–64.

52. Skirboll SS, Ojemann GA, Berger MS, et al. Functional cortex and subcortical white matter located within gliomas. Neurosurgery 1996;38(4):678–84 [discussion: 84–5].

53. Ulmer JL, Salvan CV, Mueller WM, et al. The role of diffusion tensor imaging in establishing the proximity of tumor borders to functional brain systems: implications for preoperative risk assessments and postoperative outcomes. Technol Cancer Res Treat 2004;3(6):567–76.

54. Petrella JR, Shah LM, Harris KM, et al. Preoperative functional MR imaging localization of language and motor areas: effect on therapeutic decision making in patients with potentially resectable brain tumors. Radiology 2006;240(3):793–802.

55. Lurito JT, Dzemidzic M. Determination of cerebral hemisphere language dominance with functional magnetic resonance imaging. Neuroimaging Clin N Am 2001;11(2):355–63.

56. Wada J, Rasmussen T. Intracarotid injection of sodium amytal for the lateralization of cerebral speech dominance. J Neurosurg 1960;17:266–82.

57. Benson RR, FitzGerald DB, LeSueur LL, et al. Language dominance determined by whole brain functional MRI in patients with brain lesions. Neurology 1999;52(4):798–809.

58. Desmond JE, Sum JM, Wagner AD, et al. Functional MRI measurement of language lateralization in Wada-tested patients. Brain 1995;118(Pt 6):1411–9.

59. Duffau H, Lopes M, Arthuis F, et al. Contribution of intraoperative electrical stimulations in surgery of low grade gliomas: a comparative study between two series without (1985–96) and with (1996–2003) functional mapping in the same institution. J Neurol Neurosurg Psychiatr 2005; 76(6):845–51.

60. Ilmberger J, Ruge M, Kreth FW, et al. Intraoperative mapping of language functions: a longitudinal neurolinguistic analysis. J Neurosurg 2008;109(4): 583–92.

61. Haglund MM, Berger MS, Shamseldin M, et al. Cortical localization of temporal lobe language sites in patients with gliomas. Neurosurgery 1994; 34(4):567–76 [discussion: 76].

62. Chang S, Parney IF, McDermott M, et al. Perioperative complications and neurological outcome of first versus second craniotomy among patients enrolled in the glioma outcomes project. J Neurosurg 2003;98:1175–81.

63. Clark CA, Barrick TR, Murphy MM, et al. White matter fiber tracking in patients with space-occupying lesions of the brain: a new technique for neurosurgical planning? Neuroimage 2003;20(3): 1601–8.

64. Field AS, Alexander AL, Wu YC, et al. Diffusion tensor eigenvector directional color imaging patterns in the evaluation of cerebral white matter tracts altered by tumor. J Magn Reson Imaging 2004;20(4):555–62.

65. Mori S, Frederiksen K, van Zijl PC, et al. Brain white matter anatomy of tumor patients evaluated with diffusion tensor imaging. Ann Neurol 2002;51(3): 377–80.

66. Nimsky C, Ganslandt O, Hastreiter P, et al. Intraoperative diffusion-tensor MR imaging: shifting of white matter tracts during neurosurgical procedures—initial experience. Radiology 2005;234(1): 218–25.

67. Jellison BJ, Field AS, Medow J, et al. Diffusion tensor imaging of cerebral white matter: a pictorial review of physics, fiber tract anatomy, and tumor imaging patterns. AJNR Am J Neuroradiol 2004; 25(3):356–69.

68. Laundre BJ, Jellison BJ, Badie B, et al. Diffusion tensor imaging of the corticospinal tract before and after mass resection as correlated with clinical motor findings: preliminary data. AJNR Am J Neuroradiol 2005;26(4):791–6.

69. Nimsky C, Ganslandt O, Fahlbusch R. Implementation of fiber tract navigation. Neurosurgery 2007; 61(1 Suppl): 306–17[discussion: 317–8].

70. Bello L, Gambini A, Castellano A, et al. Motor and language DTI Fiber Tracking combined with intraoperative subcortical mapping for surgical removal of gliomas. Neuroimage 2008;39(1):369–82.

71. Bello L, Gallucci M, Fava M, et al. Intraoperative subcortical language tract mapping guides surgical removal of gliomas involving speech areas. Neurosurgery 2007;60(1):67–82.

72. Dejerine J, Dejerine-Klumpke A. Anatomies des centres nerveux. Paris: Rueff et Cie; 1895.

73. Petrides M, Pandya DN. Association fiber pathways to the frontal cortex from the superior temporal region in the rhesus monkey. J Comp Neurol 1988;273:52–66.

74. Petrides M, Pandya DN. Dorsolateral prefrontal cortex: comparative cytoarchitectonic analysis in the human and the macaque brain and corticocortical connection patterns. Eur J Neurosci 1999; 11(3):1011–36.

75. Catani M, Jones DK, Ffytche DH. Perisylvian language networks of the human brain. Ann Neurol 2005;57(1):8–16.

76. Lawes IN, Barrick TR, Murugam V, et al. Atlas-based segmentation of white matter tracts of the human brain using diffusion tensor tractography and comparison with classical dissection. Neuroimage 2008;39(1):62–79.

77. Catani M, Howard RJ, Pajevic S, et al. Virtual in vivo interactive dissection of white matter fasciculi in the human brain. Neuroimage 2002;17(1):77–94.

78. Duffau H, Gatignol P, Mandonnet E, et al. New insights into the anatomo-functional connectivity of the semantic system: a study using cortico-subcortical electrostimulations. Brain 2005;128(Pt 4): 797–810.

79. Mandonnet E, Nouet A, Gatignol P, et al. Does the left inferior longitudinal fasciculus play a role in

language? A brain stimulation study. Brain 2007; 130(Pt 3):623–9.

80. Adcock JE, Wise RG, Oxbury JM, et al. Quantitative fMRI assessment of the differences in lateralization of language-related brain activation in patients with temporal lobe epilepsy. Neuroimage 2003;18(2):423–38.

81. Amunts K, Schleicher A, Bürgel U, et al. Broca's region revisited: cytoarchitecture and intersubject variability. J Comp Neurol 1999;412(2):319–41.

82. Geschwind N, Levitsky W. Human brain: left-right asymmetries in temporal speech region. Science 1968;161(837):186–7.

83. Liegeois-Chauvel C, de Graaf JB, Laguitton V, et al. Specialization of left auditory cortex for speech perception in man depends on temporal coding. Cereb Cortex 1999;9(5):484–96.

84. Cantalupo C, Hopkins WD. Asymmetric Broca's area in great apes. Nature 2001;414(6863):505.

85. Cantalupo C, Oliver J, Smith J. The chimpanzee brain shows human-like perisylvian asymmetries in white matter. Eur J Neurosci 2009;30(3):431–8.

86. Rizzolatti G, Arbib MA. Language within our grasp. Trends Neurosci 1998;21(5):188–94.

87. Gannon PJ, Holloway RL, Broadfield DC, et al. Asymmetry of chimpanzee planum temporale: humanlike pattern of Wernicke's brain language area homolog. Science 1998;279(5348):220–2.

88. Toga AW, Thompson PM. Mapping brain asymmetry [review]. Nat Rev Neurosci 2003;4(1):37–48.

89. Paus T, Zijdenbos A, Worsley K, et al. Structural maturation of neural pathways in children and adolescents: in vivo study. Science 1999; 283(5409):1908–11.

90. Galuske RA, Schlote W, Bratzke H, et al. Interhemispheric asymmetries of the modular structure in human temporal cortex. Science 2000;289(5486): 1946–9.

91. Barrick TR, Lawes IN, Mackay CE, et al. White matter pathway asymmetry underlies functional lateralization. Cereb Cortex 2007;17(3):591–8.

92. Büchel C, Raedler T, Sommer M, et al. White matter asymmetry in the human brain: a diffusion tensor MRI study. Cereb Cortex 2004;14(9):945–51.

93. Glasser MF, Rilling JK. DTI tractography of the human brain's language pathways. Cereb Cortex 2008;18(11):2471–82.

94. Matsumoto R, Okada T, Mikuni N, et al. Hemispheric asymmetry of the arcuate fasciculus: a preliminary diffusion tensor tractography study in patients with unilateral language dominance defined by Wada test. J Neurol 2008;255(11):1703–11.

95. Nucifora PGP, Verma R, Melhem ER, et al. Leftward asymmetry in relative fiber density of the arcuate fasciculus. Neuroreport 2005;16(8):791–4.

96. Vernooij MW, Smits M, Wielopolski PA, et al. Fiber density asymmetry of the arcuate fasciculus in relation to functional hemispheric language lateralization in both right- and left-handed healthy subjects: a combined fMRI and DTI study. Neuroimage 2007;35(3):1064–76.

97. Parker GJM, Luzzi S, Alexander DC, et al. Lateralization of ventral and dorsal auditory-language pathways in the human brain. Neuroimage 2005; 24(3):656–66.

98. Powell HWR, Parker GJ, Alexander DC, et al. Hemispheric asymmetries in language-related pathways: a combined functional MRI and tractography study. Neuroimage 2006;32(1):388–99.

99. Schmahmann JD, Pandya DN, Wang R, et al. Association fibre pathways of the brain: parallel observations from diffusion spectrum imaging and autoradiography. Brain 2007;130(Pt 3):630–53.

100. Catani M, Allin MP, Husain M, et al. Symmetries in human brain language pathways correlate with verbal recall. Proc Natl Acad Sci U S A 2007; 104(43):17163–8.

101. Cao Y, Whalen S, Huang J, et al. Asymmetry of subinsular anisotropy by in vivo diffusion tensor imaging. Hum Brain Mapp 2003;20(2):82–90.

102. Rodrigo S, Naggara O, Oppenheim C, et al. Human subinsular asymmetry studied by diffusion tensor imaging and fiber tracking. AJNR Am J Neuroradiol 2007;28(8):1526–31.

103. Friederici AD. Syntactic, prosodic, and semantic processes in the brain: evidence from event-related neuroimaging. Jpn Psychol Res 2001;30(3):237–50.

104. Saur D, Lange R, Baumgaertner A, et al. Dynamics of language reorganization after stroke. Brain 2006; 129(Pt 6):1371–84.

105. Kimura D. Manual activity during speaking. II. Lefthanders. Neuropsychologia 1973;11(1):51–5.

106. Kimura D. Manual activity during speaking. I. Righthanders. Neuropsychologia 1973;11(1):45–50.

107. Celsis P, Boulanouar K, Doyon B, et al. Differential fMRI responses in the left posterior superior temporal gyrus and left supramarginal gyrus to habituation and change detection in syllables and tones. Neuroimage 1999;9(1):135–44.

108. Butz M, Worgotter F, van Ooyen A. Activity-dependent structural plasticity. Brain Res Rev 2009;60(2): 287–305.

109. Hess G, Donoghue JP. Long-term depression of horizontal connections in rat motor cortex. Eur J Neurosci 1996;8(4):658–65.

110. Farkas T, Perge J, Kis Z, et al. Facial nerve injury-induced disinhibition in the primary motor cortices of both hemispheres. Eur J Neurosci 2000;12(6):2190–4.

111. Gowers WR. Lectures on the diagnosis of diseases of the brain. 2nd edition. In: Gowers WR, editor. London: J & A. Churchill; 1887.

112. Blasi V, Young AC, Tansy AP, et al. Word retrieval learning modulates right frontal cortex in patients with left frontal damage. Neuron 2002;36(1):159–70.

113. Flitman SS, Grafman J, Wassermann EM, et al. Linguistic processing during repetitive transcranial magnetic stimulation. Neurology 1998;50(1):175–81.

114. Naeser MA, Martin PI, Nicholas M, et al. Improved picture naming in chronic aphasia after TMS to part of right Broca's area: an open-protocol study. Brain Lang 2005;93(1):95–105.

115. Damasio H, Damasio AR. Lesion analysis in neuropsychology. Oxford: Oxford University Press; 1989.

116. Thiel A, Herholz K, Koyuncu A, et al. Plasticity of language networks in patients with brain tumors: a positron emission tomography activation study. Ann Neurol 2001;50(5):620–9.

117. THn Lucas, Drane DL, Dodrill CB, et al. Language reorganization in aphasics: an electrical stimulation mapping investigation. Neurosurgery 2008;63(3):487–97.

118. Desmurget M, Bonnetblanc F, Duffau H. Contrasting acute and slow-growing lesions: a new door to brain plasticity. Brain 2007;130(Pt 4):898–914.

119. Robles SG, Gatignol P, Lehéricy S, et al. Long-term brain plasticity allowing a multistage surgical approach to World Health Organization Grade II gliomas in eloquent areas. J Neurosurg 2008;109(4):615–24.

120. Springer JA, Binder JR, Hammeke TA, et al. Language dominance in neurologically normal and epilepsy subjects: a functional MRI study. Brain 1999;122(Pt 11):2033–46.

121. Sabsevitz DS, Swanson SJ, Hammeke TA, et al. Use of preoperative functional neuroimaging to predict language deficits from epilepsy surgery. Neurology 2003;60(11):1788–92.

122. Powell HWR, Parker GJ, Alexander DC, et al. Imaging language pathways predicts postoperative naming deficits. J Neurol Neurosurg Psychiatr 2008;79(3):327–30.

123. Rodrigo S, Oppenheim C, Chassoux F, et al. Language lateralization in temporal lobe epilepsy using functional MRI and probabilistic tractography. Epilepsia 2008;49(8):1367–76.

Intraoperative Mapping for Tumor Resection

Lorenzo Bello, MD[a,*], Enrica Fava, MD[a], Giuseppe Casaceli, MD[a],
Giulio Bertani, MD[a], Giorgio Carrabba, MD[a],
Costanza Papagno, MD[b], Andrea Falini, MD[c,d],
Sergio M. Gaini, MD[a]

KEYWORDS

- Gliomas • Intraoperative mapping
- Cortical and subcortical stimulation • DTI • Neurophysiology

Intraoperative mapping refers to a group of techniques that allow for safe and effective removal of lesions located in so-called eloquent or functional areas. Although the entire brain can be inferred as eloquent, the eloquent areas are usually involved in motor, language, visual, or visuospatial control. The surgical removal of lesions in or close to those areas or pathways aims to maximize surgical removal and to minimize postoperative morbidity. These results can be achieved by the identification and preservation during surgery of the cortical and subcortical sites involved in specific functions. Detecting and preserving the essential functional cortical and subcortical sites have recently been defined as surgery according to functional boundaries, and is performed using the brain-mapping technique.

Brain-mapping techniques are generally applied to the surgical resection of intrinsic lesions, such as gliomas., They can occasionally be used during removal of cavernoma or meningioma, when these lesions are located in or close to functional areas of the brain. However, these techniques have been developed and used mainly for the surgical resection of low-grade gliomas.

Low-grade glioma refers to a series of primary brain tumors characterized by benign histology and aggressive behavior related to the slowly progressive invasion of the normal brain parenchyma.[1–5] These neoplasms are classified as grade II (of IV) by the World Health Organization classification of brain tumors and include grade II astrocytoma (further divided into fibrillary and protoplasmic), grade II oligoastrocytoma and grade II oligodendroglioma.[6,7] Pilocytic astrocytomas, or grade I astrocytomas, are occasionally referred to as low-grade gliomas but because of their peculiar behavior, they require separate considerations. Low-grade gliomas are slow-growing tumors, typically affecting younger individuals (median age 35 years), mainly men (male/female ratio 1.5), which clinically present with seizures (often partial seizures).[8] Headache, personality changes, and focal neurologic deficits are the other most common symptoms. The neurologic symptoms include motor/sensory deficits, dysphasia/aphasia, disinhibition, apathy, and visuospatial disturbances, according to the tumor location and size.[1,9,10] Low-grade gliomas mainly occur in eloquent areas or in their proximity,[11] and grow diffusely, along short and long white-matter tracts. They grow continuously, and the speed of growth as measured on magnetic resonance (MR) images has been advocated as an important prognostic factor. In addition, these tumors systematically evolve toward a more

[a] Department of Neurological Sciences, Università degli Studi di Milano, Via Francesco Sforza 35, 20122. Milano, Italy
[b] Department of Psychology, Università Milano Bicocca, Pz Ateneo Nuovo, 1, 20126. Milano, Italy
[c] Department of Neuroradiology, Università Vita e Salute, Istituto Scientifico San Raffaele, via Olgettina 60, 20130. Milano, Italy
[d] Neuroradiology, Ospèdale San Raffaele, Via Olgettina 60, 20130. Milano, Italy
* Corresponding author. Neurochirurgia, Dipt di Scienze Neurologiche, Università degli Studi di Milano, Via Francesco Sforza 35, 20122. Milano, Italy.
E-mail address: lorenzo.bello@unimi.it (L. Bello).

Neuroimag Clin N Am 19 (2009) 597–614
doi:10.1016/j.nic.2009.08.011
1052-5149/09/$ – see front matter © 2009 Elsevier Inc. All rights reserved.

malignant phenothype: so-called malignant transformation. Overall, the median survival of low-grade gliomas is about 10 years and well-defined negative prognostic factors include older age (>40 years old), larger size (>5 cm), eloquent location, and reduced Karnofsky performance status. The optimal treatment of those tumors that are no longer indolent has yet to be determined. Watchful observation, needle biopsy, open biopsy, and surgical resection have all been advocated by different investigators.[2,12–21] Surgical resection of low-grade gliomas is still a matter of debate but recent studies have increasingly supported resection.[12,14,22–26] Surgery can achieve multiple aims: a more reliable histologic diagnosis with eventual molecular profiling (eg, 1p/19q loss and methyl guanine methyl transferase [MGMT] status); symptom relief; a beneficial effect on seizure control; and a decrease in the rate of recurrence and of malignant transformation, as confirmed by recent studies.[22,23,26] Nevertheless, surgery carries risks, which although low can permanently affect the patient's quality of life. Considering the behavior of low-grade glioma and the possibility of treatment, the modern surgical approach to low-grade gliomas is to resect the tumor mass maximally, and at the same time to minimize postoperative morbidity to preserve the patient's functional integrity.[14,22,23,26] Because the natural history of the tumor can be long (with or without surgery), the conservation of simple and complex neurologic functions of the patients is mandatory.

High-grade gliomas are a larger group of intrinsic brain tumors, which include anaplastic tumors (such as oligodendrogliomas or astrocytomas) and glioblastomas. They can be classified as primary, when they are discovered and diagnosed de novo, or they can come from the transformation and evolution of low-grade gliomas. They are highly infiltrative neoplasms, invading along white-matter tracts and vessels. In addition, they are characterized by an elevated tumor cell proliferation, which results in the formation of a large, densely cellulated tumor mass, with high vascularization. Less frequently than low-grade gliomas, these tumors may develop within or close to eloquent areas or pathways. In such cases, as with low-grade gliomas, surgical removal should involve amaximal tumor removal, which is associated with the best oncologic result, while still maintaining the patient's total functional integrity, which allows the patient rapid access to adjuvant treatments.

To achieve the goal of a satisfactory tumor resection associated with the full preservation of the patient's abilities, a series of neuropsychological, neurophysiologic, neuroradiological, and intraoperative investigations have to be performed. This article describes the rationale, the indications, and the modality for performing safe and effective surgical removal of tumors located within functional brain areas.

RATIONALE AND INDICATIONS

The major aims of surgical treatment are: (1) to obtain adequate specimens and representative tissue to reach a correct histologic and molecular diagnosis; (2) to achieve a maximal cytoreduction to decrease the rate of recurrence and malignant transformation for low-grade gliomas, and increase the effect of adjuvant therapies for high-grade gliomas, in both cases possibly prolonging patient survival; (3) to improve the neurologic symptoms of the patients; and (4) to obtain better seizure control. These goals can be reached by tailoring the surgical approach to the particular features of location, modality of growth, and behavior of the tumor.

Surgery for gliomas aims to remove the tumor mass maximally and to preserve the patient's functional integrity. This policy applies to the resection of any glioma but more specifically to those located close to or within eloquent areas. The concept of eloquence refers not only to those areas that are involved in motor, language, or visuospatial functions but also, more widely, to any area affecting the well-being of the individual (eg, memory, socioaffective behavior, specific task performance). In all these cases, extensive resection and maximal functional integrity can still be achieved through the intraoperative use of brain-mapping techniques.[13–15,23,26–29]

THE BRAIN-MAPPING TECHNIQUE

Brain mapping requires a series of preoperative evaluations and intraoperative facilities that involve different specialists. A complete neuropsychological evaluation is generally the first step of the process, to select suitable patients and individualize intraoperative testing. In addition, sophisticated imaging techniques, including functional magnetic resonance imaging (fMRI) and diffuse tensor imaging, fiber tracking techniques (DTI-FT), help with surgical strategies. These images can be loaded into the neuronavigation system and are thus available peri- and intraoperatively for orientation. Intraoperative MR can also be used. A series of neurophysiologic techniques are employed at the time of surgery to guide the surgeon precisely in the tumor removal. These techniques include cortical and subcortical direct electrical stimulation (DES), motor evoked potentials (MEPs), multichannel electromyography (EMG), electroencephalography (EEG), and electrocorticography (ECoG) recordings. These techniques are detailed in the next section. For reasons of simplicity, the management protocol is divided into 3 parts: preoperative, perioperative, and postoperative.

PREOPERATIVE PROTOCOL

The preoperative part includes the neuropsychological and neuroradiological evaluation, which completes the standard neurologic examination. A neuroanesthesiologic evaluation should be performed also for the selection and preparation of the patients from this perspective.

Neuropsychology

Neuropsychological evaluation is composed of a large number of tests for the assessment of various neurologic functions, such as the cognitive, emotional, intelligence, and basic language functions. This broad-spectrum evaluation provides information on how the tumor has affected the social, emotional, and cognitive life of the patient, who is frequently intact or only mildly impaired at the neurologic examination. Test area should be as large as possible because a tumor that grows along fiber tracts may alter the connectivity between separate areas of the brain, resulting in the impairment of functions that might not be documented if the examination is limited to those functions strictly related to the area of the brain in which the tumor has grown.[23,27,30] When this extensive testing is administered, some alteration in the neuropsychological examinations can be documented in more than 90% of patients with low-grade gliomas, and in more than 70% with high-grade gliomas.[23,27] These data represent the baseline against which future treatment should be compared. In addition, when the tumor involves language or visuospatial areas or pathways, a more extensive specific evaluation should also be performed. In addition to better defining the preoperative status of patients, the neuropsychological assessment is a series of tests, composed of various items, which are used intraoperatively for the evaluation and brain mapping of various functions, of which memory, language, and visuospatial orientation are some of the most important. For language evaluation, patients are submitted preoperatively to extensive language testing from a battery of tests aimed at evaluating oral language production and comprehension, together with repetition.[27,29,31,32] Hemispheric language dominance is evaluated

through the Edinburgh Inventory Questionnaire and fMRI. The following tasks are usually performed: spontaneous speech; oral controlled association by phonemic cue; famous face naming; object picture naming; action picture naming; word comprehension; sentence comprehension; transcoding tasks. The token test, the digit span, and counting are also performed. Ideomotor apraxia and face apraxia are assessed. Most of the tests used have been standardized on the normal population. In addition, different tests aimed at studying the previous aspects of language can be found and adjusted according to the nationality of the patient. Qualitative and quantitative tests should be included in the battery, and normative data must be available for the quantitative procedure. A speech therapist and a neuropsychologist should manage the assessments. Preoperative language evaluation is used in a series of tests intraoperatively for the assessment of language; object naming is probably the most important. In patients with a tumor located in dominant or parietal areas, number recognition and reading, calculation, or writing should be added to the preoperative testing and considered for the intraoperative evaluation.[33–35] When the patient is bilingual or speaks more than 2 languages, the preoperative testing should include extensive evaluation of the various languages.[36–39] The patient can be defined as early or late bi- or multilingual, depending on the time at which he or she has learned the various languages. A multilingual assessment is generally recommended.

Visuospatial functions are usually evaluated for tumor located in the parietal lobe, generally on the right side.[23] Unilateral spatial neglect is a complex and disabling syndrome that typically results from right-hemisphere damage, and it is characterized by an impairment of awareness of the contralesional left half of space, objects, and mental images. These patients are given various tests such as the line bisection test or the star cancellation test to evaluate their spatial awareness.

Imaging and Neuroradiology

The neuroradiological examination is composed of basic examinations, such as morphologic T1, T2, and fluid attenuated inversion recovery (FLAIR) images, and postcontrast T1 images. These images together with volumetric sequences provide information on the site and location of the tumor, and allow determination of its relationship with various structures, such as major vessels, and measurement of tumor volume. With low-grade gliomas, additional MR studies such as MR spectroscopy or MR perfusion can be performed. MR spectroscopy, which provides information on the metabolic characteristics of the tumor, allows design of a map of areas within the tumor in which tumor metabolism is more or less pronounced (a multipixel MR spectroscopy map).[40,41] This helps with tissue sampling during surgery for histologic and molecular purposes. In addition, perfusion MR studies are useful for designing perfusion maps, or maps in which the blood flow is depicted in the different tumor areas.[42–46] Because regional blood flow is dependent on tumor angiogenesis, these maps provide additional and complementary information on the biologic behavior of the tumor and help with collection of tissue during surgery for histologic and molecular examination.[47] Metabolic information may be also obtained by performing single photon emission computed tomography (SPECT) or positron emission tomography (PET), and these data may be incorporated into the navigation system for surgical guidance. PET with fluorodeoxyglucose (FDG) is generally used for high-grade gliomas, and metionine for low-grade tumors.

The neuroradiological investigations include functional studies, such as fMRI, and anatomic studies such as DTI-FT. The former provides functional information on the location of cortical sites that activates in response to motor tasks or various language tasks.[48] Motor fMRI is generally used to design a map of the cortical motor sites and to establish their relationship with the tumor.[49] fMRI for language provides a map of the cortical sites that activate during various language tasks, such as denomination (object naming), verb generation, and verbal fluency.[50,51] All these data are pooled to form a complex map of how the various components of language are organized at the cortical level, and establish the spatial relationship between these cortical areas of language activation and the tumor mass. It is usually recommended that language fMRI is performed with the same tests that are used for language evaluation to increase its reliability.

The DTI-FT techniques allow the connectivity around and inside a tumor to be depicted, by reconstructing and visualizing the fiber tracts that run around or inside the tumor mass.[52,53] A deterministic DTI-FT approach is generally used for clinical purposes. DTI-FT provides anatomic information on the location of motor tracts, mainly the corticospinal tract and various language tracts.[54–58] The basic DTI-FT map includes the corticospinal tract (CST) for the motor part, and the superior longitudinalis (SLF), which includes the fasciculus arcuatus, and the inferior frontooccipital (IFO) tract for the language part.[29,31,54] The SLF is the basic tract involved in the phonologic component of language; the IFO is the basic tract involved in the semantic component of language. Additional tracts that can be reconstructed are the uncinatus (UNC) and the inferior longitudinalis (ILF) tracts, which provide information on the semantic and phonologic component of language in the frontal and temporal lobe, or the subcallosum fasciculus, involved in the phonologic component of language, sited in the lateral border of the lateral ventricle. Generally, preoperative DTI-FT shows that in low-grade gliomas most of the tracts involved in language or motor function are located within the tumor mass, and infiltrated or interrupted by the tumor. In high-grade gliomas most of the tracts are located in the tumor periphery and dislocated by the tumor mass. Although DTI-FT maps are only anatomic and do not provide any functional information, they can be used to predict resectability of a tumor. Preoperative neuroimaging produces a large amount of information concerning the anatomic and functional boundaries of the lesion to be resected. Together with the volumetric morphologic images, the DTI-FT images are usually loaded into the neuronavigation system, and help in the perioperative period in performing the resection. However, the imaging gives information based on probabilistic measurements, and although they may have a high sensitivity or specificity, they still carry the potential for error, which is not efficient for performing a safe and effective resection. For this reason the neuroradiological information loaded into the neuronavigation system has to be supported during surgery by the results of the brain mapping. Only intraoperative brain mapping by electrical stimulation allows the surgeon to identify functional regions, which may be displaced and infiltrated by the tumor at a cortical and a subcortical level, and thus to define the strategy of resection to maximize the extent of tumor removal and reduce the risks of permanent neurologic deficits.

Anesthesiology

Besides the standard anesthesiological work-up, the patient should be examined for his or her capacity for intraoperative awake monitoring. Preparation and selection of the patients by anesthesiologists with expertise in surgery in an awake patient is recommended.[59,60] In the authors' institution, the only absolute contraindications to awake surgery are lack of cooperation from patients, patients older than 65 years, obese patients, patients with difficult airways, or patients affected by severe cardiovascular or respiratory diseases, common contraindications to any general anesthesia regimen, communication difficulties (moderate-to-severe aphasia), psychological imbalance (extreme anxiety), prone position, and inability to lie still for many hours.

Once the preoperatory work-up (according to the site and the characteristics of the tumor), the neuropsychological evaluation, and the functional and anatomic imaging are completed, each patient is offered an individualized surgical and monitoring strategy, which can be summarized as follows:

1. Lesions in the nondominant hemisphere, away from eloquent areas and with no relationship with areas of activation according to fMRI: motor monitoring (optional).
2. Lesions in the nondominant hemisphere, in central or precentral area or in relationship with the CST (eg, insular, temporomesial tumors) and small central lesions in the dominant hemisphere: motor mapping and monitoring.
3. Lesions in the nondominant hemisphere, in the postcentral region: motor mapping and monitoring, visuospatial mapping.
4. Lesions in the dominant hemisphere: motor mapping and monitoring, language mapping ± visuospatial mapping for parietal lesions.

INTRAOPERATIVE PROTOCOL

The general policy in surgical treatment is to remove the maximal amount of tumor and to preserve the functional integrity of the patient, by removing the tumor according to anatomic and functional boundaries. The anatomic boundaries can be defined by using neuronavigation or intraoperative MR; sonography can also be used. The functional boundaries can be defined by using neurophysiologic and neuropsychological adjuncts. The intraoperative protocol includes anesthesia modalities, neurophysiology, neuropsychology, and intraoperative imaging (neuronavigation and intraoperative MR).

Anesthesia

The patient can be kept awake during surgery, or awakened for the phase during which the mapping is performed.[26,27,29,33,54,59–62] Total intravenous anesthesia with propofol and remifentanil is used in the authors' institution for performing these procedures. Newer drugs, such as dexmedetomidine, are emerging as effective and safe in achieving sedation without inducing respiratory depression or affecting electrophysiologic

monitoring. In the authors' institution, patients requiring only motor mapping are intubated through the nose and a light surgical anesthesia is maintained throughout the procedure. No muscle relaxants are employed during surgery to allow the neurophysiologic assessment. When the language or the visuospatial functions have to be tested intraoperatively, the patients receive a laryngeal mask, which is maintained until after dural opening.[63] At this point, the patients are awakened, and adequate analgesia is maintained to allow functional monitoring. The anesthesiologist should keep the patient awake during the entire subcortical mapping, and particularly during long operations this may require alternating periods of resting with periods during which the patient is fully awake and responsive. Fatigue is observed in most patients, and its appearance correlates with the duration of the mapping and the difficulties of testing (extensive language and visuospatial mapping).[36,40,64] Seizure is the most important complication during the awake time of the surgery, and can be controlled either by cold saline irrigation or by the infusion of a small bolus (1 mL) of propofol. Vomiting is a rare complication, and can be controlled by the administration of antiemetics at the beginning of the mapping phase.[65]

Neurophysiology

The major components of the neurophysiologic protocol are EEG, ECoG, EMG, DES, and MEP techniques. The protocol includes mapping (DES) and monitoring (EEG, ECoG, MEP) procedures.[13,66–72]

EEG/ECoG

In the authors' institution, EEG activity is recorded bilaterally by 4 subdermal needle electrodes, providing 4 bipolar leads. EEG is registered to monitor brain activity when ECoG is not available, at the beginning and the end of surgery, when it is particularly useful for titrating the level of anesthesia. Moreover, it allows assessment of brain activity at a distance from the operating area, such as in the contralateral hemisphere.

ECoG activity is recorded from a cortical region adjacent to the area being stimulated, by means of subdural strip electrodes with 4 to 8 contacts, in a monopolar array, connected to a midfrontal electrode. Cerebral activity is recorded with a bandpass of 1.6 to 320 Hz, and displayed with a sensitivity of 50 to 100 µ/cm for EEG and 200 to 400 µ/cm for ECoG. Continuous electrocorticographic recordings (Comet, Grass Technologies, West Warwick, RI, USA) are used throughout the procedure to monitor the brain basal electrical activity and the level of anesthesia, to define the working current (detection of afterdischarges), and to monitor for the occurrence of afterdischarges, electrical seizures, or clinical seizures during the resection. Because of this, EEG and ECoG recordings should be maintained throughout the operation.

EMG

Continuous multichannel EMG recording (Comet, Grass Technologies) is used throughout the procedure. Several separate muscles (agonist and antagonist muscles) can be monitored in the contralateral or ipsilateral body. Motor responses are collected by pairs of subdermal hooked needle electrodes inserted into the contralateral muscles from face to foot. Each pair of electrodes records 2 different muscles in the same body segment, to sample as many muscles as possible (ie, a flexor and an extensor muscle in the forearm). On average, 16 channels are used for each procedure. The most used setting comprises the face (upper and lower face), neck, arm, forearm, hand, upper leg, and lower leg. A computerized video and image capturing system is continuously coupled with the EMG recordings (Comet, Grass Technologies), to further monitor and register the motor activity. In addition to EMG recordings, motor activity is also evaluated clinically.

MEP

Continuous monitoring of motor function is performed through MEP recording. The "train of 5 technique," which was introduced for surgery in anesthetized patients, has been described as sensitive for detecting imminent lesions of the motor cortex and the pyramidal pathways.[73] A strip electrode containing 4 to 8 electrodes is placed over the precentral gyrus. In awake patients a single stimulus or a double-pulse stimulus (individual pulse width 0.3–0.5 ms, anodal constant current stimulation, interstimulus interval 4 milliseconds, stimulation intensity close to motor threshold) is usually delivered. The muscle MEPs have to be recorded with needle or (more conveniently in patients who are awake) with surface EMG electrodes. MEP recording is usually alternated with direct cortical and subcortical motor mapping. MEP monitoring is useful because it provides real-time information on the integrity of the motor pathways during the resection of large parts of the tumor not closely related to the functional structures. In addition, MEP provides warnings of impending brain ischemia, caused by critical vessel interruption, mostly in deep temporal or insular regions.[74]

DES

DES for cortical and subcortical mapping is performed with a bipolar hand-held stimulator,[66] with 1-mm electrode tips, 5 mm apart, connected to an Ojemann Cortical Stimulator (Integra Neuroscience, Plainsboro, NJ, USA) or an Osiris stimulator (Inomed, Teningen, Germany). The stimulator delivers biphasic square wave pulses, each phase lasting 1 millisecond, at 60 Hz in trains lasting 1 second for cortical mapping and 1 to 2 seconds for subcortical mapping. Subcortical mapping is alternated back and forth with the resection. Subcortical mapping is performed using the same current threshold applied for cortical mapping.

In mapping performed under general anesthesia, the current intensity ranges from 5 to 15 mA. In patients who are awake, a current intensity ranging from 2 to 8 mA is usually enough to evoke motor responses. In these patients, no electrodes are placed in the mouth, and the activity of the muscles of this region can be checked by monitoring the responses of the patients and by overt inspection. Patients who are awake are asked to relax before and during stimulation, and to assist in the description of induced movements or sensory changes.

The purpose of the mapping procedure is to test motor, language, and cognitive function reliably. At the beginning of the mapping procedure, the initial concern is to define the stimulation parameters. A low frequency of 60 Hz is used to establish the working current. It is advisable to start the procedure with the mapping of motor functions. Once determined, the same intensity of stimulating current is used in most cases throughout the procedure, and for the mapping of cognitive and language functions. Initially, a low-current intensity (2 mA) is used, which is progressively increased until a movement is induced. A stimulus duration of 1 or 2 seconds is usually enough to generate a motor response. At this point, it is good practice to stimulate the areas close to that in which the current induced the movement, to map them, and to check if the current evokes motor responses in these zones. If not, the current intensity may be increased and adjusted to evoke appreciable motor responses. It is also recommended to check with the ECoG if the applied current induces afterdischarges in the nearby brain areas. Only the current that is immediately below the one that induces afterdischarges has to be used for mapping. If afterdischarges are seen, the current should be set at least 0.5 mA less than the previous one. Because only the responses evoked in the absence of afterdischarges are considered to be trustworthy, continuous ECoG recording is used to check the appearance of afterdischarges during the mapping, to maintain the reliability of the test.

For language mapping, the initial test used is counting. The current is usually applied onto the premotor cortex related to the face, and the test aims to check if the current stops the patient counting. This test should be repeated several times, and counting stopped at least 3 times, to be reliable.[32] If not, the current intensity is increased until this is produced. When the current is established, DES is applied to the whole exposed surface of the brain, and the occurrence of afterdischarges checked in the ECoG. The duration of the stimulus is between 3 and 4 seconds. Only the current that is not inducing afterdischarges in the entire stimulated cortex is used for mapping. In afterdischarges, the current intensity is decreased at least by 0.5 mA.

For subcortical mapping, either the same current used for cortical mapping or a current increased by 2 mA is applied, and the stimulus is continuously alternated with the resection. When a response is induced at a subcortical level, the authors perform an intensity-response curve, to assess the maintenance of the response at low current intensity levels. This action can help in estimating the distance between the point of stimulation and the functional tract. During subcortical mapping, ECoG is continuously monitored to look for afterdischarges and seizures, to verify the reliability of the responses.

The resection margin is usually kept at least 5 mm away from functional areas, and may come close to subcortical pathways.

POSTOPERATIVE PROTOCOL

When resection is performed to functional boundaries, most patients develop postoperative deficits. Patients during the postoperative phase are submitted to neuropsychological evaluation (at 3 and 7 days) and to motor rehabilitation, to follow deficit recovery. MR studies, inclusive of volumetric T1, post-Gd T1-weighted images, and volumetric FLAIR images, are also performed. Neuroradiological studies should be performed within 24 to 48 hours of surgery.

RESULTS OF THE MAPPING OR MONITORING PROCEDURES
Motor Mapping

The authors usually map motor responses in patients with tumors located in the rolandic, premotor, or parietal region. Motor mapping is also applied at the cortical and subcortical levels for lesions located in the insula or deep temporal region, in which motor pathways can be encountered during resection. For lesions located in the nondominant hemisphere, the patient is kept under general anesthesia, and the tube positioned through the nose, which allows the placement of a series of electrodes in the inner palate and pharyngeal muscles, and in the tongue, which are useful for detecting responses from these muscles (Fig. 1). For lesions close to or within visuospatial or language areas of pathways, the patient is always awakened during the procedure. In awake and asleep settings, a stimulation duration of 1 or 2 seconds is usually enough to generate a motor response. At cortical stimulation the authors observed different morphologies of EMG responses: cortically evoked responses showed great variations in amplitude, but they always appeared as continuous, tonic bursts of activity, often incrementing during stimulation. The smallest amplitudes were observed in the neck and the shoulder, or in the mouth. Occasionally in patients under general anesthesia who are taking several antiepileptic medications, it might be difficult to evoke cortical motor responses, even after the current intensity has been increased to one that might induce afterdischarges. In these patients, MEP recording can be useful for identifying the location of the motor cortex and to plan the site of incision, allowing continuing resection. During subcortical stimulation, motor responses appeared as focal (few muscles) when the tract was stimulated close to the surface, although they appeared on multiple muscle groups with deep stimulation. Subcortical stimulation evoked tonic bursts and on-off activity (ie, an M-shaped response), peaking at the onset and the end of stimulation. For resection of tumors located in the premotor cortex, the placement of electrodes in the ipsilateral muscles allows responses coming from these segments to be detected during resection. In addition, when resection is approaching the deep portion of the tumor, subcortical stimulation allows the detection of small motor responses without overt muscle activity, which indicates that the resection is close to motor pathways. When these warning responses are identified, resection in this region should be particularly cautious and can proceed until more pronounced motor responses are identified, usually when the tip probe is touching and stimulating the motor pathways. The identification of such pathways is therefore particularly useful for performing an effective resection (see Fig. 1).

The simultaneous use of a cavitron ultrasonic surgical applicator (CUSA) and DES at the

A

Localization of pathological tissue

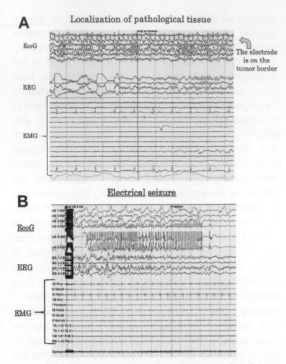

Fig. 1. (A) ECoG allows the identification of spikes in a cortical area close to the tumor border. This area of pathologic electrical activity was resected because it was recognized as not functional at the motor and language mapping. (B) ECoG shows the occurrence of an electrical seizure, without EMG abnormalities.

subcortical level close to the corticospinal tract may abolish previously evident motor responses. This abolition is generally fully reversible after turning off the CUSA. An analogous pattern of inhibition of motor responses is also evident when the DES is applied cortically and CUSA used subcortically close to motor pathways. This interference with motor mapping may be interpreted as a transitory inhibition of axonal conduction and should be kept in mind by the surgeon during resection using both tools.[75]

Motor Monitoring

For continuous motor monitoring with MEP, a second ECoG strip electrode is placed over M1, delivering monopolar pulses to elicit MEPs in a few target muscles: MEPs are monitored throughout the surgery, except when the surgeon needs direct subcortical mapping for mapping purposes. MEP monitoring is useful because it provides online information of the integrity of the motor pathways during resection of a large part of the tumor not closely located to functional

structures. In addition, MEP provides warnings of impending brain ischemia, caused by critical vessel interruption, mostly in deep temporal or insular regions.[74]

Language and Visuospatial Monitoring

Each of the stimulations should start before the presentation of the material, and should be followed by at least 1 task without stimulation; 2 tasks are the standard. If the stimulation lasts longer than the motor mapping (4 seconds vs 1–2 seconds), repetitive stimulation might trigger afterdischarges or seizures. The stimulus is applied immediately before the item is presented to the patient, and a neuropsychologist who is present in the operating room evaluates the performance of the patient during the various tests administered at cortical and subcortical level to maintain the patient's language integrity. Various types of mistake can be encountered during the performance of the tests. The ECoG and EEG should be checked during each test for afterdischarges or electrical seizures. Only mistakes in the absence of ECoG disturbances are reliable. In addition, a site can be defined as essential for language when it produces language disturbances at least 3 times in various nonconsecutive stimulations. Cortical language sites coding for object naming, verb generation, face naming, word or sentence comprehension, numbers, or colors can be identified in several regions in the frontal, temporal, or parietal lobe, with a distribution that differs according to patient and patient gender.[27,76] For subcortical language mapping, the patient is asked to perform an object-naming and a verb-generation task during which the surgeon can continue to perform resection alternated with stimulaton. When language disturbance is produced, the site is carefully tested for the occurrence of semantic or phonemic paraphasia. Each tract can be recognized at a subcortical level by the appearance of semantic (inferior frontooccipital tract, UNC) or phonemic (superior longitudinalis, ILF) paraphasia associated with typical language disturbances, such as speech arrest for the subcallosum. During subcortical mapping it is also possible to evoke motor responses, as a result of the identification and stimulation of motor fibers belonging to the premotor component of the face, which induce anarthya, or to the corticospinal tract, which induce various type of muscle activation depending on the location and depth of stimulation.

Visuospatial mapping is performed usually in patients with lesions located in the parietal lobe, and in a dominant location it is intermingled with language mapping. The patient is usually requested to look at a line on a touch screen and to bisect the line by touching its center with a pen. A deviation toward the right or left of more than 2 cm is usually considered as pathologic, and associated with interference in the visuospatial function. The current intensity is the same as for cortical motor mapping. Subcortical visuospatial mapping identified a small and discrete tract usually running along the lateral midborder of the tumor involved in this function. The preservation of this tract and of the cortical sites prevents neglect postoperatively.

EEG and ECoG Monitoring

EEG and ECoG recordings should be maintained during the procedure to monitor afterdischarges, electrical seizures, or clinical seizures. Afterdischarges are common during these procedures, and the main objective of monitoring is to recognize those that occur in response to stimulation, to maintain the reliability of the testing (Fig. 2). A group of ECoG spikes or electrical seizures occur in up to 30% to 40% of patients, which may or may not be related to the stimulation. When they appear, it is recommended that the cortex and the surgical cavity be irrigated with cold saline; this controls and reverses the situation in most patients. Clinical seizures occur in 8% of patients, and most of them are focal seizures. In these patients, EEG is useful to locate diffusion of the seizure, either in the same or in the contralateral hemisphere. The few clinical seizures observed by the authors appeared most frequently at the end of the resection, when cortical stimulation was applied to assess the integrity of the motor pathway. The current was subsequently reduced, and seizure was no longer elicited. At the end of the surgical resection, it might be necessary to reduce the intensity of the current, because of the reduction of the mass effect exerted by the tumor mass on the surrounding functional parenchyma. In selected patients, ECoG can be used to detect the generation of spikes in specific areas of the cortex, close to or far away from the tumor mass, which are responsible for sustained electrical activity. ECoG is also used to titrate and monitor the level of anesthesia, particularly in patients who are asleep. A continuous trace recording is usually recommended in this setting to assure an optimal response to cortical and subcortical stimulation.

RESULTS OF INTRAOPERATIVE IMAGING

Morphologic volumetric T1 and T2 images, along with motor and language fMRI and DTI-FT images,

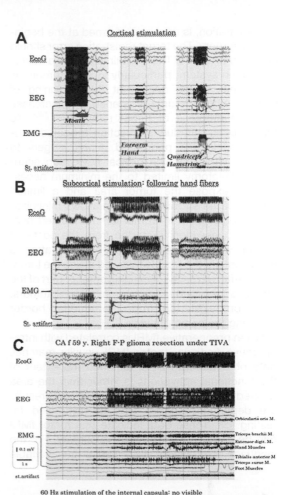

Fig. 2. Examples of motor responses during cortical and subcortical motor mapping (A) Cortical stimulation (60 Hz, 4 mA). EMG shows that stimulation induced responses in the mouth, forearm, and quadriceps and hamstring, allowing identification of the major components of the motor homunculus. (B) Subcortical stimulation (60 Hz, 6 mA). EMG shows that stimulation induces responses in the hand and that hand fibers were followed until the deeper part of resection. (C) Subcortical stimulation in an anesthesized patient (60 Hz, n). EMG shows response in several muscles caused by the stimulation of the corticospinal tract at the level of the internal capsule; no overt movements were observed clinically.

are usually loaded into the neuronavigation system. Neuronavigation helps during surgery to localize the tumor, and to define the relationship between the tumor and the surrounding functional and anatomic structures, at the cortical and subcortical level. As an estimate of the clinical navigation accuracy, the target registration error localizing a separate fiducial, which is not used for registration, is usually performed at the beginning of surgery. The target registration error should be less than 2 mm. The main limitation of a neuronavigation system, particularly in large tumors, is brain shift, which occurs at the beginning of surgery, when the dura is opened, and increases with the progress of tumor removal.[54,77–80] To reduce brain shift during resection, repeated landmark checks are performed during surgery to ensure overall ongoing clinical navigation accuracy; craniotomy limited to the minimum necessary to expose the tumor area and a limited portion of the surrounding brain allows minimization of brain shift; in frontal tumors located near the CST, resection is started from the posterior border, where the CST is located, and, after its identification, the tract is followed inside the tumor mass. Afterwards the remaining anterior part of the tumor is removed. Similarly, in parietal tumors, resection is started from the anterior border following the same principle.

When preoperative fMRI is correlated with intraoperative findings, motor fMRI usually matches data obtained with DES, although the extent of the functional activations is larger than the area defined with intraoperative mapping, and results are dependent on the type of task used for testing.[48,81] These data indicate that motor fMRI can be safely used for planning surgery. For the language correlation, the results are variable according to series. Naming and verb-generation tasks are most widely used for language fMRI studies. Generally, language fMRI data obtained with naming or verb-generation tasks were imperfectly correlated with intraoperative brain-mapping results (sensitivity 59% and specificity 97% when the 2 fMRIs are combined).[50,51,82] Generally, fMRI shows larger activation than those observed with direct cortical mapping, which demonstrates only essential language sites. In the authors' experience, the sensitivity can be increased up to 72% by using in the fMRI naming tasks the same figures used during surgery. Nevertheless, false-negative results are documented in up to 8% of patients. Therefore, language fMRI should not be used to make critical decisions in absence of direct brain mapping. Language fMRI is useful for establishing language laterality and can effectively replace the Wada test.

Preoperative DTI-FT showed that in most high-grade gliomas, tracts are extensively dislocated and infiltrated by the tumor. In addition, most of these tracts are located at the tumor periphery, outside the enhancing tumor area. In low-grade gliomas, tracts are less frequently dislocated, most frequently infiltrated ,and located inside the tumor mass. In DES in clinical use, DTI-FT provides anatomic information, whereas subcortical mapping provides functional information.[54,55]

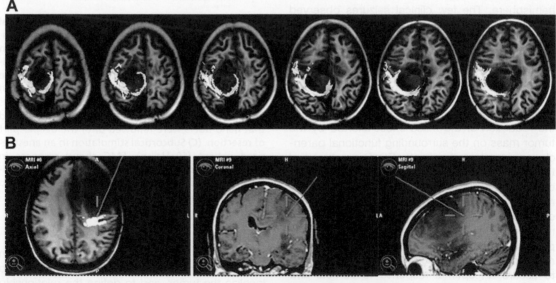

Fig. 3. DTI-FT and subcortical motor mapping. (A) DTI-FT reconstruction (FA 0.1) for CST was fused with T1-weighted images, in a right frontal grade II oligodendroglioma. CST was located inside the peripheral portion of the tumor, and highly infiltrated. (B) DTI-FT images for CST were fused with T1-weighted MR images in a left grade II astrocytoma, and loaded into the neuronavigation system. The panels show an intraoperative snapshot from the neuronavigation system, which indicates the location where subcortical stimulation induced arm and hand responses.

This is relevant to CST (Fig. 3), and of particular relevance for language tracts, in which the anatomic distribution of the tract as depicted by DTI is larger than the functional distribution obtained with mapping. Therefore, large part of tracts as depicted by DTI-FT can be removed because it is not functional for the function tested. Additional problems may come from the fractional anisotropy (FA) that is used for tract reconstruction, which may vary inside the same tumor according to grade of heterogeneity. In high-grade gliomas, subcortical mapping detect tracts at the tumor periphery, as DTI-FT does. In low-grade gliomas located in rolandic or supplementary motor areas, DTI-FT may fail in reconstructing portions of CST, particularly in areas of extensive tumor infiltration. The anatomic distribution of the SLF tract is usually larger than the functional distribution when language subcortical mapping is performed, particularly in frontal and temporal tumors. The anatomic distribution of the IFO tract is small and usually corresponds to the functional distribution depicted by subcortical mapping (Fig. 4). Some problems may occur for F3 low-grade gliomas in which DTI-FT may fail to reconstruct the more superior part of the tract at the inferior border of the tumor, when the tumor infiltration in this area is extensive. As for the UNC, the anatomic distribution of this tract is small and usually corresponds to the functional distribution depicted by subcortical mapping. The

reconstruction of this tract in F3 tumors requires the placement of an additional region of interest at this level. In F3 low-grade gliomas, the tract is usually inside the tumor mass, and the depicted fibers are usually found to be functional by subcortical mapping. In temporal low-grade gliomas, the tract is still described as inside the tumor mass, but the fibers are extensively infiltrated and interrupted, and not functional.

FUNCTIONAL RESULTS OF SURGERY

Resection margins are usually kept 5 mm apart from essential cortical sites, and are usually coincident with subcortical sites. When this is achieved, motor or language deficits develop in the immediate postoperative period in 72.8% and 65.4% of cases, respectively. When no subcortical sites are identified, this risk is low (3%–5%).[15,27,29,31,54,83] In the authors' experience, most of the deficits were transient and disappeared within 1 month of surgery. Overall, in the group of patients in which a subcortical functional site was identified during the resection, the likelihood of developing a permanent deficit was 3.8%, independently from histology and location. This percentage reached 7% in patients with a preexisting motor or language deficit. In contrast, when no subcortical sites were found at the time of surgery, the chance of inducing permanent deficit was even lower (2%). These results

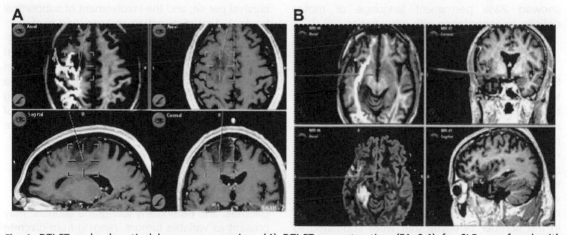

Fig. 4. DTI-FT and subcortical language mapping. (A) DTI-FT reconstruction (FA 0.1) for SLF was fused with T1-weighted MR images in a left frontal grade II oligodendroglioma and loaded into the neuronavigation system. The tract is inside the peripheral portion of the tumor. The panels show an intraoperative snapshot from the neuronavigation system, which indicates the location of a subcortical site where phonemic paraphasias were evoked. (B) DTI-FT reconstruction (FA 0.1) for IFO was fused with T1-weighted MR images in a left temporal recurrent grade II oligodendroglioma and loaded into the neuronavigation system. The tract is located at the periphery of the tumor mass, and constitutes the upper medial margin of the lesion. The panels show an intraoperative snapshot from the neuronavigation system, which indicates the location of a subcortical site where semantic paraphasias were evoked.

further reinforce the concept that when a subcortical site is found, the surgeon is close to the subcortical pathway. Therefore, when a subcortical response is reliably detected, the resection has to be stopped and should be continued in the adjacent structures, because there is a high risk of damaging functional structures.[27,31,83] If no subcortical structures are found, the resection can be continued, because the chance of damaging essential structures is low. These data indicate subcortical stimulation as a reliable tool for guiding surgical resection, and at the same time predicting the likelihood of deficit developing postoperatively. Postoperative deficits in patients in whom no subcortical tracts were identified is usually caused by vascular damage and the development of ischemic areas. MEP monitoring can help in monitoring and preventing the appearance of motor deficits caused by vascular injury,[75] and to further decrease its incidence.

When the authors considered the results of the long-term postoperative neuropsychological evaluation, 79.5% of patients were found to have long-term postoperative normal language, 18.6% showed mild disturbances still compatible with normal daily life, and only 2.3% showed long-term impairment. Similar figures were observed for the resection of gliomas close to motor areas or pathways. These functional results were different from those obtained when subcortical stimulation was not applied. Analysis of patients with high- or low-grade gliomas operated on in the authors' institution before the use of DES showed 23% permanent language or motor deficits, in accordance with other series.[15,27,84]

ONCOLOGICAL RESULTS OF SURGERY

Surgery performed with the aid of brain-mapping techniques allows several oncological end-points to be reached, particularly in low-grade gliomas and helps the pathologist with histologic and molecular diagnosis. In addition, it increases the number of patients submitted for surgery; in accordance with previous reports, this percentage in the authors' series increased from 11% of cases when mapping was not available to 81% when mapping was applied, with a significant decrease in the number of cases that were submitted to biopsy only.[15,27,84] It decreased the percentage of postoperative permanent deficits from 33% to 2.3%, for language or motor functions. Another important effect is the decrease in the incidence of seizures, particularly in patients with low-grade glioma who have a long history of epilepsy and are affected by insular tumors. Seizure control is more likely after gross-total resection than after subtotal resection/biopsy alone. When total or subtotal resection is achieved, in more than 80% of patients a positive impact on seizures is documented, with reduction in the number of automated external defibrillators (AEDs) administered. In addition, suppression of AEDs is possible in 30% of cases.[31] These techniques have an effect on the extent of resection. The use of brain-mapping techniques increased the percentage of patients in which a total and subtotal resection was achieved. This is particularly evident in low-grade gliomas. In the authors' series of low-grade gliomas, the percentage of total and subtotal resections increased from 11% when no mapping was available to 69.8% when brain-mapping techniques were applied. These figures are in accordance with the results of other groups. A large number of class III and II tumors suggests that more extensive resection at initial diagnosis may be a favorable prognostic factor for this type of tumor.[12,14,15,20,22,24–26,85,86] The evaluation of the extent of resection is usually performed on postoperative FLAIR volumetric images, with semiautomatic segmentation software.[87,88] Achieving a complete resection (no abnormalities seen on postoperative FLAIR images) or subtotal resection (a postoperative volume on volumetric postoperative FLAIR images less than 10 mL) is influenced by the preoperative tumor volume and by tumor involvement of eloquent tissue, particularly at the subcortical level.[26] Preoperative tumor volume is a significant predictor of patient survival and progress-free survival per se, and the involvement of subcortical tracts. Extent of resection and pre- and postoperative tumor volume strongly influence progression-free survival and time to malignant transformation. In addition, extent of resection also influences patient survival. The smaller the tumor the better the patient outcome, and delaying surgical intervention may increase the risk of malignant transformation. Efforts should be made to increase the extent of resection.[26]

STRATEGY FOR DIFFUSE TUMORS: THE CONCEPT OF BRAIN PLASTICITY

Gliomas, and particularly low-grade gliomas, may present as variable tumors, ranging from discrete and apparently well-defined lesions to diffuse and less discrete lesions. The therapeutic strategies for the more defined tumors are those described earlier, which can also be applied to high-grade tumors. Large diffuse tumors are a challenge. Most of them are histologically diffuse astrocytomas, and contain functional subcortical tracts. In these tumors, a total or subtotal resection as an initial strategy is difficult. Although partial removal may still be beneficial,[26] particularly in those tumors in which a mass effect is present, most of these patients underwent stereotactic biopsy only, usually guided by spectroscopy MR images followed by adjuvant treatments. A recent strategy to increase the rate of resection in these tumors is upfront preoperative chemotherapy. Temazapam administered upfront up to a period of 6 months in a limited group of patients decreased tumor cell invasion, and reduced tumor cell infiltration along large fiber tracts, which helps achieve a greater percentage of tumor removal.[16] Alternatively, chemotherapy may be used as an adjuvant treatment, after partial removal, and in these patients it may further decrease postoperative tumor volume.[89-92] In addition, in large tumors, a 2-time surgical strategy may be chosen, particularly in large tumors involving language areas or pathways. In these patients, in whom surgery indicates a long collaboration period, the initial surgery is continued until patient collaboration and responsiveness are maintained and is resumed from 1 week to several months later. The authors' institution adopted the policy that 4 to 6 months is needed before submitting the patient to further surgery, to allow the patient to recover from the initial surgery, and to allow brain plasticity.[31]

The phenomenon of brain plasticity helps in planning surgery.[23] Cerebral plasticity could be defined as the continuous processing that allows short-, mid-, and long-term remodeling of neuronosynaptic organization.[23] Plasticity may occur in the preoperative period in low-grade gliomas as a result of progressive functional brain reshaping induced by these slow-growing lesions.[23] The postoperative period is most important in brain plasticity, as has been shown by submitting patients who have recovered from postoperative deficit status to functional neuroimaging studies some months after surgery; a recovery demonstrates the activation of different areas of the brain, close to or remote from those involved in the preoperative period.[93] Plasticity may occur at a cortical level or less frequently at a subcortical level, where it can be explained by the recruitment or unmasking of parallel and redundant subcortical circuits.[94] Compensation is of particular relevance because it extends surgical indications. It extends the initial surgery until functional boundaries are encountered and allows the patient to recover in the postoperative period because of the activation of redundant functional areas, when the essential areas are preserved at the cortical or subcortical level. The functional reshaping induced by the initial surgery can be used to perform further surgery to remove areas of the brain initially essential for function, and which are no longer essential in terms of function because of the functional reshaping induced by the initial surgery or because of the continuous slow growth of the tumor. Functional reshaping can be observed up to 6 months after the initial surgery, and allows more radical further surgery with an increase in oncological benefit to the patient.

SUMMARY

The purpose of brain-mapping techniques is to identify and preserve at the time of surgery the cortical and subcortical sites essential for maintaining function. In the authors' experience, in most low-grade gliomas motor or language disturbances were induced either inside the tumor mass or at the tumor margins, because most of the essential sites, particularly at the subcortical level, were located within the tumor or adjacent to it. In most high-grade gliomas, functional tracts were induced at the tumor border. In both cases, the resection was stopped when language, motor, visuospatial, cortical, or subcortical areas were encountered, resulting in a low percentage of postoperative permanent neurologic deficits. In particular, the preservation of subcortical tracts seemed to be critical for long-term patient integrity.[12,27,29,32,84,95] Postoperative deficits in patients in whom no subcortical tracts were identified was usually caused by vascular damage and development of ischemic areas. MEP monitoring can help prevent motor deficits caused by vascular injury,[17] and may further decrease their incidence.

The systematic use of brain-mapping techniques reduced the incidence of postoperative deficits to less than 3%, which differs from the 23% in the authors' institution when these techniques were not applied. These figures are similar to those reported by other groups.[29,32,96] Brain mapping did not negatively affect ability to perform an extensive resection in a high percentage of patients; on the contrary, the percentage of total and subtotal resections significantly improved in comparison with the time when DES was not applied. The improvement in surgical resections further influences seizure outcome and various oncological end-points, such as progression-free survival, overall survival, and, in low-grade gliomas, malignant transformation.

Nevertheless, brain mapping and monitoring is a demanding technique. In surgery on patients who are awake, close collaboration between neurosurgeon, neuropsychologist, and neurophysiologist is required. The neuropsychologist and neurophysiologist should be present in the operating room and work as a team to assist the surgeon in combining the neurophysiology information with the interpretation of the language disturbances, and to compare these data with the surgical anatomy. In addition, a well-trained anesthesiologist is essential, to titrate the sedation and the analgesics to keep the patient calm and without pain but fully awake and able to perform the tasks reliably. Excessive sedation or anxiety and pain may reduce the compliance of the patient and compromise the results of the tests. In anesthesia in patients who are awake, the patients need to be prepared for the awakening phase and the performance of tasks in the operating room; these events can be particularly stressful, and only patients who are properly instructed and motivated are able to tolerate the operative environment and to focus on the tests. During mapping, a high level of interaction within the operating team is the key to obtaining an accurate evaluation of each task and a precise definition of the functional sites. Extensive training of each team member and familiarity with working together are important to save time and better assist the surgeon. Brain mapping can be particularly time-consuming when the results of mapping are unsatisfactory and additional or repeated testing is required, which may result in extra stress for the patient and a need for rest, with further prolongation of surgical times. Moreover, a tired patient is prone to poorer performance in the tests. If the compliance of the patient is compromised because of excessive duration of the procedure, it is recommended to stop surgery and to plan a second intervention in 2 or 3 months. This surgery can be scheduled in advance, according to the preoperative size and characteristics of the tumor.[97]

Along with the issues described earlier, brain mapping is intrinsically limited because only the functions that are specifically tested are preserved. This limitation is important for simple functions, such as the motor function, and is particularly relevant for complex cognitive functions. As already mentioned, time affects the quality of mapping and means that a limited number of well-selected tests can be administered to the patient; this should be kept in mind when dealing with large tumors located in the dominant hemisphere in areas densely filled with functional sites, such as the temporoparietal junction or the precentral area.[61,98] In such regions careful selection of the tasks and systematic mapping are crucial to save the basic cognitive functions, but it may not be possible to investigate other superior functions, such as calculation, writing, reading, and second languages.[9,18,43,52,64,74,99] The

surgeon should plan preoperatively, according to tumor size and location, which information should be obtained during the mapping procedure, and should inform the patient about the possible limitations of each approach.

Another critical technical issue is the relationship between the intensity of the stimulating current and the distance from the functional site, in particular when subcortical mapping is performed. In the literature there are no available studies of the penetration distance of subcortical bipolar stimulation in white matter, although the range of bipolar stimulation on the cortex has been observed to be approximately 2 to 10 mm.[13,100] In the authors' experience, when a response was induced at a subcortical level, an intensity-response curve was used to assess the maintenance of the response at low current intensity levels. This procedure can help in estimating the distance between the point of stimulation and the functional tract. When the authors reached the functional fibers, the resection was stopped, preserving the functional pathways in most cases. In addition, the authors observed that, towards the end of the resection, a lower current intensity was needed to induce a response. Applying the same current intensity used at the beginning of resection induces more marked responses and carries a higher risk of inducing seizures. Functional structures may regain their normal excitability threshold once the mass effect exerted by the tumor is relieved. Anaesthesiological factors may also play a role (eg, progressive clearance of anesthetic drugs). To maintain the reliability of the mapping and to avoid false-positive findings, which could lead to premature interruption of the resection, it is recommended that the working current is verified and reduced once a large part of the tumor has been removed. Further studies are needed to clarify this point.

SUMMARY

Surgical removal of lesions in eloquent areas requires the combined efforts of a multidisclipinary team of neurosurgeons, neuroradiologists, neuropsychologists, neurophysiologists, and neurooncologists who together define the location, extension, and extent of functional involvement that a specific lesion has induced in a particular patient. Each tumor induces specific changes in the functional network that varies among patients. Each treatment plan should be tailored to the tumor and to the patient. Surgery should be performed according to functional and anatomic boundaries, and should aim for maximal resection with maximal preservation of function in the patient. These goals can be achieved at initial surgery, depending on the functional organization of the brain, or may require additional surgery, combined with adjuvant treatments. Brain-mapping techniques extend surgical indications and improve the extent of resection with greater oncological impact, minimization of morbidity, and increase in quality of life.

REFERENCES

1. Cavaliere R, Lopes MB, Schiff D. Low-grade gliomas: an update on pathology and therapy. Lancet Neurol 2005;4:760–70.

2. Johannesen TB, Langmark F, Lote K. Progress in long-term survival in adult patients with supratentorial low-grade gliomas: a population-based study of 993 patients in whom tumors were diagnosed between 1970 and 1993. J Neurosurg 2003;99: 854–62.

3. Lote K, Egeland T, Hager B, et al. Survival, prognostic factors, and therapeutic efficacy in low-grade glioma: a retrospective study in 379 patients. J Clin Oncol 1997;15:3129–40.

4. Peraud A, Ansari H, Bise K, et al. Clinical outcome of supratentorial astrocytoma WHO grade II. Acta Neurochir (Wien) 1998;140:1213–22.

5. Stupp R, Janzer RC, Hegi ME, et al. Prognostic factors for low-grade gliomas. Semin Oncol 2003; 30:23–8.

6. Kleihues P, Burger PC, Collins P, et al. In: Kleihues P, Cavenee W, editors. Pathology and genetics of tumours of the nervous system. Lyon: International Agency for Research on Cancer Press; 2000. p. 29–39.

7. Kleihues P, Louis DN, Scheithauer BW, et al. The WHO classification of tumors of the nervous system. J Neuropathol Exp Neurol 2002;61:215–29.

8. Leighton C, Fisher B, Bauman G, et al. Supratentorial low-grade glioma in adults: an analysis of prognostic factors and timing of radiation. J Clin Oncol 1997;15:1294–301.

9. Nikas DC, Bello L, Zamani AA, et al. Neurosurgical considerations in supratentorial low-grade gliomas: experience with 175 patients. Neurosurg Focus 1998;4(4):e4.

10. Pignatti F, van den Bent M, Curran D, et al. European Organization for Research and Treatment of Cancer Brain Tumor Cooperative Group. European Organization for Research and Treatment of Cancer Radiotherapy Cooperative Group. Prognostic factors for survival in adult patients with cerebral low-grade glioma. J Clin Oncol 2002;20: 2076–84.

11. Duffau L, Capelle L. Preferential brain locations of low-grade gliomas. Cancer 2004;100:2622–6.

12. Berger MS, Deliganis AV, Dobbins J, et al. The effect of extent of resection on recurrence in patients with low grade cerebral hemisphere gliomas. Cancer 1994;74:1784–91.

13. Berger MS. Functional mapping-guided resection of low-grade gliomas. Clin Neurosurg 1995;42: 437–52.

14. Berger MS, Rostomily RC. Low grade gliomas: functional mapping resection strategies, extent of resection and outcome. J Neurooncol 1997;34: 85–101.

15. Duffau H, Lopes M, Arthuis F, et al. Contribution of intraoperative electrical stimulations in surgery of low grade gliomas: a comparative study between two series without (1985–96) and with (1996–2003) functional mapping in the same institution. J Neurol Neurosurg Psychiatr 2005;76:845–51.

16. Duffau H, Taillandier L, Capelle L. Radical surgery after chemotherapy: a new therapeutic strategy to envision in grade II glioma. J Neurooncol 2006; 80(2):171–6.

17. Laws ER, Shaffrey ME, Morris A, et al. Surgical management of intracranial gliomas–does radical resection improve outcome? Acta Neurochir Suppl 2003;85:47–53.

18. Nakamura M, Konishi N, Tsunoda S, et al. Analysis of prognostic and survival factors related to treatment of low-grade astrocytomas in adults. Oncology 2000;58:108–16.

19. Papagikos MA, Shaw EG, Stiebert VW. Lessons learned from randomised clinical trials in adult low grade glioma. Lancet Oncol 2005;6:240–4.

20. Rostomily RC, Keles GE, Berger MS. Radical surgery in the management of low-grade and high-grade gliomas. Baillieres Clin Neurol 1996;5:345–69.

21. van Veelen ML, Avezaat CJ, Kros JM, et al. Supratentorial low grade astrocytoma: prognostic factors, dedifferentiation, and the issue of early versus late surgery. J Neurol Neurosurg Psychiatr 1998;64:581–7.

22. Claus EB, Horlacher A, Hsu L, et al. Survival rates in patients with low-grade glioma after intraoperative magnetic resonance image guidance. Cancer 2005;103:1227–33.

23. Duffau H. New concepts in surgery of WHO grade II gliomas: functional brain mapping, connectionism and plasticity–a review. J Neurooncol 2006; 79(1):77–115.

24. Keles GE, Lamborn KR, Berger MS. Lowgrade hemispheric gliomas in adults: a critical review of extent of resection as a factor influencing outcome. J Neurosurg 2001;95:735–45.

25. Sanai N, Berger MS. Glioma extent of resection and its impact on patient outcome. Neurosurgery 2008; 62(4):753–64 [discussion: 264–6].

26. Smith JS, Chang EF, Lamborn KR, et al. Role of extent of resection in the long-term outcome of low-grade hemispheric gliomas. J Clin Oncol 2008;26(8):1338–45.

27. Bello L, Gallucci M, Fava M, et al. Intraoperative subcortical language tract mapping guides surgical removal of gliomas involving speech areas. Neurosurgery 2007;60(1):67–80 [discussion: 80–2].

28. Black PM, Ronner SF. Cortical mapping for defining the limits of tumor resection. Neurosurgery 1987; 25:786–92.

29. Duffau H, Capelle L, Sichez N, et al. Intraoperative mapping of the subcortical language pathways using direct stimulations. An anatomo-functional study. Brain 2002;125:199–214.

30. Duffau H. Lessons from brain mapping in surgery for low-grade glioma: insights into associations between tumour and brain plasticity. Lancet Neurol 2005;4:476–86.

31. Duffau H, Gatignol P, Mandonnet E, et al. New insights into the anatomo-functional connectivity of the semantic system: a study using cortico-subcortical electrostimulations. Brain 2005;128: 797–810.

32. Ojemann J, Ojemann G, Lettich E, et al. Cortical language localization in left, dominant hemisphere. An electrical stimulation mapping investigation in 117 patients. J Neurosurg 1989;71: 316–26.

33. Duffau H, Denvil D, Lopes M, et al. Intraoperative mapping of the cortical areas involved in multiplication and subtraction: an electrostimulation study in a patient with a left parietal glioma. J Neurol Neurosurg Psychiatr 2002;73:733–8.

34. Gasparini FM, Cohen L, Lopes M, et al. A clinical study of the number processing system: decimal size effects on reading numbers in patients with left parieto-occipital gliomas. Rev Neurol (Paris) 2005;161:427–35.

35. Roux FE, Boetto S, Sacko O, et al. Writing, calculating, and finger recognition in the region of the angular gyrus: a cortical stimulation study of Gerstmann syndrome. J Neurosurg 2003;99:716–27.

36. Bello L, Acerbi F, Giussani C, et al. Intraoperative language localization in multilingual patients with gliomas. Neurosurgery 2006;59(1):115–25.

37. Giussani C, Roux FE, Lubrano V, et al. Review of language organisation in bilingual patients: what can we learn from direct brain mapping? Acta Neurochir (Wien) 2007;149(11):1109–16 [discussion: 1116].

38. Lucas TH, McKhann GM, Ojemann GA. Functional separation of languages in the bilingual brain: a comparison of electrical stimulation language mapping in 25 bilingual patients and 117 monolingual control patients. J Neurosurg 2004;101: 449–57.

39. Roux FE, Tremoulet M. Organization of language areas in bilingual patients: a cortical stimulation study. J Neurosurg 2002;97:857–64.

40. Galanaud D, Chinot O, Nicoli F, et al. Use of proton magnetic resonance spectroscopy of the brain to differentiate gliomatosis cerebri from low-grade glioma. J Neurosurg 2003;98:269–76.

41. Guillevin R, Menuel C, Duffau H, et al. Proton magnetic resonance spectroscopy predicts proliferative activity in diffuse low-grade gliomas. J Neurooncol 2008;87(2):181–7.

42. Benard F, Romsa J, Hustinx R. Imaging gliomas with positron emission tomography and single-photon emission computed tomography. Semin Nucl Med 2003;33:148–62.

43. De Witte O, Levivier M, Violon P, et al. Prognostic value positron emission tomography with [^{18}F]fluoro-2-deoxy-D-glucose in the low-grade glioma. Neurosurgery 1996;39:470–6.

44. Kuznetsov YE, Caramanos Z, Antel SB, et al. Proton magnetic resonance spectroscopic imaging can predict length of survival in patients with supratentorial gliomas. Neurosurgery 2003;53:565–76.

45. Meyer PT, Sturz L, Schreckenberger M, et al. Preoperative mapping of cortical language areas in adult brain tumor patients using PET and individual non-normalised SPM analyses. Eur J Nucl Med Mol Imaging 2003;30:951–60.

46. Minn H. PET and SPECT in low-grade glioma. Eur J Radiol 2005;56:171–8.

47. Cha S, Tihan T, Crawford F, et al. Differentiation of low-grade oligodendrogliomas from low-grade astrocytomas by using quantitative blood-volume measurements derived from dynamic susceptibility contrast-enhanced MR imaging. AJNR Am J Neuroradiol 2005;26(2):266–73.

48. Bogomolny DL, Petrovich NM, Hou BL, et al. Functional MRI in the brain tumor patient. Top Magn Reson Imaging 2004;15:325–35.

49. Holodny AI, Schulder M, Liu WC, et al. The effect of brain tumors on BOLD functional MR Imaging activation in the adjacent motor cortex: implications for image-guided neurosurgery. AJNR Am J Neuroradiol 2000;21:1415–22.

50. Roux FE, Boulanouar K, Lotterie JA, et al. Language functional magnetic resonance imaging in preoperative assessment of language areas: correlation with direct cortical stimulation. Neurosurgery 2003;52:1335–45.

51. Rutten GJ, Ramsey NF, van Rijen PC, et al. Development of a functional magnetic resonance imaging protocol for intraoperative localization of critical temporoparietal language areas. Ann Neurol 2002;51:350–60.

52. Basser PJ, Pajevic S, Pierpaoli C, et al. In vivo fiber tractography using DT-MRI data. J Magn Reson Imaging 2000;44(4):625–32.

53. Catani M, Howard RJ, Pajevic S, et al. Virtual in vivo interactive dissection of white matter fasciculi in the human brain. NeuroImage 2002;17:77–94.

54. Bello L, Gambini A, Castellano A, et al. Motor and language DTI Fiber Tracking combined with intraoperative subcortical mapping for surgical removal of gliomas. Neuroimage 2008;39(1):369–82.

55. Berman JI, Berger MS, Mukherjee P, et al. Diffusion-tensor imaging-guided tracking of fibers of the pyramidal tract combined with intraoperative cortical stimulation mapping in patients with gliomas. J Neurosurg 2004;101(1):66–72.

56. Clark CA, Barrick TR, Murphy MM, et al. White matter fiber tracking in patients with space-occupying lesions of the brain: a new technique for neurosurgical planning? NeuroImage 2003; 20(3):1601–8.

57. Gossl C, Fahrmeir L, Putz B, et al. Fiber tracking from DTI using linear state space models: detectability of the pyramidal tract. Neuroimage 2002; 16:378–88.

58. Jbabdi S, Mandonnet E, Duffau H, et al. Diffusion tensor imaging allows anisotropic growth simulations of low grade gliomas. Magn Reson Med 2005;54:616–24.

59. Danks RA, Rogers M, Aglio LS, et al. Patient tolerance of craniotomy performed with the patient under local anesthesia and monitored conscious sedation. Neurosurgery 1998;42:28–36.

60. Danks RA, Aglio LS, Gugino LD, et al. Craniotomy under local anesthesia and monitored conscious sedation for the resection of tumors involving eloquent cortex. J Neurooncol 2000;49:131–9.

61. Ebel H, Ebel M, Schillinger G, et al. Surgery of intrinsic cerebral neoplasms in eloquent areas under local anesthesia. Minim Invasive Neurosurg 2000;43:192–6.

62. Sarang A, Dinsmore J. Anesthesia for awake craniotomy – evolution of a technique that facilitates awake neurological testing. Br J Anaesth 2003;90:161–5.

63. Fukaya C, Katayama Y, Yoshino A, et al. Intraoperative wake-up procedure with propofol and laryngeal mask for optimal excision of brain tumor in eloquent areas. J Clin Neurosci 2001;8:253–5.

64. Ebeling U, Schmid UD, Ying H, et al. Safe surgery of lesions near the motor cortex using intraoperative mapping techniques: a report on 50 patients. Acta Neurochir (Wien) 1992;119:23–8.

65. Manninen PH, Tan TK. Postoperative nausea and vomiting after craniotomy for tumor surgery: a comparison between awake craniotomy and general anesthesia. J Clin Anesth 2002;14:279–83.

66. Berger MS, Ojemann GA, Lettich E. Neurophysiological monitoring during astrocytoma surgery. Neurosurg Clin N Am 1990;1:65–70.

67. Branco DM, Coelho TM, Branco BM, et al. Functional variability of the human cortical motor map: electrical stimulation findings in perirolandic epilepsy surgery. J Clin Neurophysiol 2003;20: 17–25.

68. Carrabba G, Fava E, Giussani C, et al. Cortical and subcortical motor mapping in rolandic and perirolandic glioma surgery: impact on postoperative morbidity and extent of resection. J Neurosurg Sci 2007;51(2):45–51.

69. Cedzich C, Taniguchi M, Schaffer S, et al. Somatosensory evoked potential phase reversal and direct motor cortex stimulation during surgery in and around the central region. Technical application. Neurosurgery 1996;38:962–71.

70. Reijneveld JC, Sitskoorn MM, Klein M, et al. Cognitive status and quality of life in patients with suspected versus proven low-grade gliomas. Neurology 2001;56:618–23.

71. Romstock J, Fahlbusch R, Ganslandt O, et al. Localisation of the sensorimotor cortex during surgery for brain tumours: feasibility and waveform patterns of somatosensory evoked potentials. J Neurol Neurosurg Psychiatr 2002;72:221–9.

72. Yingling CD, Ojemann S, Dodson B, et al. Identification of motor pathways during tumor surgery facilitated by multichannel electromyographic recording. J Neurosurg 1999;91:922–7.

73. Szelényi A, Kothbauer KF, Deletis V. Transcranial electric stimulation for intraoperative motor evoked potential monitoring: stimulation parameters and electrode montages. Clin Neurophysiol 2007; 118(7):1586–95 [Epub 2007 May 15].

74. Neuloh G, Schramm J. Motor evoked potential monitoring for the surgery of brain tumours and vascular malformations. Adv Tech Stand Neurosurg 2004;29:171–228.

75. Carrabba G, Fava E, Mandonnet E, et al. Transient inhibition of motor function induced by Cavitron ultrasonic surgical aspirator during brain mapping. Neurosurgery 2008;63(1):E178–9 [discussion: E179].

76. Sanai N, Mirzadeh Z, Berger MS. Functional outcome after language mapping for glioma resection. N Engl J Med 2008;358(1):18–27.

77. Kamada K, Todo T, Masutani Y, et al. Combined use of tractography-integrated functional neuronavigation and direct fiber stimulation. J Neurosurg 2005;102(4):664–72.

78. Keles GE, Lamborn KR, Berger MS. Coregistration accuracy and detection of brain shift using intraoperative sononavigation during resection of hemispheric tumors. Neurosurgery 2003;53: 556–64.

79. Nimsky C, Ganslandt O, Fahlbusch R. Implementation of fiber tract navigation. Neurosurgery 2006; 58(4 Suppl 2):ONS292–303 [discussion: ONS303–4].

80. Reinges MH, Nguyen HH, Krings T, et al. Course of brain shift during microsurgical resection of supratentorial cerebral lesions: limits of conventional neuronavigation. Acta Neurochir (Wien) 2004;146: 369–77.

81. Lehericy S, Duffau H, Cornu P, et al. Correspondence between functional magnetic resonance imaging somatotopy and individual brain anatomy of the central region: comparison with intraoperative stimulation in patients with brain tumors. J Neurosurg 2000;92:589–98.

82. Petrovich N, Holodny AI, Tabar V, et al. Discordance between functional magnetic resonance imaging during silent speech tasks and intraoperative speech arrest. J Neurosurg 2005;103:267–74.

83. Keles GE, Lundin DA, Lamborn KR, et al. Intraoperative subcortical stimulation mapping for hemispherical perirolandic gliomas located within or adjacent to the descending motor pathways: evaluation of morbidity and assessment of functional outcome in 294 patients. J Neurosurg 2004;100: 369–75.

84. Duffau H, Capelle L, Sichez J, et al. Intraoperative direct electrical stimulations of the central nervous system: the Salpêtrière experience with 60 patients. Acta Neurochir (Wien) 1999;141:1157–67.

85. Capelle L, Duffau H, Lopes M, et al. WHO grade 2 gliomas in adults: a study of prognostic factors with special emphasis on the role of surgery. J Neurooncol 2002;4:S17–69.

86. Mariani L, Siegenthaler P, Guzman R, et al. The impact of tumour volume and surgery on the outcome of adults with supratentorial WHO grade II astrocytomas and oligoastrocytomas. Acta Neurochir (Wien) 2004;146:441–8.

87. Keles GE, Chang EF, Lamborn KR, et al. Volumetric extent of resection and residual contrast enhancement on initial surgery as predictors of outcome in adult patients with hemispheric anaplastic astrocytoma. J Neurosurg 2006;105(1):34–40.

88. Mandonnet E, Jbabdi S, Taillandier L, et al. Preoperative estimation of residual volume for WHO grade II glioma resected with intraoperative functional mapping. Neuro Oncol 2007;9(1):63–9.

89. Hoang-Xuan K, Capelle L, Kujas M, et al. Temozolomide as initial treatment for adults with low-grade oligodendrogliomas or oligoastrocytomas and correlation with chromosome 1p deletions. J Clin Oncol 2004;22:3133–8.

90. Kaloshi G, Benouaich-Amiel A, Diakite F, et al. Temozolomide for low-grade gliomas: predictive impact of 1p/19q loss on response and outcome. Neurology 2007;68(21):1831–6.

91. Quinn JA, Reardon DA, Friedman AH, et al. Phase II trial of temozolomide in patients with progressive low-grade glioma. J Clin Oncol 2003;21:646–51.

92. Ricard D, Kaloshi G, Amiel-Benouaich A, et al. Dynamic history of low-grade gliomas before and after temozolomide treatment. Ann Neurol 2007; 61(5):484–90.

93. Krainik A, Duffau H, Capelle L, et al. Role of the healthy hemisphere in recovery after resection of the supplementary motor area. Neurology 2004; 62:1323–32.

94. Duffau H, Khalil I, Gatignol P, et al. Surgical removal of corpus callosum infiltrated by low-grade glioma: functional outcome and oncological considerations. J Neurosurg 2004;100:431–7.

95. Duffau H, Capelle L, Denvil D, et al. Functional recovery after surgical resection of low grade gliomas in eloquent brain: hypothesis of brain compensation. J Neurol Neurosurg Psychiatr 2003;74:901–7.

96. Desmurget M, Bonnetblanc F, Duffau H. Contrasting acute and slow-growing lesions: a new door to brain plasticity. Brain 2007;130(Pt 4):898–914.

97. Pace A, Vidiri A, Galie E, et al. Temozolomide chemotherapy for progressive low-grade glioma: clinical benefits and radiological response. Ann Oncol 2003;14:1722–6.

98. Nimsky C, Ganslandt O, Hastreiter P, et al. Intraoperative diffusion-tensor MR imaging: shifting of white matter tracts during neurosurgical procedures–initial experience. Radiology 2005;234(1): 218–25.

99. Klein M, Heimans JJ. The measurement of cognitive functioning in low-grade glioma patients after radiotherapy. J Clin Oncol 2004; 22:966–7.

100. Goldstein B, Obrzut JE, John C, et al. The impact of frontal and non-frontal brain tumor lesions on Wisconsin card sorting test performance. Brain Cogn 2004;54:110–6.

Quantitative Sodium MR Imaging and Sodium Bioscales for the Management of Brain Tumors

Keith R. Thulborn, MD, PhD*, Aiming Lu, PhD,
Ian C. Atkinson, PhD, Fred Damen, MS,
John L. Villano, MD, PhD

KEYWORDS

- Brain tumor • Sodium MR imaging • Tissue viability
- Bioscales • Treatment protocols
- Imaging treatment response

The standard of care for the comprehensive treatment of high-grade primary brain tumors includes surgery, radiation treatment, and chemotherapy. MR imaging is involved in the initial diagnosis for detection and characterization of the lesion, focusing on size, location, and its effect on surrounding brain, and then on the heterogeneity of the signal characteristics, the presence of hemorrhage, magnetic resonance (MR) perfusion characteristics, and integrity of the blood-brain barrier. These imaging properties have been correlated with tumor grade that has prognostic significance. Functional MR imaging can be used for presurgical planning and for image guidance of the surgical procedures (biopsy, resection) to minimize disruption of eloquent cortex. The surgical debulking is not considered curative for high-grade tumors but a preliminary step toward improving response to the subsequent treatments. After a short recovery period to allow some degree of healing of the surgical site, radiation treatment planning begins. The radiation planning uses the radiography attenuation coefficients from CT scans to design the distribution of the radiation used in the treatment plan. Advantage is taken of the better display of tumors on MR imaging by fusing the MR and CT scan images. The course of radiation involves fractionated targeted radiation projected along multiple beams at many angles to achieve high dose over the tumor volume and margins while minimizing the dose to surrounding normal brain. The radiation is fractionated, usually administered for 5 days per week over about 6 weeks to a total dose of about 55 Gy. Imaging is not routinely performed during radiation treatment. Symptoms of brain swelling are controlled by use of oral steroids. Chemotherapy at low dose may be delivered during radiation treatment. Full-dose, single-agent chemotherapy follows the completion of radiation and is administered over multiple cycles to maintain tumor control. Follow-up MR imaging studies begin after radiation treatment is completed and are then performed every few months or more frequently depending on the clinical status of the patient. Although this protocol has been developed based on experience from large numbers of patients in multicenter trials, the prognosis has not changed in 3 decades (20% survival at 2 years).[1] This extremely poor success rate for a significant

The authors acknowledge funding support from PHS RO1 CA1295531A1 and PHS RO1 CA63661.
Center for Magnetic Resonance Research, University of Illinois at Chicago, Room 1307, OCC, MC707, 1801 West Taylor Street, Chicago, IL 60612, USA
* Corresponding author.
E-mail address: kthulbor@uic.edu (K.R. Thulborn).

Neuroimag Clin N Am 19 (2009) 615–624
doi:10.1016/j.nic.2009.09.001
1052-5149/09/$ – see front matter © 2009 Published by Elsevier Inc.

neoplasm, despite this, comprehensive protocol after decades of experience, suggests that there is a fundamental oversight in the current treatment of this disease. This article provides an imaging perspective of how regional responses of primary brain tumors may be examined during treatment to guide a flexible treatment plan to the response of each patient's tumor, rather than using a fixed rigid protocol based on population studies. Sodium imaging provides a direct measurement of cell density that can be used to measure regional cell kill during treatment. These bioscales of regionally and temporally sensitive biologic-based parameters may be helpful to measure tumor responsiveness that the oncologists can use to guide treatment for each patient. The suggestions are speculative and still being examined experimentally but are presented to challenge the medical community to be receptive to changes in the standard of care when that standard continues to fail.

The conventional imaging workup for a brain tumor is a proton MR imaging examination with and without gadolinium contrast enhancement. The standard T1- and T2-weighted images define the location and dimensions of the mass. Diffusion-weighted imaging defines the extent of vasogenic edema while excluding cytotoxic edema. Perfusion imaging defines the regions of tumor with high vascularity on the relative cerebral blood volume map consistent with high-grade tumor (Fig. 1). The role of perfusion imaging in tumor grading is discussed in another article elsewhere in this issue.

These anatomic characteristics are important in defining the proximity of eloquent cortex that should be mapped with functional MR (fMR) imaging before biopsy and surgical resection. The fMR imaging study is best done with fiducial markers in place over the head so that accurate anatomic registration of the patient's head with the images can be achieved on the neurosurgical workstation to guide the location and size of the craniotomy (Fig. 2). The functional maps are best registered over the contrast-enhanced images to aid in distinguishing tumor margins from eloquent cortex. Functional mapping for presurgical planning is also discussed in more detail in another article elsewhere in this issue.

Once surgical resection is accomplished, a few weeks are allowed for healing and anatomic stabilization before beginning radiation planning. The radiation treatment uses a CT scan for establishing radiation attenuation coefficients but requires a new MR imaging study to be merged with the CT scan to delineate the margins of the surgical bed and residual tumor and regions of normal brain. Radiation exposure to normal brain should be minimized while dose to the tumor bed should be maximized (Fig. 3). The functional maps could also be used in this setting, but this is rarely done.

Once radiation treatment commences, a CT scan is used to ensure that the alignment of the radiation distribution is accurately maintained. MR imaging is rarely done during radiation treatment unless there is a dramatic clinical change that requires specific evaluation. After radiation treatment is completed, there is a baseline MR imaging study to which all subsequent imaging is referred. The full-dose chemotherapy begins after radiation is completed and is used across multiple cycles. All follow-up MR examinations should include perfusion imaging (as discussed elsewhere in this issue), but this is still not done universally. The issue of pseudoprogression (Fig. 4, consequence of combined radiation and chemotherapy) with worsening gadolinium contrast enhancement but reduced cerebral blood volume in the few weeks to months after radiation with subsequent resolution is also discussed elsewhere in this issue.[2]

Given the comprehensive nature of this combined treatment protocol extending over months to years, why has the prognosis for brain tumors not improved? This poor outcome surely reflects the failure to gain control over the tumor in the initial stages of treatment. Cancer stem cells or residual malignant cells with longer cell cycle times that make them less vulnerable to even fractionated therapy may initiate recurrence. Radiation damages DNA, but radiation sensitivity decreases as the oxygen concentration in the tissue decreases.[3] Thus, poorly vascularized tissue is less sensitive to radiation damage than normal tissues. Necrotic areas of tumors are, by definition, poorly vascularized and may contain cells that are less sensitive to treatment. Surgical debulking attempts to remove these regions. The radiation sensitivity is greatest at the mitotic phase of the cell cycle.[3] In other phases of the cell cycle the radiation damage is repaired before the cell is required to undergo mitosis. Such cells proliferate to produce the tumor recurrence observed later by imaging. Multiple mechanisms of different radiobiological sensitivities, heterogeneity of cell types, and variable microenvironments presumably underlie current treatment failure.

For a more successful treatment protocol to be found, it would seem reasonable that the variability of each tumor for each patient must be considered. This customization of treatment to the heterogeneity of response promotes the need for rapid feedback about the tumor response across the spatial distribution of the tumor and a need

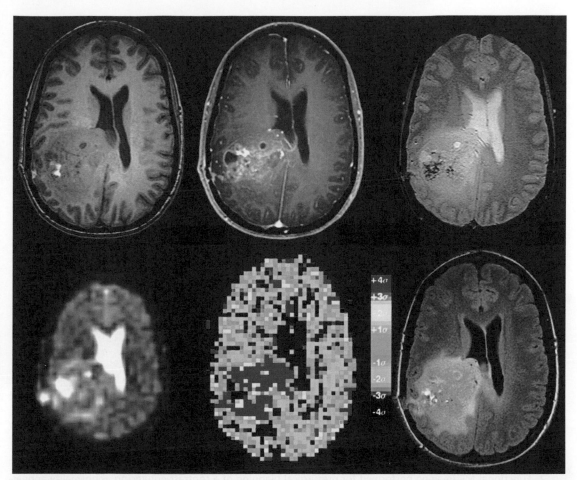

Fig. 1. Representative MR images from the 3.0 Tesla clinical examination of a patient with a large right hemispheric high-grade glioneuroma before treatment. Images are from the following acquisition sequences. *Top left:* non-contrast-enhanced T1-weighted 3-dimensional (D) inversion recovery gradient echo. *Top middle:* contrast-enhanced T1-weighted 3D inversion recovery gradient echo. *Top right:* magnetic susceptibility-sensitive 2D gradient echo. *Bottom left:* 3D quantitative 3D sodium image at a nominal resolution of 5 x 5 × 5 mm³ acquired in under 10 minutes. *Bottom middle:* relative cerebral blood volume map from a dynamic susceptibility contrast MR perfusion study. *Bottom right:* 2D T2-weighted FLAIR propeller. The interpretation is a large, heterogeneous mass with cystic and hemorrhagic components and markedly increased (*red*) relative cerebral blood volume centered in the right parietotemporal region. The lesion has been biopsied. Surgical resection was not considered as an option.

to treat the tumor of each patient individually and flexibly. The current use of a standard rigid protocol for each patient is to deny the nature of the tumor biology. The current approach of a standard protocol for a particular tumor grade and cell type is a product of multicenter trials taking many years and patients to attempt to reach statistical significance for finding small differences in the average survival of patients. Such protocols are exceedingly difficult and expensive to establish and, at the end, only provide average effects across a still very heterogeneous patient group.[4,5] The impact of this epidemiologic approach to finding the appropriate treatment is, as can be expected for a heterogeneous disease,

disappointing.[1] In contrast, adaptive treatment in which the radiation distribution is sculptured to the ongoing tumor responses has much to be recommended in that responsive areas are not over treated and unresponsive areas are provided with additional treatment. Boosted radiation doses could be directed objectively rather than prescribed subjectively by the radiation oncologist.

What means are available to achieve such response monitoring? Clearly, a change in tumor size and texture are usually late events on MR imaging and unsatisfactory for this goal. The desired parameter should be a measure of tissue viability, which may be reflected in metabolic

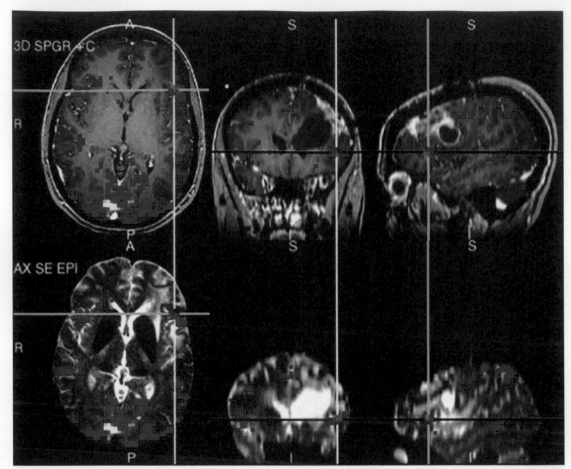

Fig. 2. Functional MR imaging performed for presurgical planning of a contrast-enhancing abnormality appearing in the surgical bed years after treatment for a brain tumor in the left frontal lobe. The activation map from the fMR imaging using the reading language comprehension paradigm is presented superimposed over the contrast-enhanced 3D T1-weighted inversion recovery gradient echo images (3D SPGR +C, *top row*) and over the T2-weighted spin-echo, echo-planar images (AX SE EPI, *bottom row*) in the axial (*left column*), coronal (*middle column*) and sagittal (*right column*) planes. The planes are cross-referenced with colored lines (*blue*, axial; *green*, coronal; *yellow*, sagittal). The Broca area is cross-referenced (intersection of planes) and is anterior and inferior to the lesion, but in close proximity to it so that the surgeon was aware of the potential of producing an aphasia. This location of function was confirmed by intraoperative cortical mapping. The lesion was primarily radiation necrosis as predicted by the low relative cerebral blood volume.

parameters. Glucose use such as reflected in 18-fluoro-deoxy-glucose positron emission tomography may be suggested but this requires that the tumor have a different metabolic rate from surrounding brain tissue. As brain uses glucose as its primary substrate, discrimination may not be achieved.[6] Another metabolic parameter is tissue sodium concentration (TSC) that reflects sodium ion homeostasis. If a cell looses its ability to maintain a sodium ion gradient across its cell membrane, it ceases to be viable. Thus, TSC can be used as an operational definition of tissue viability. The TSC is the volume-fraction–weighted mean of the intracellular sodium concentration (ICC~10–12 mM) and the extracellular sodium

concentration (ECC~145–150 mM).[7] The interstitial volume of the brain is small at about 0.2, leaving a cell volume fraction (CVF) of 0.8.[8]

$$TSC = ICC.CVF + (1-CVF).ECC \qquad (1)$$

After correction for the fractional average water content of normal brain as 0.8, the simple Equation (1) gives the TSC as about 45 mM. This value is measured experimentally in normal human brain tissue.[9–12] This expression can be rearranged in the form of CVF, that is, cell density as:

$$CVF = (TSC - ECC)/(ICC - ECC) \qquad (2)$$

These parameters of TSC and CVF are termed bioscales in that they are quantitative parameters

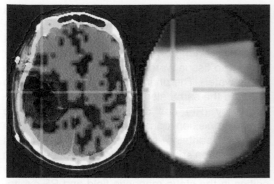 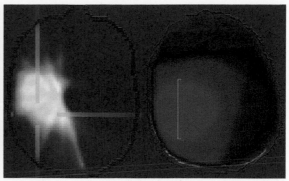

Fig. 3. The radiation treatment planning fuses the CT scans and MR imaging studies (*left*), especially the perfusion study for high-grade tumors, to generate a radiation distribution (*middle*) that covers the tumor while minimizing the dose to normal brain. The contour of the head is drawn as the *blue* outline. The base dose (*middle left*) is supplemented by an additional boost to the tumor (*middle right*). The radiation plan (*red*) can then be superimposed over the contrast-enhanced MR image. The large enhancing tumor in the right temporal lobe is well covered but there is still considerable exposure to the rest of the brain despite targeted treatment.

with a spatial distribution that can be displayed as a map of the underlying anatomy. The term bioscale emphasizes the quantitative nature of these parameters as compared with the term biomarker, which is often only a binary indicator of disease being present or not and has no connotation of spatial distribution. When cells fail to maintain ion homeostasis as is reflected in the TSC bioscale,

the intracellular compartment is breached and becomes continuous with the extracellular compartment. This interstitial compartment is maintained at high sodium concentration by the entire systemic homeostatic mechanisms of ion balance through tissue perfusion and diffusion. The increasing TSC bioscale indicates loss of tissue viability and the CVF bioscale reflects the

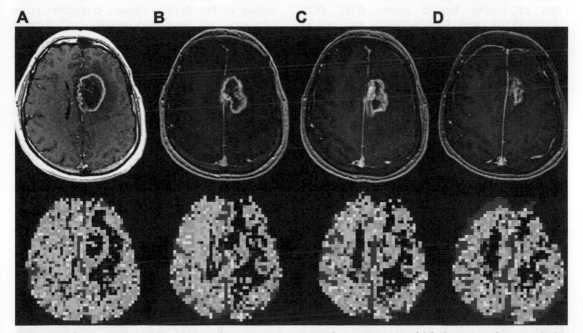

Fig. 4. Pseudoprogression is demonstrated in a patient across early treatment in which the tumor shows variation in enhancement (*top row*) and the relative cerebral blood volume (rCBV) map (*bottom row*). (*A*) Prior to surgery and radiation treatment, there is a thin rim of enhancement and increased rCBV. (*B*) After resection, radiation, and low-dose chemotherapy, there is increasingly thickened enhancement that subsequently resolves while the rCBV shows continuous monotonically decreasing rCBV. (*B, C, D*) Follow-up studies were done every 2 to 3 months after radiation treatment was completed.

concomitant decrease in cell density. These trends in the bioscales have been used to document loss of tissue viability in the clinical settings of stroke and brain tumors.[9–14]

The sodium nucleus has an MR signal that can be imaged, albeit challenging because of the low concentration of tissue sodium (~45 mM) compared with protons in tissue water (80 M) used by conventional clinical MR imaging of the brain. Another challenge for sodium MR imaging is the lower intrinsic sensitivity (gyromagneto ratio of the sodium nucleus is about one quarter of that of the proton nucleus) of the sodium nucleus. Additionally, the rapid nuclear relaxation properties of sodium (biexponential T2 with a fast T2 component of less than 3 ms and a long T2 component of less than 15 ms compared with the monoexponential T2 of brain water protons of about 80 ms) owing to its quadrupolar nuclear spin of 3/2 require different imaging strategies from protons. These were formidable technical challenges when sodium MR imaging was first proposed for clinical applications in the mid 1980s,[15] but these challenges have been surmounted over the last two decades and clinical applications have been demonstrated.[16,17] Although the role of sodium MR imaging in treatment response assessment of brain tumors remains under investigation through National Institutes of Health funded grants (PHS RO1 CA1295531A1 and RO1CA63661), this article summarizes current preliminary findings to prepare clinicians for future options that may improve their care of patients who currently confront the grim prognosis of high-grade brain tumors.

An example of the sodium images, with corresponding TSC and CVF bioscale maps and the calibration phantom at 3.0 Tesla is shown in Fig. 5 for a normal human subject.

The TSC bioscale is derived from the sodium image by using the sodium MR imaging of a calibration phantom under equivalent conditions as the patient to convert arbitrary MR signal intensities into voxel concentrations (mmoles/L wet tissue) or after correction for the tissue water content to tissue water concentrations (mmoles/L tissue water). The phantom has been designed to produce the same electrical loading on the radiofrequency (RF) coil and is imaged under the same acquisition conditions as the patient. The phantom contains samples of known sodium concentration spanning the biologic concentration range. Appropriate corrections for the inhomogeneities in the static magnetic field and RF excitation field are made to the images of both the patient and the phantom. As expected, the calibration curve is linear (Fig. 6). The method at 3.0 Tesla has an error across repeated independent measurements of less than 3% for young normal adults. The value of TSC~45 mM gives a CVF of ~80% leaving an interstitial compartment of 0.2, which matches well with known value for normal brain.[18]

The feasibility of routine sodium imaging in conjunction with the conventional proton MR imaging at 3.0 Tesla was illustrated in Fig. 1 for a patient with a brain tumor. The full display of the sodium imaging and its TSC bioscale for this same patient are displayed in Fig. 7 to illustrate human imaging at 9.4 Tesla.[19] The technical details of the flexible twisted projection pulse sequence are described elsewhere.[16] Sodium imaging at 3.0 and 9.4 Tesla are similar but with improved spatial resolution possible at the increased sensitivity of higher field at 9.4 Tesla. The nominal resolution of $5 \times 5 \times 5$ mm^3 is achieved in less than 9 minutes at 3.0 Tesla, whereas a resolution of $3 \times 3 \times 3$ mm^3 can be obtained in the same time at 9.4 Tesla. However, it is important to emphasize that the sodium imaging technology is available commercially on current 3.0 Tesla clinical scanners with multi-nuclear capabilities. This 3.0 Tesla resolution is probably

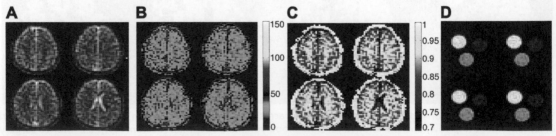

Fig. 5. Sodium imaging and its derived metabolic bioscales in a normal subject. (A) Four partitions from a 3D sodium imaging dataset. (B) TSC map derived from (A). (C) CVF map derived by applying Equation (2) to the TSC map. (D) Calibration phantom image used to calibrate the sodium signal intensity into a TSC value. These measurements were performed at 3.0 Tesla at a resolution of $5 \times 5 \times 5$ mm^3 in less than 10 minutes.

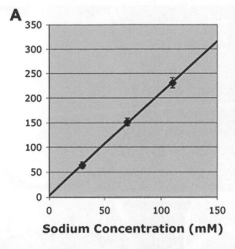

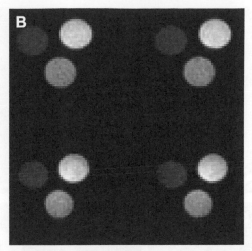

Fig. 6. (A) Linear calibration curve for the conversion of the intensity (arbitrary scale) from the sodium MR signal to a tissue sodium concentration (mM). The phantom has the same electrical loading on the RF coil as the human head and is corrected for static magnetic field and RF excitation field inhomogeneities. Similar calibration curves are obtained at 3.0 and 9.4 Tesla. (B) Four partitions of an image through the phantom showing the three calibration tubes with different concentrations (30, 70, 110 mM).

adequate for sampling the spatial distribution of responses of tumors to treatment.

The application of TSC mapping during radiation is shown for another patient with a right temporal glioblastoma multiforme (GBM) in **Fig. 8**. The clinical imaging indicated that residual tumor was present after surgery.

The standard radiation treatment plan used was about 55 Gy to the tumor as shown in **Fig. 3**. Quantitative sodium imaging was performed before and weekly during the radiation treatment as shown in **Fig. 9**. The images were aligned to the preradiation

images in postprocessing at subvoxel accuracy so that the time courses of TSC could be examined in each voxel across the brain. The realignment was performed in k-space rather than the image domain to avoid blurring of the images. Representative time courses shown in **Fig. 10** illustrate TSC responses.

Although these investigations are preliminary, several points are already evident. The TSC bioscale is responsive to radiation effects on a weekly time scale. The responsive regions (pattern C), showing increases in TSC as the cell density

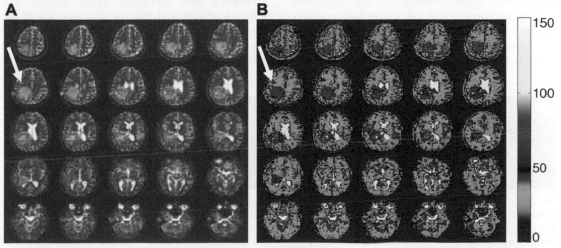

Fig. 7. (A) Sodium images showing the high sodium concentration in the large tumor (arrow) in the right hemisphere of the same patient as in **Fig. 1**. (B) The color bioscale shows TSC from 0 to 150 mM with normal brain shown as green (cell density = 0.8) and the tumor as pink indicating a lower cell density (cell density ~0.4–0.6). These images were acquired at 9.4 Tesla at a nominal resolution of $3 \times 3 \times 3$ mm^3 in less than 10 minutes.

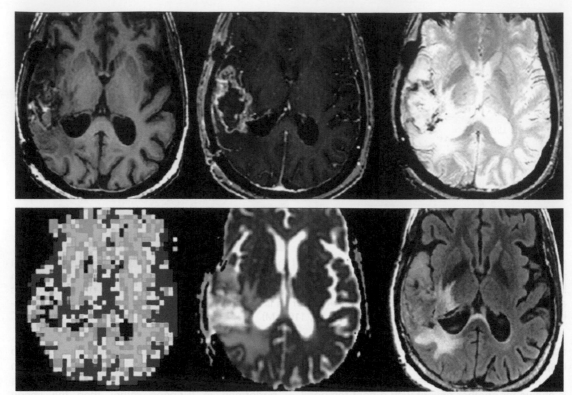

Fig. 8. Conventional proton MR images of a patient after resection of a right temporal GBM. *Top left:* T1-weighted gradient echo image without gadolinium contrast enhancement. *Top middle:* T1-weighted gradient echo image with gadolinium contrast enhancement. *Top right:* magnetic susceptibility-sensitive T2-weighted gradient echo image. *Bottom left:* relative cerebral blood volume (rCBV) map showing residual areas of increased rCBV. *Bottom middle:* apparent diffusion coefficient map. *Bottom right:* T2-weighted FLAIR image.

decreases, have completed responding by 3 weeks, well before the end of treatment. The unresponsive regions (pattern B) never become responsive. These observations are consistent with the suggestion that the spatial heterogeneity may well be the basis of the failure of standardized protocols. This patient expired from the tumor within a few months of radiation treatment, after requesting that chemotherapy be stopped because of side effects. The perfusion maps over these months confirmed increasing vascularity consistent with continued tumor growth. The adverse effects and the low success rate of the standard treatment should encourage examination of such rigid treatment protocols. Adaptive treatment protocols should be considered if

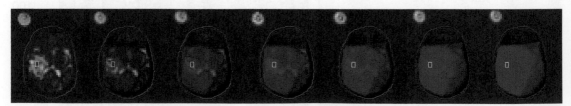

Fig. 9. Realigned sodium images showing the superimposed accumulated radiation dose (*red*) for the same patient in Figs. 3 and 8. The left image is before radiation and each subsequent image to the right is another week of radiation therapy with the far-right image being after completion of treatment. The images have been coregistered in postprocessing to ensure alignment. The realignment is performed within k-space to avoid blurring that would occur if performed in image space, an important advantage of 3D datasets. The two tubes anterior to the brain are calibration phantoms placed within the field of view to demonstrate reproducible signal intensity. These can be used for quantification but with less accuracy than obtained with a separate calibration phantom.

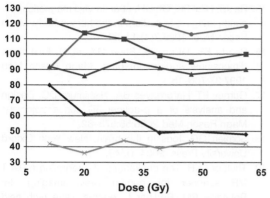

Fig. 10. Voxelwise classification of temporal responses of TSC during radiation therapy covering the center of the surgical bed of the lesion of the patient in **Figs. 3, 8,** and **9.** The five categories of responses: contralateral hemisphere with normal TSC values (*green star*), no response with elevated TSC (*red solid triangle*), desirable response with cell death shown by increasing TSC (*orange solid circle*), decreasing edema with elevated TSC decreasing back toward normal TSC (*blue solid diamond*), and elevated TSC decreasing but toward tumor TSC values (*magenta solid square*). Each voxel can be classified into these responses and related to the subsequent follow-up change in relative cerebral blood volume that revealed recurrence many weeks later. Response patterns B (*red triangle*) and E (*magenta square*) are hypothesized to be predictive of recurrence as they are incomplete responses.

sodium MR imaging proves to be an effective method for monitoring early tumor response.

One advantage of voxelwise analysis of tumor response is that many voxels can be assessed to provide regional tissue survival statistics for each patient. Such tissue survival characteristics can use the same radiobiologic models used for multicenter trials in which patient survival is used as the outcome. Thus, imaging results from each patient may be able to provide sufficient information to guide the treatment of each tumor. Such personalized care may avoid the use of rigid standard protocols based on mean population statistics and capitalize on individual sensitivity characteristics of each patient's tumor. In some cases, the lack of response may reduce unsuccessful treatment to avoid the adverse effects of those treatments.

SUMMARY

Sodium MR imaging, with its TSC and CVF bioscales, has a direct interpretation in terms of tissue viability. These bioscales can monitor the spatial distribution of tissue responses to radiation treatment on at least a weekly basis. Such rapid feedback could be used to guide adaptive radiation treatment for each patient and avoid excessive radiation when no response can be achieved. This approach can potentially minimize unnecessary treatment to avoid adverse effects for the patient. Similar responses can be monitored for chemotherapy. Although these hypotheses remain under investigation, it is imperative that new strategies be considered for high-grade brain tumors where the prognosis remains grim.

REFERENCES

1. Ries LAG, Harkins D, Krapcho M, et al. editors. SEER cancer statistics review, 1975–2003, National Cancer Institute. Bethesda (MD). Available at: http://seer.cancer.gov/csr/1975_2003/. Based on November 2005 SEER data submission, posted to the SEER web site, 2006.
2. Fabi A, Russillo M, Metro G, et al. Pseudoprogression and MGMT status in glioblastoma patients: implications in clinical practice. Anticancer Res 2009;29(7):2607–10.
3. Hall EJ, Cox JD. Physical and biologic basis of radiation therapy. In: Moss WT, Cox JD, editors. Radiation oncology. 6th edition. St Louis: Mosby; 1989. Chapter 1. p. 1–57.
4. Cairncross G, Berkey B, Shaw E, et al. Phase III trial of chemotherapy plus radiotherapy compared with radiotherapy alone for pure and mixed anaplastic oligodendroglioma: intergroup radiation therapy oncology group trial 9402. J Clin Oncol 2006; 24(18):2707–14.
5. Gilbert MR, Lang FF. Anaplastic oligodendroglial tumors: a tale of two trials. J Clin Oncol 2006; 24(18):2689–90.
6. Pauleit D, Stoffels G, Bachofner A, et al. Comparison of (18)F-FET and (18)F-FDG PET in brain tumors. Nucl Med Biol 2009;36(7):779–87.
7. Christensen JD, Barrère BJ, Boada FE, et al. Quantitative tissue sodium concentration mapping of normal rat brain. Magn Reson Med. 1996;36:83–9.
8. Neeb H, Ermer V, Stocker T, et al. Fast quantitative mapping of absolute water content with full brain coverage. Neuroimage 2008;42.1094–109.
9. Thulborn KR, Davis D, Snyder J, et al. Sodium MR imaging of acute and subacute stroke for assessment of tissue viability. Neuroimaging Clin N Am 2005;15:639–53.
10. Thulborn KR, Gindin TS, Davis D, et al. Comprehensive MRI protocol for stroke management: tissue sodium concentration as a measure of tissue viability in a non-human primate model and clinical studies. Radiology 1999;139:26–34.
11. Thulborn KR, Davis D, Adams H, et al. Quantitative tissue sodium concentration mapping of the growth

of focal cerebral tumors with sodium magnetic resonance imaging. Magn Reson Med 1999;41:351–9.

12. Thulborn KR. Clinical sodium MR imaging of the brain. In: Latchaw RE, Kucharczyk J, Moseley ME, editors. Diagnostic and therapeutic imaging of the nervous system. Philadelphia (PA): Elsevier; 2004, Chap 14 and CD.

13. Kline RP, Wu EX, Petrylak DP, et al. Rapid in vivo monitoring of chemotherapeutic response using weighted sodium magnetic resonance imaging. Clin Cancer Res 2000;5:2146–56.

14. Sharma R, Kline RP, Wu EX, et al. Rapid in vivo Taxotere quantitative chemosensitivity response by 4.23 Tesla sodium MRI and histo-immunostaining features in N-Methyl-N-nitrosourea induced breast tumors in rats. Cancer Cell Int 2005;5:26.

15. Ra JB, Hilal SK, Oh CH, et al. In vivo magnetic resonance imaging of sodium in the human body. Magn Reson Med. 1988;7(1):11–22.

16. Boada FE, Gillen JS, Shen GX, et al. Fast three dimensional sodium imaging. Magn Reson Med 1997;37:706–15.

17. Gurney PT, Hargreaves BA, Nishimura DG. Design and analysis of a practical 3D cones trajectory. Magn Reson Med 2006;55:575–82.

18. Somjen GG. Ions in the brain. New York: Oxford University Press; 2004. p. 49.

19. Thulborn KR. The challenges of integrating a 9.4 T MR scanner for human brain imaging. In: Robitaille PM, Berliner L, editors. Ultra high field magnetic resonance imaging. New York: Springer; 2007. Chapter 5. p. 104–26.

Molecular Imaging (PET) of Brain Tumors

Sandip Basu, MBBS (Hons), DRM, DNB, MNAMS[a],
Abass Alavi, MD, PhD (Hon), DSc (Hon)[b],*

KEYWORDS

- Brain tumor • Positron emission tomography (PET)
- Single photon emission computed tomography (SPECT)
- Computed tomography (CT)
- Magnetic resonance imaging (MRI) • PET/CT • PET/MRI

CLASSIFICATION, EPIDEMIOLOGY, MANAGEMENT, AND OUTCOME OF BRAIN TUMORS: THE SALIENT POINTS

Intracranial brain neoplasms can be classified as primary brain tumors and metastatic neoplasms from primary extracranial malignancies. The latter is far more common than the former; according to an American Cancer Society estimate,[1] more than 100,000 people die every year with symptomatic intracranial metastases while death occurs due to primary brain tumors in approximately 12,760 of the 20,500 new cases diagnosed. Primary central nervous system (CNS) tumors account for about 1% to 2% of all malignancies. The basic classification of primary brain neoplasms by the World Health Organization (WHO) relies on their cellular origin.[2] The incidence of primary brain neoplasms varies among subtypes, with the most common primary brain neoplasms in adults being gliomas, which account for about 45% to 50%, and meningiomas, comprising about 15% of all primary brain tumors, all other types being less common.

Gliomas are classified into astrocytomas, oligodendrogliomas, mixed oligoastrocytomas, ependymal tumors, and tumors of the choroid plexus based on histologic characteristics. Grade of malignancy is generally assigned according to the WHO criteria, which are primarily based on nuclear atypia, mitotic activity, endothelial/ microvascular proliferation, and necrosis.[2,3] The prognosis of primary brain tumors is primarily based on 3 factors: (1) histologic characteristics (subtype and grade of the tumor), (2) age, and (3) performance status. The other poor prognostic parameters for gliomas include presence of focal neurologic deficits, mental changes, seizure, symptoms of neoplastic expansion, and contrast enhancement on computed tomography (CT). However, the precise value of some of these factors is still unclear. Therefore, using an objective marker to determine patient's prognosis is beneficial, as this helps guide therapeutic decision making for this unpredictable malignancy.

Low-grade gliomas histopathologically encompass pilocytic astrocytoma (a grade I tumor), astrocytoma (a grade II tumor), and oligodendroglioma (a grade II tumor). In general, the low-grade tumors affect younger patients (mean age: fourth decade) compared with the high-grade gliomas (mean age of presentation at the sixth decade of life). The most fatal and common primary brain neoplasm is the glioblastoma multiforme (GBM), which accounts for 45% to 50% of all gliomas and corresponds to WHO grade IV. Despite aggressive multimodal treatment regimens of conventional therapies (surgery, radiation, and chemotherapy), the disease invariably leads to death over months or years, with a median survival of 1 year. Combination of radiotherapy and chemotherapy with temozolomide has recently

[a] Radiation Medicine Centre (BARC), Tata Memorial Hospital Annexe, Parel, Bombay 400012, India
[b] Division of Nuclear Medicine, Department of Radiology, University of Pennsylvania School of Medicine, Hospital of the University of Pennsylvania, 3400 Spruce Street, Philadelphia, PA 19104, USA
* Corresponding author.
E-mail address: abass.alavi@uphs.upenn.edu (A. Alavi).

Neuroimag Clin N Am 19 (2009) 625–646
doi:10.1016/j.nic.2009.08.012

been shown to improve survival in patients with newly diagnosed glioblastoma, with a 2-year survival rate of 26.5% with radiotherapy plus temozolomide and 10.4% with radiotherapy alone. The remaining high-grade tumors include anaplastic tumors (astrocytoma and oligodendroglioma) and correspond to grade III, with a median survival of 2 to 3 years.

A complex series of molecular events occur during tumor growth resulting in deregulation of the cell cycle, alterations in apoptosis and cell differentiation, neovascularization, and tumor cell migration and invasion into the normal brain parenchyma. Genetic alterations also play an important role in the development of glioma including a loss, mutation, or hypermethylation of a tumor suppressor gene such as PTEN or p53, or other genes involved in the regulation of the cell cycle. During progression from low-grade to high-grade, stepwise accumulation of genetic alteration occurs. Growth of certain tumors seems to be related to the presence of viruses and familial diseases that accelerate the progression of molecular alterations, or to exposure to environmental chemicals, pesticides, herbicides, and fertilizers.[4,5]

POSITRON EMISSION TOMOGRAPHY IN BRAIN TUMORS: WHAT DO THE ONCOLOGISTS DESIRE?

The exact delineation of the tumor volume, the characterization of the important tumor characteristics in its entirety, and assessment of the tumor response to the ongoing treatment regimen are necessary for successful management of these patients. In the current practice, initial imaging is usually done with contrast/enhanced CT or magnetic resonance (MR) imaging, which provides excellent information about lesion anatomy. However, follow-up of primary brain tumors after

surgery, chemotherapy, and particularly radiation is often difficult, as these morphologic imaging modalities are usually not able to differentiate recurrent tumor and radiation necrosis. In all tumor types, diagnosing radiation injuries and differentiating them from tumor recurrence pose a potential diagnostic challenge because the accurate diagnosis has important implications for the patient's management. Also, an optimal understanding of tumor biology is crucial for the development of specific molecular therapies that specifically target the neoplasm and reduce patient morbidity and mortality.

POSITRON EMISSION TOMOGRAPHY: HOW HAS IT ADDRESSED THESE NEEDS?

The interest in positron emission tomography (PET) in brain tumor stems from its potential ability to image a wide range of biochemical processes that are critical for understanding the pathophysiology of brain neoplasms, and thereby can play a significant role in developing and monitoring targeted therapies. Different radiotracers have been used with PET to help in the diagnosis and management of patients with brain neoplasms,[6–10] and these are summarized in Table 1.

Depending on the radiotracer, various molecular processes can be visualized and quantified by PET, which makes it an attractive modality for studying tumor biology of gliomas and other brain neoplasms. Radiolabeled 2-[^{18}F]fluoro-2-deoxy-D-glucose (FDG), methyl-[^{11}C]-L-methionine (MET), and 3-deoxy-3-[^{18}F]fluoro-L-thymidine (FLT) are taken up by proliferating gliomas depending on tumor grade as a reflection of increased activity of membrane transporters for glucose, amino acids, and nucleosides, respectively. More recently, methyl-[^{11}C]choline (CHO) has been introduced as a novel tracer to evaluate

Table 1
PET tracers investigated for brain tumor imaging

	Principal Class of PET Tracer and Molecular Mechanism Involved	Name of Tracer
A	Glucose metabolism	Fluorodeoxyglucose (FDG)
B	Amino acid analogues	[^{11}C]Methionine (MET), fluoroethyl-L-tyrosine (FET) and L-3, 4-dihydroxy-6-[^{18}F]fluorophenylalanine (FDOPA), L-1-[^{11}C]tyrosine (TYR), and L-3-[^{18}F]fluoro-α-methyltyrosine (FMT)
C	Radiolabeled cell membrane components	[^{11}C]Choline PET (CHO)
D	Radiolabeled nucleosides	[^{18}F]Fluorothymidine (FLT)
E	Hypoxia Imaging Tracers	[^{18}F]Fluoromisonidazole, [^{18}F]EF5
F	Somatostatin receptor imaging tracers	[^{68}Ga]DOTA-TOC PET

proliferating cell membrane, as is discussed later in this article.[11,12] PET has been also used to assess the expression of endogenous or exogenous genes coding for enzymes or receptors by measuring the accumulation or binding of the respective enzyme substrates or receptor binding compounds.[13,14]

Continuous developments in PET provide new insights into the diagnosis, classification, and pathophysiology of brain neoplasms. As such, PET has played an increasingly important role in the staging of brain neoplasms, image-guided therapy planning, and treatment monitoring. Multimodality imaging has brought about a new perspective into neuro-oncology, as PET complements the conventional anatomic imaging modalities of CT and MR imaging. In selected situations, PET is used in conjunction with CT[15] and MR imaging[16,17] to better define the extent of neoplasm.

Recent research has concentrated on the fusion of PET and MR imaging technologies into one single machine. The goal of this development is to integrate the PET detectors into the MR imaging scanner, which would allow simultaneous data acquisition, resulting in combined functional and morphologic images with excellent soft tissue contrast, spatial and temporal resolution, and improved coregistration of the fused images. Because advanced MR imaging techniques, such as perfusion weighted imaging, diffusion weighted imaging (DWI), blood oxygenation level dependent (BOLD) imaging, and proton magnetic resonance spectroscopy (MRS) provide physiologic and metabolic information, fusion of PET with MR imaging may provide more insight into the pathophysiology of brain neoplasms in vivo.[18,19]

The following discussion addresses the most commonly used agents in PET imaging of brain tumors.

FLUORODEOXYGLUCOSE

Although there are certain advantages for newer radiotracers, the vast majority of clinical PET studies are still based on administering FDG, an analogue of glucose. Because of its relatively simple synthesis, long half-life (approximately 2 hours), and well-understood mechanism of uptake, FDG is the radiotracer commonly used in neuro-oncology.

Malignant cells generally have enhanced glucose metabolism compared with nonmalignant cells, and therefore exhibit increased glycolytic activity.[20] The increase in glucose metabolic rate is not simply related to the accelerated tumor growth but also to malignant transformation[21] and increased membrane glucose transport capability.[22] There is a significant increase in the number of functional glucose transporters at the transformed cell's surface, and nearly all mitogens and cellular oncogenes activate glucose transport.[23] Six mammalian glucose transporters have been identified, and overexpression of both GLUT-1 and GLUT-3 has been demonstrated in brain tumors, with a higher ratio of GLUT-3 seen in more aggressive neoplastic lesions.[24]

FDG is metabolized similarly to glucose, and as FDG enters a cell via glucose transporter proteins, it competes with glucose for hexokinase and is phosphorylated. In contrast to glucose-6-phosphate, however, FDG-6-phosphate is metabolically trapped within tumor cells in proportion to the glucose metabolic rate, and thus PET can detect its accumulation in these cells over time. The FDG uptake into malignant cells is a consequence of a tumor cell's increased expression of glucose transport and glycolytic activity.

CLINICAL APPLICATIONS OF FDG-PET IN NEURO-ONCOLOGY
Tumor Detection with FDG-PET

Distinguishing nonneoplastic from neoplastic lesions can be challenging when based on anatomic imaging. Due to its poor spatial resolution, FDG-PET has been shown to be of limited value in distinguishing between neoplastic and nonneoplastic ring-enhancing intracranial lesions, as observed on MR imaging. High FDG uptake may occur in cases of neoplasm, brain abscess, and in acute inflammatory demyelination.[25] Multiple reports have shown that lesions with a high concentration of inflammatory cells, such as neutrophils and activated macrophages, also show increased uptake of FDG that can be mistaken for malignant neoplasm.[26] In general, inflammatory cells often exhibit lower levels of FDG uptake compared with malignant cells. However, despite low levels of FDG uptake by inflammatory cells in the resting state, glucose metabolic activity of these cells can increase dramatically in the activated state, making the distinction from tumor difficult. In addition to the neoplastic cells, inflammatory cells also have increased expression of glucose transporters, particularly after cellular stimulation by multiple cytokines.[27-30] Cytokines and growth factors have been shown to acutely increase the affinity of glucose transporters in inflammatory cells to deoxyglucose, and this upregulation involves both tyrosine kinases and protein kinase C activity.[31] It is postulated that the newly formed granulation tissue around a neoplasm contains high concentrations of macrophages and thus can show a higher uptake of FDG than the viable neoplastic cells.

Delineation of Tumor

Both high-grade gliomas and gray matter structures take up FDG avidly. Thus, when tumors are in or near gray matter, it may be difficult to distinguish between the two.[32] Two maneuvers seem to greatly enhance the performance of FDG-PET imaging in brain tumors: (1) coregistration with MR imaging and (2) delayed PET Imaging. An MR image delineates the area of interest precisely, and any increased uptake more than that of background in this region should be considered to reflect an active process. The importance of delayed imaging has recently been stressed when it was observed that FDG-PET imaging 3 to 8 hours after injection can improve the distinction between tumor and normal gray matter.[32,33] The rational approach to interpreting brain FDG-PET is detailed later in this article. It has been demonstrated that the rate constant of FDG-6-phosphate degradation was not significantly different between tumor and normal brain tissue at early imaging times, but was lower in tumor than normal brain tissue at extended time intervals between FDG administration and PET data acquisition. This finding suggests that greater FDG-6-phosphate degradation at delayed time points may be responsible for higher elimination of FDG from normal tissue relative to

neoplasm, which improves the contrast between the tumor and the background activity (**Fig. 1**).

In a group of 10 patients with astrocytomas (WHO grade II and III), Herholz and colleagues[34] found that cell density, but not nuclear polymorphism, correlated significantly with FDG uptake. Standardized uptake values (SUV) in the brain do not correlate well with regional metabolic rates of glucose use (MRGlu), and are less effective in characterizing primary brain neoplasms than neoplasm-to-white matter or neoplasm-to-cortex ratios.[35]

As noted earlier, FDG uptake is not specific for cancer, as FDG accumulation has been observed in inflammatory cells and granulation issue.[27] However, it must be noted that FDG uptake is decreased in the gray matter adjacent to the brain tumor on PET images due to surrounding edema (**Figs. 2** and **3**).

Tumor Grading with FDG-PET

Although some studies have failed to show a relationship between FDG uptake and Ki-67 index, a histologic index for cell proliferation,[36,37] in general, low-grade gliomas and high-grade gliomas demonstrate different degrees of FDG uptake. A glioma-to-white matter ratio of greater than 1.5 and a glioma-to-gray matter ratio of greater than 0.6 have been found to indicate high-grade gliomas with high sensitivity (94%) and limited specificity (77%).[38] In general, the low-grade and high-grade glioma have FDG metabolic activity similar to white matter and gray

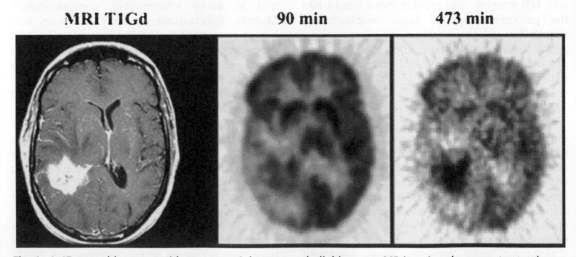

Fig. 1. A 45-year-old woman with recurrent right temporal glioblastoma. MR imaging shows contrast enhancement. Tumor to gray matter contrast is more pronounced at a later time image (*at 473 minutes*) than at an early scan (*at 90 minutes*). (*Reproduced from* Spence AM, Muzi M, Mankoff DA, et al. [18F]FDG-PET of gliomas at delayed intervals: improved distinction between tumor and normal gray matter. J Nucl Med 2004;45(10):1653–9; with permission.)

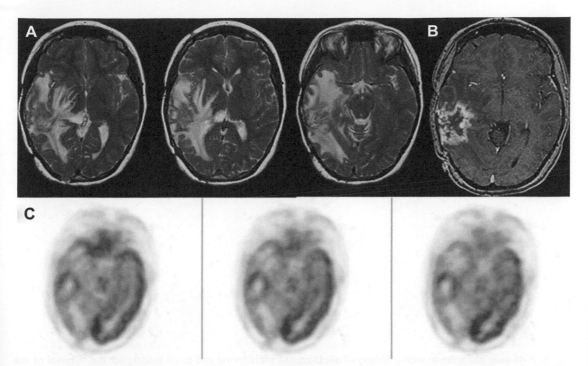

Fig. 2. Anaplastic astrocytoma grade 3 brain tumor treated with radiation, then removed surgically. Following surgery, the patient received another course of radiation therapy and subsequent chemotherapy. (A) T2-weighted image reveals significant edema, which appears to involve most of the right hemisphere extending to the visual cortex. (B) Contrast-enhanced T1-weighted image demonstrates a donut-shaped area of enhancement located in the right temporal lobe. (C) Corresponding FDG-PET images demonstrate a metabolically active tumor corresponding to the areas of enhancement in shape and size. In addition, the entire cortex and the adjacent gray matter structures appear hypometabolic; this is a common observation and is due the adverse effects of edema on the adjacent cortex. Note the loss of function in the ipsilateral visual cortex, which frequently is associated with homonymous hemianopsia. (Reprinted from Hustinx R, Pourdehnad M, Kaschten B, et al. PET imaging for differentiating recurrent brain tumor from radiation necrosis. Radiol Clin North Am 2005;43(1):35–47; with permission.)

matter, respectively. Kaschten and colleagues[39] proposed a cutoff value of 0.8 and 1.1 for tumor-to-mean cortical uptake to differentiate grade II from grade III and grade III from grade IV gliomas, respectively. Several other reports[39,40] have also shown significant correlation between glioma grade and FDG uptake, whereas others have failed to show such an association.[36,37,41] The underlying mechanisms leading to glucose hypermetabolism in high-grade gliomas are likely related to increased energetic demands related to proliferative processes,[34] increased expression of glucose transporters In response to oncogene expression, or the deregulation of the hexokinase enzymatic activity.[42,43] Oligodendroglial tumors harboring combined 1p and 19q chromosomal deletions are characterized by a favorable prognosis and response to treatment. In a recent study, investigators reported the potential of FDG uptake to predict 1p/19q loss preoperatively. Positive FDG uptake was identified in 6 of 8 grade II gliomas

with 1p/19q loss, but in none of the 8 grade II gliomas without 1p/19q loss.[44] This finding needs to be investigated in a larger sample of patients.

Disease Prognosis with FDG-PET

FDG-PET imaging of brain neoplasms provides important information on neoplastic grade and patient prognosis. High FDG uptake in a previously known low-grade tumor is a reliable indicator of anaplastic transformation. In high-grade gliomas, some studies have claimed that FDG-PET has predictive value of survival independent from the histologic classification.[45–47] Di Chiro[45] examined 45 patients with proven high-grade brain tumors after surgery, radiation, and chemotherapy. Poorly differentiated tumors showed significantly higher glucose metabolism than more differentiated ones. The calculation of the ratio of metabolic values (tumor compared with the contralateral normal brain parenchyma) revealed that a ratio of

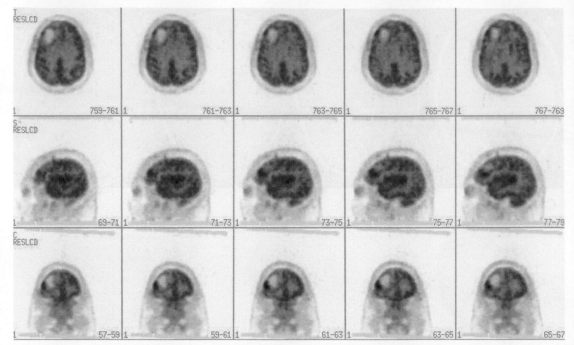

Fig. 3. A 45-year-old woman with a history of glioblastoma multiforme and brain surgery for the removal of the tumor. She also had received and chemotherapy during the course of the disease. MR imaging demonstrated right frontal craniotomy and a large area with signal abnormality in the right frontal lobe, with overall decrease in mass effect and surrounding T2 signal abnormality that could represent any combination of tumor, radiation change, and edema without definitive diagnosis. FDG-PET study showed an intense focus at the lateral aspect of a negative defect (likely related to fluid collection following surgery) suggestive of an active disease despite these therapeutic interventions.

greater than 1.4 was associated with a poor prognosis (median survival 5 months), whereas patients with a ratio of less than 1.4 had a median survival of 19 months. Alavi and colleagues[46] came to similar conclusions using ^{18}FDG-PET in 29 patients with primary brain tumors. Patients with hypermetabolic tumors had a median survival of 7 months after PET scan, compared with 33 months for those with hypometabolic lesions on FDG-PET ($P = .0007$). Of the 23 patients with high-grade tumors, 9 patients with hypometabolic lesions had a 1-year survival of 78%, whereas the group with hypermetabolic lesions had a 1-year survival of only 29%. These investigators concluded that glucose metabolic studies may provide an independent measure of the aggressiveness of a brain tumor, and may supplement pathologic grading. In another study[47] of a pediatric population, 38 children with primary brain tumors were evaluated. Four grade IV tumors had a mean index of 4.27 ± 0.5, 4 grade III tumors had a mean index of 2.47 ± 1.07, 10 grade II tumors had a mean index of 1.34 ± 0.73, and 8 of 12 grade I tumors had a mean index of −0.31 ± 0.59. Eight patients with no histologic confirmation had a mean index of 1.04. For these 34 tumors,

FDG uptake was positively correlated with the grade of malignancy ($n = 34$; $r = 0.72$; $P<.01$), and for the 26 histologically classified tumors ($n = 26$; $r = 0.89$; $P<.01$).

Barker and colleagues[48] studied the prognostic value of FDG-PET in 55 patients with malignant glioma. In univariate analysis, the FDG-PET score was a significant predictor of survival time after FDG-PET scanning ($P = .005$). Median survival was 10 months for patients with FDG-PET uptake scores of 2 or 3 and 20 months for those with low uptake scores of 0 or 1. Padma and colleagues[49] also observed similar findings, and the median survival of patients with high uptake scores in their study was 11 months as compared with 28 months in patients with low uptake scores. Survival differed significantly between patients with low versus high uptake of FDG ($P = .001$).

Other groups have reported significant correlation between FDG-PET score and survival in patients with malignant gliomas imaged at various times in the course of their disease. Patronas and colleagues[50] reported median survival of 5 and 19 months in patients with hypermetabolic and hypometabolic lesions, respectively ($P<.001$). Not all studies have confirmed the high predictive ability of FDG-PET with regard to grade of pathology or survival. Tyler and colleagues[51] found variable FDG uptake rates without correlation to neoplastic grade and size, and low FDG uptake in several patients with high-grade gliomas. Janus and colleagues[32] found that decreased uptake of FDG suggested prolonged survival in their study of 30 patients with primary brain neoplasms, but that increased uptake of FDG did not predict survival. Rozenthal and colleagues[52] found that neither the baseline glucose uptake ratio nor the visual tumor grade accurately predicted length of survival. This lower sensitivity and specificity of FDG-PET in the prediction of pathologic grade and survival may be due volume averaging from necrotic portions of a heterogeneous neoplasm and surrounding edema. Moreover, cystic and calcified regions are also hypovascular.

Differential Diagnosis of Enhancing Brain Neoplasms with FDG-PET and Other PET Tracers

The role of FDG-PET is limited in the differential diagnosis of solitary intracranial ring-enhancing lesions. FDG is nonspecific in that its uptake is increased in inflammatory/infectious lesions as well as in certain benign lesions like pituitary adenomas and choroid plexus papillomas.[53] Also, metastases from various non-CNS primary tumors appear to have more variable FDG uptake. A negative FDG-PET could be helpful to exclude a glioblastoma. The diagnostic value of O-2-[^{18}F]fluoroethyl-L-tyrosine (FET)-PET and MET-PET does not seem to be superior to that of FDG-PET, both of which have been reported to show uptake in the area of macrophage infiltration at the rim of brain abscesses. A single study[54] has demonstrated a significant difference in fluorocholine uptake between benign lesions, high-grade glioma, and the metastatic lesions. The other relatively benign neoplasms with a high FDG uptake include pilocytic astrocytoma and ganglioglioma. Pilocytic astrocytomas have a good prognosis despite exhibiting high FDG uptake due to the presence of metabolically active fenestrated endothelial cells.

It is also possible to differentiate grade I from grade II to III meningiomas using FDG-PET.[55] Meningiomas are usually benign, curable neoplasms but can occasionally recur and demonstrate aggressive behavior.[56] Di Chiro[45] found that the glucose metabolism of meningiomas correlates with tumor growth and aggressive behavior. In this study an atypical meningioma had the highest metabolic rate greater than that of cerebral cortex. Hemangiopericytomas are richly vascularized mesenchymal tumors that are derived from pericytes. Kracht and colleagues[57] observed low glucose use in a case of hemangiopericytoma despite high cellularity and proliferation rate.

Efficacy of Therapy: Differentiating Post-Therapy Radiation Necrosis from Residual/Recurrent Brain Tumor

Differentiation of post-therapy radiation necrosis from residual/recurrent brain neoplasm remains a challenging task. This differential diagnosis seems particularly critical in the early and late phases after the completion of radiation therapy. The effect of radiation appears more pronounced when it is combined with chemotherapy for treating high-grade gliomas. A wide range of FDG-PET performance has been reported in different studies in differentiating radiation necrosis from recurrent tumor, and this can be primarily attributed to the following: (a) timing of PET study following radiation (Table 2), (b) type of radiation administered; and (c) type of tumor. All these factors can lead to considerable overlap of FDG uptake between these 2 entities. Residual/recurrent neoplasm can have similarly varied degrees of metabolic activity that also can frequently be lower than that of normal brain. The accuracy appears better in gliomas compared with metastatic lesions and is worse in lesions treated with stereotactic radiosurgery. Whereas there is no clear-cut guideline with regard to optimal time for performing FDG-PET after radiation, the general recommendation is that FDG-PET should not be performed before 6 weeks after the completion of radiation treatment for this purpose.

Varying degrees of background metabolic activity can be observed in the area of treated brain as well as the recurring tumors, and hence in the lesion to contralateral normal brain tissue uptake ratio or the absolute uptake value. This factor has led to decidedly mixed results in various studies.[58–61] Whereas in some studies FDG-PET has been found not to be ideal to evaluate residual/recurrent neoplasm after therapy,[62] others have reported promising results[61,63] using receiver operating characteristics analysis. In an early report, Patronas and colleagues[63] demonstrated that metabolic imaging with FDG can differentiate recurrent brain tumor from radiation necrosis. The same group, in another study with brain tumors, demonstrated the feasibility of brain tumor imaging with FDG-PET and showed that it is more accurate than contrast CT for tumor grading.[50] The effects of radiation and chemotherapy can be visualized by FDG-PET only after

Table 2
The different pathologic processes occurring after irradiation of the CNS along with their time course

Types of Radiation Injuries			
Type of Injury	Time Interval after Irradiation	Pathology	Prognosis
Acute	Hours to weeks	Tumor swelling Edema of the surrounding brain	Good (reversible)
Early delayed	Weeks to months	Demyelination	Good (spontaneously reversible)
Late	Months to years	Liquefactive or coagulative necrosis	Usually irreversible Clinical severity variable

Reprinted from Hustinx R, Pourdehnad M, Kaschten B, et al. PET imaging for differentiating recurrent brain tumor from radiation necrosis. Radiol Clin North Am 2005;43(1):35–47; with permission.

several weeks,[60] with a possible transient increase of FDG uptake in the initial phase, most likely due to infiltration of macrophages.[64,65] At further follow-up, however, recurrent neoplasm and progression from low-grade to high-grade glioma can be visualized by the appearance of new hypermetabolic sites.[66,67] Glantz and colleagues[67] demonstrated that FDG-PET imaging in brain tumor patients was not only superior to contrast CT in identifying early recurrence but also a better predictor of outcome than surgical biopsy results. In this study the vast majority of patients (19 of 20) with hypermetabolic lesions in areas of prior resection had early tumor recurrence. All 12 patients with hypometabolic abnormalities revealed radiation necrosis.

Overall performance that has been reported indicates that FDG-PET had a sensitivity of 81% to 86% and a specificity of 40% to 94% for distinguishing between radiation necrosis and residual/recurrent neoplasm.[63] It should be emphasized that in patients receiving corticosteroids, evaluation with FDG-PET might be hampered by a generalized reduction in cerebral metabolic rate for glucose.[68] Coregistration of FDG-PET images with MR imaging and delayed imaging greatly improves the accuracy of FDG-PET in this setting (**Fig. 4**), and this is addressed in detail later in this article.[69–71]

FDG-PET Imaging for Planning Stereotactic Biopsy

In the histologically heterogeneous gliomas, stereotactic biopsy aims for tumor sites with the highest tumor grade. FDG-PET guided stereotactic brain biopsy has proven to be useful for improved delineation of anaplastic regions[72–75] and better identification of neoplastic residues,[45]

thereby increasing the diagnostic yield of brain biopsy. It is well known that low-grade and high-grade regions may be present within the same tumor, with components that include varying degrees of cellular and nuclear pleomorphism, mitotic activity, vascular proliferation, and necrosis.[2,3] These regional variations cannot be reliably distinguished on conventional anatomic imaging such as MR imaging or CT, even with intravenous contrast administration.[72] Accurate grading and diagnosis are especially important for directing the therapeutic approach and providing the prognosis in patients with nonresectable neoplasms.[73–75] Several novel approaches have been investigated, including: (a) combined structure-function approach using PET and MR imaging; (b) combining FDG and an amino acid tracer (like [11C]methionine); and (c) using coregistered MR imaging and amino acid tracers like FET. All these multimodality approaches are useful in accurately defining the disease extent and viability. Integration of MR imaging with PET provides complementary information that helps in the assessment of neoplastic extent and surgical planning better than either technique alone. This combined information has been exploited in accomplishing maximum neoplastic resection.[17,76] Also, at follow-up, recurrent neoplasm and progression from low-grade to high-grade glioma can be visualized by the new appearance of hypermetabolism,[66,67] and this can aid in guiding the site of biopsy.

FDG-PET in Central Nervous System Lymphoma

Primary CNS lymphomas, like the other extracerebral types, are highly proliferative and untreated tumors show avid FDG uptake. However, prior

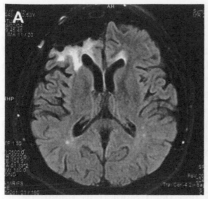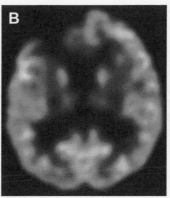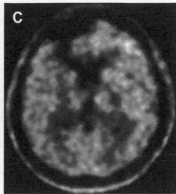

Fig. 4. Right frontal oligodendroglioma (WHO grade III) treated 2 years earlier by surgery and radiotherapy. (*A*) T2-weighted MR imaging shows a hyperintense signal just behind the surgical site of resection. PET shows no uptake of FDG (*B*) or F-TYR (*C*) in this region, suggesting postradiation therapy changes. A 9-month follow-up was negative. (*Reprinted from* Hustinx R, Pourdehnad M, Kaschten B, et al. PET imaging for differentiating recurrent brain tumor from radiation necrosis. Radiol Clin North Am 2005;43(1):35–47; with permission.)

chemotherapy as well as dexamethasone treatment can cause substantial reduction in the FDG uptake and should be borne in mind while interpreting scan in this setting.[77] In human immunodeficiency virus–infected patients, FDG-PET can help to discriminate CNS lymphoma from toxoplasmosis[78] with a high degree of accuracy (80%–95%).

Pitfalls of FDG-PET in Brain Tumors and Improving the Accuracy of Interpretation: The Rational Approach

Compared with other organ systems, the brain presents unique challenges because of the high background glucose metabolism of normal gray matter structures. As noted earlier, the diagnostic limitations of FDG-PET related to the high physiologic glucose metabolism of normal brain tissue can lead to low sensitivity for detecting low-grade tumors and recurrent high-grade tumors in posttreatment settings. Uptake can at times be similar or even less than the normal gray matter. Hence, attempts have been made to improve the sensitivity of FDG-PET for lesion detection. Two steps seem critical for improving the accuracy of interpretation: (a) MR imaging coregistration and (b) delayed imaging whereby the tumor to normal brain uptake ratio increases with time following injection. Coregistration of FDG-PET images with MR imaging greatly improves the performance of FDG-PET. If the PET/MR imaging coregistration software is not available, it is important to review MR imaging along with the FDG-PET images at the same time.[69] Because residual/recurrent neoplasm may show FDG uptake equal to or lower than that of the normal cortex, reference to the MR

imaging delineates the area of interest and aids in improved accuracy. A reasonable approach for interpretation that can be useful is that in the area of interest on MR imaging, any FDG uptake higher than the expected background level in the adjacent brain may be considered recurrent neoplasm, even though the uptake may be equal to or less than that in normal cortex.[70] In addition, with delayed imaging there is enhanced tumor to normal brain uptake ratio compared with the baseline image, which can further substantiate the presence of disease. A recent report has also advocated the use of coregistered FDG-PET and MR imaging to determine the residual/recurrent neoplasm viability by enhancing regions of the tumor.[71] Another major limitation of PET is its relatively low specificity.

Promising "Non-FDG" PET Tracers for Brain Tumor Imaging and Their Current Status with Regard to Clinical Applications

In the past few years there have been an increasing number of brain tumor PET studies to circumvent the shortcomings of FDG-PET imaging, which apply other positron labeled radiotracers. These studies are enumerated in **Table 1**.

The most significant advantage of these tracers is related to the markedly lower background activity in normal brain tissue compared with FDG, and relatively avidity toward the brain neoplasms that enables the detection of smaller and low-grade tumors (primary or recurrent). Among these tracers the labeled methionine, tyrosine, and thymidine tracers are relatively more widely investigated, as are the hypoxia imaging tracers, owing to their ability to define tumor biology and thereby guide the course of therapy.

Promising Role of Amino Acid PET Tracers

Proteins play a critical role in nearly every biologic process within the body. Amino acids, the building blocks of proteins, are either produced via metabolic processes or obtained via dietary ingestion. Fundamental to their ability to be a target of metabolic imaging, they can serve as components in metabolic cycles, many of which are upregulated in cells with increased proliferative activity, such as in the setting of cancer. Amino acids enter cells either through passive diffusion or, more commonly, active diffusion, particularly via the L-amino acid transporter. What makes amino acids attractive for the most common form of radiolabeling is that the substitution of [11C] for a nonradioactive [12C] carbon atom does not alter the amino acid's chemical characteristics. Certain amino acids have gained more popularity than others as metabolic imaging agents because of differences in relative ease and cost of production, biodistribution, and formation of radiolabeled metabolites. Positron labeled amino acid analogues have in general a low background uptake in gray and white matter, which allows easier detection of tumors (especially small ones).

Whereas the most studied radiolabeled amino acid for PET imaging of brain tumors is MET, other [18F]-labeled aromatic amino acid analogues have been developed recently for tumor imaging including FET and L-3,4-dihydroxy-6-[18F]fluorophenylalanine (FDOPA), because of the short half-life of [11C] (20 minutes) that requires an onsite cyclotron. The other radiolabeled amino acid PET tracers include L-1-[11C]tyrosine (TYR), and L-3-[18F]fluoro-α-methyltyrosine (FMT).

MET-PET

MET-PET has been one of the most popular amino acid imaging modalities in neuro-oncology, although its use is restricted to PET centers with an in-house cyclotron facility. This popularity is largely due to its relative ease of production that lacks complicated purification steps.

The precise underlying molecular mechanisms this methionine dependence remains yet to be completely elucidated. Methionine, a sulfur-containing essential amino acid, is transported mainly through Na^+-independent system L (leucine preferring) and Na^+-dependent systems A (alanine preferring) and ASC (alanine, serine, cysteine). LAT1 (high substrate affinity), 1 of the 2 membrane-spanning proteins belonging to system L, is strongly expressed in malignant glioma cells,[79] and there is enhanced facilitated transport of amino acids in the supporting vasculature of the tumors due to upregulation of amino acid transporter expression.[79,80] The rates of transmethylation are frequently increased in human tumor cells, and this can lead to the "methionine dependence" observed in vitro tumor cell lines.[81] Overall, the increased uptake of methionine in cancer cells caused by increased in fluxes of the amino acids (mediated largely by the L system of transport), enhanced the pathways of protein synthesis, transmethylation, and transsulfuration.[79–81]

MET-PET has been studied to determine its value in a variety of roles in the evaluation of brain neoplasms, including: detection and delineation of tumor, tumor grading, prognosis, and effectiveness of therapy.

Detection and Delineation of Tumor Extent with MET-PET

MET-PET has been demonstrated by multiple studies to be a sensitive tool for detection of brain neoplasms.[39,82–86] The overall sensitivity of MET-PET for malignant gliomas (both low and high grades) has been higher compared with FDG-PET (Fig. 5), ranging from 76% to 95%, with higher rates for higher grade neoplasms.[85] In low-grade gliomas, the range of reported sensitivities lies between 65% and 85%.[85,87] In one study,[86] the utility of MET-PET in 45 brain lesions that were iso- or hypometabolic on FDG-PET was evaluated. MET demonstrated increased uptake in 31 of 35 tumors with 89% sensitivity. For 24 gliomas, MET demonstrated a positive uptake in 22 with a sensitivity of 92%. All 10 benign lesions (cysticercosis, radiation necrosis, tuberculous granuloma, hemangioma, organized infarction, and benign cyst) showed normal or decreased MET uptake (100% specificity), whereas false-negative MET-PET was encountered in intermediate oligodendroglioma, metastatic tumor, chordoma, and cystic ganglioma. As is discussed in greater depth later, increased uptake of MET was also seen in neoplasms in which there was little or absent contrast enhancement on MR imaging and low uptake on FDG-PET, findings that are typically noted in the low-grade gliomas.[87]

Multiple studies have shown that MET-PET shows earlier and more accurate delineation of neoplastic extent than anatomic imaging, such as with CT or MR imaging, alone.[16,75,88–90] In a study of 10 patients with pathologically proven GBM, Miwa and colleagues[16] performed both contrast-enhanced MR imaging and MET-PET before treatment to better assess the relationship

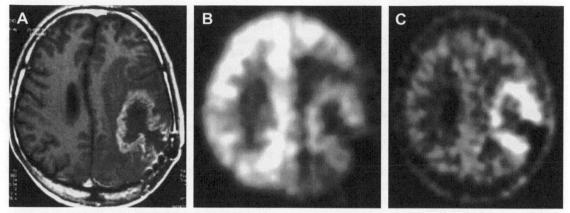

Fig. 5. Glioblastoma treated by surgery and radiotherapy 5 months before this study. (A) T1-weighted MR imaging shows a rim of contrast enhancement around the operative cavity. PET shows increased uptake of both FDG (B) and MET (C), indicating tumor recurrence, which was confirmed by a second surgery. Note that the contrast between the tumor and normal cortex is much higher on the MET image than on the FDG study. (*Reprinted from* Hustinx R, Pourdehnad M, Kaschten B, et al. PET imaging for differentiating recurrent brain tumor from radiation necrosis. Radiol Clin North Am 2005;43(1):35–47; with permission.)

between abnormalities seen on both modalities. Coregistration of the anatomic and metabolic images was performed with a commercial software package using a previously published method.[91] This study found that in 100% of cases, the area of abnormal MET uptake (MET area) was larger than the gadolinium-enhancing area (Gd area). In 90% of cases, the MET area was located within a 3-cm radius of the Gd area. This distance was positively correlated with tumor size. In 100% cases, the area of T2 prolongation surrounding the tumor was larger than the MET area, suggesting that peritumoral edema extends beyond the margins of the neoplasm. This study also showed that MET-PET was more sensitive for the earlier detection of tumor recurrence than MR imaging. Overall, this study concluded that with a better understanding of the discrepancies between MET-PET and MR imaging, the combined use of these modalities could be helpful for surgical and radiation planning.

The better sensitivity of MET-PET compared with MR imaging is likely due to the inherent differences in these modalities and the processes they image. T1-weighted MR imaging detects the morphologic abnormalities in brain structures secondary to the mass effect from a neoplasm that is relatively insensitive, especially in low-grade or infiltrative neoplasms. The addition of intravenous contrast material does not significantly increase the accuracy in assessing the extent of neoplasm, as contrast enhancement is dependent on breakdown of the blood-brain barrier, a finding usually observed in the most aggressive components of a neoplasm. T2-weighted MR imaging

shows increased signal intensity surrounding a neoplasm, which can help in defining the extent of a neoplasm, although this lacks specificity because edema can have an identical appearance. MET-PET, on the other hand, relies on the higher metabolic needs of the tumor, rather than on the associated morphologic or blood-brain barrier abnormalities, leading to more accurate delineation of the neoplasm.

Tumor Grading and Disease Prognosis with MET-PET

Many studies have investigated the possible role of MET-PET in the grading of brain neoplasms.[40,81–83,85,87,92,93] Whereas the report by Ogawa and colleagues[85] concluded it difficult to evaluate the grade of malignancy only from the degree of C-11 methionine accumulation, subsequent reports found MET-PET to be valuable for the grading of brain neoplasms.[81–83,87,92,93] MET uptake, in general, correlates with cell proliferation, in vitro Ki-67 expression, proliferating cell nuclear antigen, and microvessel density, making it a potential biomarker for active tumor proliferation.[81] The use of neoplastic grading by MET-PET has been of particular interest for low-grade tumors, which are not only difficult to detect on contrast-enhanced MR imaging and FDG-PET but also difficult to differentiate from nonneoplastic lesions. In the largest study of this topic, Herholz and colleagues[87] evaluated 196 consecutive patients suspected of having low-grade gliomas. The study found that MET-PET could differentiate between high-grade gliomas, low-grade gliomas, and chronic or subacute nonneoplastic lesions. This ability was independent from contrast enhancement on CT or MR imaging, as expected, given that MET uptake, unlike contrast enhancement, does not rely on breakdown of the blood-brain barrier.

MET-PET has also been investigated for its potential as a prognostic tool in patients with cerebral gliomas.[37,39,94–97] MET and FDG uptake as prognostic factors were directly compared in a study by Kim and colleagues[37] that found MET uptake to be an independent significant prognostic factor, whereas FDG uptake was not. In another study De Witte and colleagues[95] evaluated the role of MET-PET role in prognosis, using both a qualitative and quantitative scoring system of MET uptake; it was observed that neoplasms with higher MET-PET activity were associated with a statistically significantly shorter survival time. When both MET-PET and FDG-PET were used in the setting of suspected glioma recurrence, 2 different studies found that the combination of both radiotracers resulted in the highest prognostic accuracy; however, MET was found to be the preferred single agent, due its increased sensitivity and specificity.[39,94]

Preliminary data suggest that MET-PET also has an important role to play in determining the prognosis for patients with gliomas that are suspected or confirmed to be low grade. It is important to take into consideration the variable outcome of patients with low-grade gliomas, and there is no definitive consensus on treatment. In this scenario, the ability of MET-PET to risk stratify low-grade gliomas could play a crucial role in managing this subset of gliomas.[98]

Assessing Effectiveness of Therapy with MET-PET

Identifying posttreatment inflammatory change or radiation necrosis in the postradiation or postsurgical brain is of crucial importance, as radiation necrosis may prompt steroid therapy or debulking neurosurgery whereas a finding of neoplastic recurrence may lead to more aggressive therapy or, conversely, palliative care. The findings on contrast-enhanced MR imaging or FDG-PET can be nonspecific; at times the recurrent tumor is indistinguishable from that of posttreatment inflammatory change or radiation necrosis. The studies have shown that MET-PET is an accurate tool for the evaluation of recurrence in a previously treated brain.[59,94,99–101] In a series of 15 patients suspected of having recurrent brain tumor or radiation injury, Ogawa and colleagues[99] showed that MET-PET was useful in the early detection of

recurrent brain neoplasm whereas FDG-PET was helpful in the detection of radiation necrosis; the investigators concluded that FDG-PET and MET-PET were additive in their accuracy to distinguish radiation necrosis from recurrent/residual neoplasm. In another series, on the other hand, Van Laere and colleagues[94] showed that MET-PET had an accuracy, sensitivity, and specificity of 73%, 75%, and 70%, not significantly different to those of FDG-PET. When MET-PET and FDG-PET data were used concurrently, there was slight improvement in accuracy and sensitivity, and a slight decrease in specificity in this study.

^{18}F-Labeled Amino Acid PET Tracers in Brain Tumors

Whereas the earlier studies with radiolabeled amino acids in the evaluation of brain tumors have focused primarily on MET-PET, recent years have seen interest in ^{18}F-labeled amino acid tracers like FET and FDOPA because, as opposed to MET and other agents labeled with ^{11}C such as TYR, the former are labeled with ^{18}F, which has a longer half-life (110 minutes), obviating the need for an on-site cyclotron. These tracers, like MET, have lower uptake in normal brain tissue relative to FDG, raising the possibility of their use in the evaluation of brain tumors.[102–107] The amino acid tracers, in general, show higher sensitivities ranging from approximately 85% to 100% in detection of brain tumors. However, their exact roles in brain tumor imaging of patients continue to evolve at this point in time.[104,108]

[^{18}F]Fluoroethyl-L-tyrosine

FET, a recently introduced amino acid PET tracer for the diagnosis of brain tumors, has been shown to exhibit a similar diagnostic potential to MET, with tumor delineation appearing to be identical. FET has been shown to reliably differentiate tumor recurrence from reactive changes following various therapies, particularly external radiation therapy.[104,109] Owing to slow blood clearance and to relatively stable tumor contrast, static images from 20 to 40 minutes after injection have been recommended. Studies have shown that MET-PET and FET-PET have similar accuracies in diagnosing gliomas.[110] Furthermore, FET-PET has been shown to have value in the prognosis and evaluation of treatment in patients with gliomas.[111–113] The tumor specificity has been the major reason for the interest generated in this tracer, particularly in the setting of cerebral glioma. A potential area of interest is its usefulness in assessing tumor grading where standard evaluations have been considered of little value because of marked overlap reported between histologic grades.[104] A recent report on FET uptake kinetics in untreated glioma patients demonstrated a significant difference in the uptake values in the early phase (0–10 minutes after injection) but not in the later period (30–40 minutes after injection) between low- and high-grade gliomas.[104] From their results, the investigators hypothesized that differentiation between low- and high-grade gliomas is possible by taking into account their different kinetic behaviors in these tumors, and a kinetic analysis of FET-PET hence may provide important information in the differentiation of suspected brain lesions.[104] The factors that have been suggested to contribute to the different kinetic behavior of low- and high-grade tumors include increased angiogenesis and intratumoral microvessel density, and increased amino acid transporter expression in tumor vessels.[104,109]

In one study,[114] the added value of FET-PET was investigated in 31 patients with suspected gliomas. PET and MR imaging were coregistered and 52 neuronavigated tissue biopsies were taken from lesions with abnormal MR imaging signal and increased FET uptake (match), as well as from areas with abnormal MR imaging signal but normal FET or vice versa (mismatch). Combined use of MR imaging and FET-PET yielded a sensitivity of 93% and a specificity of 94%. The investigators concluded that combined use of MR imaging and FET-PET significantly improves the identification of tumor tissue. In a comparative study between MR imaging, FET-PET, and MR spectroscopy,[115] the predictive value of each modality was compared in 50 patients with suspected gliomas. The diagnostic accuracy of differentiating neoplastic from nonneoplastic tissue increased from 68% with MR imaging alone to 97% with MR imaging when used in conjunction with FET-PET and MR imaging spectroscopy. Sensitivity and specificity for tumor detection were 100% and 81% for MR spectroscopy, and 80% and 88% for FET-PET, respectively.

FDOPA

FDOPA is an amino acid analogue that is taken up by normal brain at the blood-brain barrier by the neutral amino acid transporter.[107,116,117] In a relatively large series of 81 patients, Chen and colleagues[107] compared FDOPA-PET to FDG-PET in the evaluation of brain neoplasms (Fig. 6). The study found that high-grade and low-grade neoplasms were well visualized with FDOPA-PET, with a significantly higher sensitivity than that of FDG-PET (96% vs 61%), whereas specificities were similar (43%). The specificity of FDOPA

brain tumor imaging could be increased by using thresholds of tumor to striatum ratio T/S of 0.75 or 1.0. FDOPA uptake, however, did not correlate with neoplastic grade, and it did not seem that FDOPA-PET could be used for this purpose. Although only 4 patients were suspected of having radiation necrosis in this study, FDOPA-PET was able to identify the one patient in this group who had recurrent neoplasm, not radiation necrosis; the investigators suggested that a dedicated study would be helpful to better evaluate the potential role of FDOPA-PET in distinguishing recurrent neoplasm from radiation necrosis.

In another study,[116] however, FDOPA-PET was found to be useful in assessing tumor grade. In this study, aimed to investigate the kinetics of FDOPA in brain tumors, 37 patients underwent 45 studies. Whereas a 2-compartment model was able to describe FDOPA kinetics in tumors in a first approximation, a 3-compartment model with corrections for metabolites and partial volume was adequately able to describe FDOPA kinetics in tumors, the striatum, and the cerebellum. From this model it was proposed that FDOPA was transported but not trapped in tumors, unlike in the striatum. The shape of the uptake curve obtained in this study appeared to be related to tumor grade. After an early maximum, high-grade tumors had a steep descending branch, whereas low-grade tumors had a slowly declining curve, like that for the cerebellum but on a higher scale.

RADIOLABELED CELL MEMBRANE COMPONENTS
Methyl-[¹¹C]Choline

Choline is a molecule normally found in blood, which enters cell membrane components. Choline is phosphorylated and then, after several biosynthetic steps, is integrated into lecithin, a component of cell membrane phospholipids. Due to a tumor cell's increased proliferation, there is increased cell membrane turnover and, therefore, a greater need for cell membrane components, such as choline. More recently, CHO has been targeted as a PET imaging molecule because of its ability to image cell membrane turnover, a likely marker of metabolic activity.[11,12,118–127]

Comparative studies have evaluated the potential role of CHO-PET in comparison with FDG-PET to determine whether it offers specific advantages over the more established tracers. Tian and colleagues,[12] in a prospective study involving 126 patients with various types of malignancy including 25 patients with brain neoplasms, compared CHO-PET to FDG-PET. For a subset of patients with brain neoplasms, CHO was

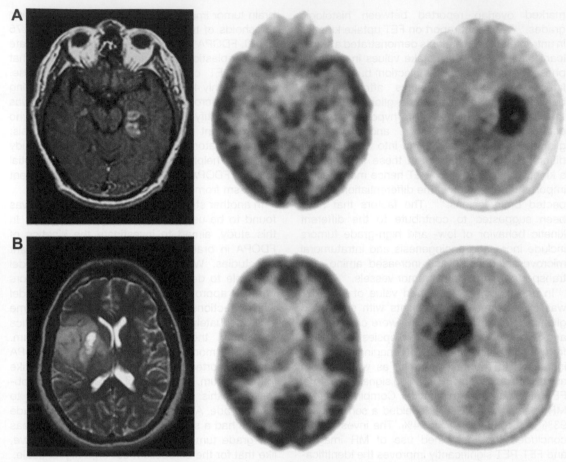

Fig. 6. MR imaging (*left*), [^{18}F]FDG-PET (*middle*), and [^{18}F]FDOPA-PET (*right*) of newly diagnosed brain tumors. (*A*) Glioblastoma. (*B*) Grade II oligodendroglioma. The FDOPA images reveal a clear-cut delineation of the tumor sites compared with FDG scans. However, the low uptake on FDG images most likely represents the lower grade associated with such tumors. In general, there is a good agreement between contrast enhancement of MR imaging and the degree of uptake amino acids on PET scans. Therefore, the latter approach may not reveal the nature of the underlying processes noted on contrast enhancement on MR images. (*Reproduced from* Chen W, Silverman DH, Delaloye S, et al. [^{18}F]FDOPA-PET imaging of brain tumors: comparison study with [^{18}F]FDG-PET and evaluation of diagnostic accuracy. J Nucl Med 2006;47(6):904–11; with permission.)

superior to FDG in delineating the true extent of the tumor. The investigators concluded that this is likely due to the brain's high baseline uptake of FDG, which likely obscures pathologic lesions and lowers sensitivity and specificity. In a recent study by Kato and colleagues[54] PET examinations using FDG, MET, and CHO were used to evaluate 96 gliomas. MR imaging was also performed, and tumor volume and degree of enhancement was assessed. Although PET images were superimposed on the anatomic MR imaging images, it seems that this was done for illustrative purposes rather than to assess the value of combining the 2 modalities. The investigators concluded that MET is the most superior and user-friendly marker for all gliomas, as it enables the straightforward localization of "hot lesions" and provides

outstanding quantitative metabolic parameters when compared with FDG and CHO, although the latter may have a role in evaluating oligodendroglial neoplasms.

Hypoxia Imaging with [^{18}F]EF5

The presence of hypoxia in solid tumors is a major cause of failure of both radiation therapy and chemotherapy, and is associated with a more aggressive tumor phenotype, increased metastatic potential, and overall a poor clinical outcome.[128–132] Hence, the presence and the magnitude of uptake of PET using fluoromisonidazole (FMISO) or other hypoxia-specific PET tracers are of potential value in therapeutic decision making and disease prognostication.

[^{18}F]EF5 (2-(2-nitro-1H-imidazol-1-yl)-N-(2,2,3,3, 3-pentafluoropropyl)-acetamide) is a 2-nitroimidazole imaging agent that has been employed to measure hypoxia in tumors (**Fig. 7**). The molecule is currently in phase 2 clinical trials using antibody techniques for the detection of hypoxic cells, and predicts radiation response in individual rodent tumors.[133–135] [^{18}F]EF5 is an etanidazole derivative and lipophilic molecule designed to have a very uniform biodistribution, a feature of obvious benefit compared with the FMISO for use in PET imaging. In humans, the biologic half-life of [^{18}F]EF5 is approximately 12 hours, and up to 70% of the administered dose is excreted unchanged in the urine.[136] Whereas the initial uptake of [^{18}F]EF5 is governed by blood flow, the uptake in the later phase is hypoxia specific. It has been predicted that 2 to 4 hours from injection would be an optimal time point for detection of specific binding of EF5 in hypoxic tissues. Preliminary results by Ziemer and colleagues[134] have suggested that [^{18}F]EF5 is a promising agent for noninvasive assessment of neoplastic hypoxia.

Role of 3-Deoxy-3-[^{18}F]Fluorothymidine PET in Brain Tumors

Uptakes of the thymidine analogue FLT, developed as a PET tracer to evaluate tumor cell proliferation, correlates with thymidine kinase-1 (TK1) activity in the cell and with proliferation index Ki-67 in tumors including the gliomas of brain. Regarding tumor detection, however, FLT-PET seems to have limited sensitivity. In one study, the potential of FLT as a prognostic marker in glioma was investigated in 19 patients[137] treated with bevacizumab and irinotecan. FLT-PET was obtained at the baseline, 1 to 2 weeks, and 6 weeks after starting treatment. A more than 25% reduction in tumor FLT uptake as measured by standardized uptake value was found to be a predictive metabolic response. Metabolic responders (9/19) lived 3 times as long as nonresponders (10.8 months vs 3.4 months). Both early and late FLT-PET responses were more significant predictors of overall survival compared with that of MR imaging responses.[137]

[^{68}Ga]DOTA-TOC Imaging in Meningioma

Meningiomas demonstrate expression of a variety of receptors, including progesterone, androgen, platelet-derived growth factor, epidermal growth factor, prolactin, dopamine, and somatostatin receptor (SSTR) subtype 2 (SSTR2). The high expression of the somatostatin receptor subtype 2 offers the possibility of receptor-targeted octreotide imaging. Differentiation between meningioma, neurinoma/neurofibromas, and metastases is often difficult with anatomic imaging modalities like CT, and MR imaging biopsy has a high risk of hemorrhage in this tumor. [^{68}Ga]DOTA-TOC shows high meningiomas to background ratios; it

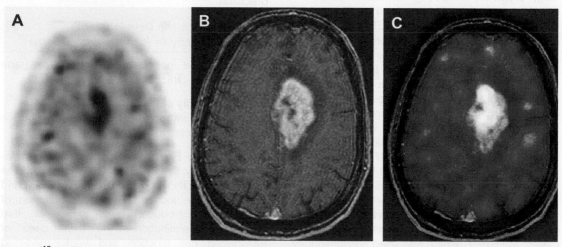

Fig. 7. [^{18}F]EF5-PET/MR imaging of malignant brain tumor hypoxia for radiation treatment planning. Axial [^{18}F]EF5 PET (*A*), axial MR (*B*), and fused PET/MR images (*C*) show uptake of [^{18}F]EF5 in anterior portion of tumor indicating intralesional hypoxia. Note discrepant findings between [^{18}F]EF5 uptake in lesion and structural appearance of lesion. Hypoxic tumors are resistant to either radiation or chemotherapy. Hypoxia agents may play a major role in selection of appropriate patients for radiation therapy planning. (*Courtesy of* Dr Cameron Koch and Dr Sydney Evans.) (*Reproduced from* Kumar R, Dhanpathi H, Basu S, et al. Oncologic PET tracers beyond [^{18}F]FDG and the novel quantitative approaches in PET imaging. Q J Nucl Med Mol Imaging 2008;52(1):50–65; with permission.)

has provided valuable additional information on the extent of meningiomas beneath osseous structures, especially at the skull base.[138] In one study,[139] the kinetic parameters of [^{68}Ga]DOTA-TOC in meningiomas determined by pharmacokinetic modeling of dynamic PET scans was found to provide a more detailed analysis of biologic properties of meningiomas.

Promising Role of Combined Anatomic and Functional Imaging Data

Multimodality image registration has been an area of active research for its implications for improving image-guided surgical resection of brain tumors and for radiation therapy treatment planning. Stereotactic radiosurgery is a technique in which multiple radiation beams are used to deliver high doses to a prescribed tumor volume while subjecting adjacent normal tissues to a much lower radiation dose. Newer PET/CT systems equipped with multidetector CT scanners also allow the possibility of dynamic CT perfusion imaging and angiographic techniques to be incorporated in PET/CT evaluation of brain tumors. However, as MR imaging remains the anatomic imaging study of choice for evaluating brain tumors, there are endeavors to fuse PET with MR imaging data that can offer "one-stop" imaging for the patient with brain tumors. The addition of metabolic imaging to the anatomic imaging of MR imaging provides valuable information for treatment planning, especially in poorly defined or infiltrative neoplasms.[140,141] Pirotte and colleagues[17] studied whether integration of PET data into neuronavigational systems for stereotactic tumor resections could lead to improved outcomes. PET scans (some of which used FDG and others which used MET) were performed on 91 patients in whom neoplasm boundaries could not be confidently determined on MR imaging for navigation-based resection. These studies were combined with MR imaging for resection navigational planning. Tumor volume based on PET was compared with tumor volume based on MR imaging, and in 80% of cases, the difference in volume led to a different final target volume for surgical resection. For the patients who underwent FDG-PET, the PET data altered surgical planning in 69% of cases. MET-PET, which was used predominantly for the low-grade gliomas, improved the tumor volume definition in 88% of low-grade gliomas and 78% of high-grade gliomas. Total resection of the area of increased metabolic activity (either FDG or MET) was accomplished in 52% of the resections. The investigators concluded that PET provided independent and complementary information about neoplastic extent and resection compared with MR imaging alone.

Potential of Novel Image Segmentation Approaches in Image-Guided Radiation Therapy for Brain Tumors

The area of image-guided radiation therapy in brain tumors continues to evolve, and this is based on 2 factors: (a) several innovative PET tracers being tested around the world that act as surrogate biomarkers for different biochemical functions, leading to better understanding of tumor biology at the molecular level; and (b) the availability of newer fusion imaging like PET-CT and the possibility of PET-MR imaging fusion in the near future.[142–145] Vees and colleagues[143] compared the various image segmentation techniques in the delineation of gross tumor volume (GTV) in patients with cerebral glioma. The results highlighted the limitations associated with some of the segmentation algorithms (eg, 2.5 SUV cutoff and the gradient finding GTV approaches) compared with the signal to background ratio (SBR)-based adaptive thresholding technique and its impact on radiotherapy planning in patients with cerebral glioma. The investigators concluded that the selection of the most appropriate FET-PET based segmentation algorithm is crucial for correct delineation of the resulting GTV. It is imperative that the application of these findings into the routine treatment planning scenario would help to define viable tumor boundaries with better precision.[142,144]

PET Imaging in the Development of Gene Therapy in Patients with Glioma

At present, the major issues for effective gene therapy in any clinical context are

1. Heterogeneity of the target tissue
2. Limitations with regard to uniform distribution vector particles throughout the tumor mass

The utility of PET imaging in this promising therapeutic modality lies in (a) accurately defining the tumor with relation to the surrounding tissue, and (b) noninvasive localization and quantitation of exogenously introduced gene expression that allows the determination of the "tissue dose" of transduced cell function and vector-mediated gene expression, which thereby can be correlated with the induced therapeutic effect. Radiolabeled 2-fluoro-2-deoxy-1-β-D-arabinofuranosyl-5-[^{124}I] iodouracil ([^{124}I]FIAU), a specific substrate for HSV-1 thymidine kinase (HSV-1-TK), and PET have been successfully used for the noninvasive localization of retroviral, adenoviral, and herpes viral vector-mediated HSV-1-TK gene expression in glioma. The similar protocol is now being tested in a prospective gene therapy trial in patients with GBM,[146] investigating the safety of intratumorally infused liposome-gene-complex followed by gancyclovir administration. It is imperative that in the future, the identification of viable target tissue and for monitoring the distribution of transgene expression over time by PET imaging will help to identify patients who are likely to benefit from gene therapy. The success of the development of standardized gene therapy protocols as well as efficient and safe vector applications in humans therefore will heavily depend on the molecular imaging techniques led by PET.

PET in Metastatic Brain Tumors

FDG-PET is usually not recommended for investigating metastatic lesions in brain, although these lesions demonstrate FDG hypermetabolism, due to the following reasons: (a) metastatic lesions, when accumulate FDG comparable to normal cortical gray matter, can be missed in the relatively high background environment of normal cerebral cortex. (b) the metastatic lesions are the result of hematogenous seeding, which usually occurs in the normal gray-white junction, making it difficult to be identified with certainty; and (c) the cytotoxic edema surrounding the metastatic lesions demonstrates relatively low FDG accumulation and may decrease the conspicuity of the lesions due to volume averaging effects. In a report by Larcos and colleagues,[147] the studies of 273 patients with various malignancies in whom both whole body and brain images were performed were reviewed. Cerebral metastases were reported in 1.5% of patients and in only 0.7% were the lesions unsuspected before the FDG-PET scan. The investigators concluded that routine screening for cerebral metastases in patients with suspected malignancy has a low yield and may not be clinically useful.

SUMMARY

Functional imaging with PET methodology provides critical information on tumor biology, heterogeneity, and the growth rate of gliomas. The authors speculate that with the advancement of molecular targeted therapies in the management of gliomas there will be further intensification of efforts to develop more appropriate PET tracers designed to demonstrate expression of functional target in vivo, which will allow greater insight into tumor type and grade, and more appropriate definition of tumor biology and extent, effectiveness of therapy, and improvement in treatment planning.

Employing fusion imaging in routine practice is likely to have a substantial impact on brain imaging, particularly in the follow-up of the disease, because metabolic changes tend to precede changes detected with structure-based imaging methods. The development of integrated MR imaging and PET systems, and evolution of appropriate image segmentation techniques would further molecular brain imaging toward achieving the "holy grail" in brain imaging that will ultimately lead to more accurate diagnoses, more informed treatment decisions, and overall improved patient outcome.

REFERENCES

1. Jemal A, Murray T, Ward E, et al. Cancer statistics. CA Cancer J Clin 2005;55:10–30.
2. Smirniotopoulos JG. The new WHO classification of brain tumors. Neuroimaging Clin N Am 1999;9(4): 595–613.
3. Louis DN, Holland EC, Cairncross JG. Glioma classification: a molecular reappraisal. Am J Pathol 2001;159(3):779–86.
4. Furnari FB, Huang HJ, Cavenee WK. Genetics and malignant progression of human brain tumours. Cancer Surv 1995;25:233–75.
5. Ichimura K, Bolin MB, Goike HM, et al. Deregulation of the p14ARF/MDM2/p53 pathway is a prerequisite for human astrocytic gliomas with G1-S transition control gene abnormalities. Cancer Res 2000; 60(2):417–24.
6. Jacobs AH, Thomas A, Kracht LW, et al. ^{18}F-fluoro-L-thymidine and ^{11}C-methylmethionine as markers of increased transport and proliferation in brain tumors. J Nucl Med 2005;46(12):1948–58.
7. Coleman RE, Hoffman JM, Hanson MW, et al. Clinical application of PET for the evaluation of brain tumors. J Nucl Med 1991;32(4):616–22.
8. Herholz K, Wienhard K, Heiss WD. Validity of PET studies in brain tumors. Cerebrovasc Brain Metab Rev 1990;2(3):240–65.
9. Price P. PET as a potential tool for imaging molecular mechanisms of oncology in man. Trends Mol Med 2001;7(10):442–6.
10. Jacobs AH, Dittmar C, Winkeler A, et al. Molecular imaging of gliomas. Mol Imaging 2002;1(4):309–35.
11. Utriainen M, Komu M, Vuorinen V, et al. Evaluation of brain tumor metabolism with [11C]choline PET and 1H-MRS. J Neurooncol 2003;62(3):329–38.
12. Tian M, Zhang H, Oriuchi N, et al. Comparison of ^{11}C-choline PET and FDG PET for the differential diagnosis of malignant tumors. Eur J Nucl Med Mol Imaging 2004;31(8):1064–72.
13. Heiss WD, Pawlik G, Herholz K, et al. Regional kinetic constants and cerebral metabolic rate for glucose in normal human volunteers determined

by dynamic positron emission tomography of [^{18}F]-2-fluoro-2-deoxy-D-glucose. J Cereb Blood Flow Metab 1984;4(2):212–23.

14. Phelps ME. PET: the merging of biology and imaging into molecular imaging. J Nucl Med 2000;41(4):661–81.

15. Kitajima K, Nakamoto Y, Okizuka H, et al. Accuracy of whole-body FDG-PET/CT for detecting brain metastases from non-central nervous system tumors. Ann Nucl Med 2008;22(7):595–602.

16. Miwa K, Shinoda J, Yano H, et al. Discrepancy between lesion distributions on methionine PET and MR images in patients with glioblastoma multiforme: insight from a PET and MR fusion image study. J Neurol Neurosurg Psychiatry 2004;75(10):1457–62.

17. Pirotte B, Goldman S, Dewitte O, et al. Integrated positron emission tomography and magnetic resonance imaging-guided resection of brain tumors: a report of 103 consecutive procedures. J Neurosurg 2006;104(2):238–53.

18. Pichler BJ, Judenhofer MS, Wehrl HF. PET/MRI hybrid imaging: devices and initial results. Eur Radiol 2008;18(6):1077–86.

19. Judenhofer MS, Wehrl HF, Newport DF, et al. Simultaneous PET-MRI: a new approach for functional and morphological imaging. Nat Med 2008;14(4):459–65.

20. Weber G. Enzymology of cancer cells (first of two parts). N Engl J Med 1977;296(9):486–92.

21. Hatanaka M, Augl C, Gilden RV. Evidence for a functional change in the plasma membrane of murine sarcoma virus-infected mouse embryo cells. Transport and transport-associated phosphorylation of ^{14}C-2-deoxy-D-glucose. J Biol Chem 1970;245(4):714–7.

22. Gallagher BM, Fowler JS, Gutterson NI, et al. Metabolic trapping as a principle of radiopharmaceutical design: some factors responsible for the biodistribution of [^{18}F] 2-deoxy-2-fluoro-D-glucose. J Nucl Med 1978;19(10):1154–61.

23. Merrall NW, Plevin R, Gould GW. Growth factors, mitogens, oncogenes and the regulation of glucose transport. Cell Signal 1993;5(6):667–75.

24. Nishioka T, Oda Y, Seino Y, et al. Distribution of the glucose transporters in human brain tumors. Cancer Res 1992;52(14):3972–9.

25. Floeth FW, Pauleit D, Sabel M, et al. ^{18}F-FET PET differentiation of ring-enhancing brain lesions. J Nucl Med 2006;47(5):776–82.

26. Zhuang H, Alavi A. 18-Fluorodeoxyglucose positron emission tomographic imaging in the detection and monitoring of infection and inflammation. Semin Nucl Med 2002;32(1):47–59.

27. Kubota R, Yamada S, Kubota K, et al. Intratumoral distribution of fluorine-18-fluorodeoxyglucose in vivo: high accumulation in macrophages and granulation tissues studied by microautoradiography. J Nucl Med 1992;33(11):1972–80.

28. Chakrabarti R, Jung CY, Lee TP, et al. Changes in glucose transport and transporter isoforms during the activation of human peripheral blood lymphocytes by phytohemagglutinin. J Immunol 1994;152(6):2660–8.

29. Gamelli RL, Liu H, He LK, et al. Augmentations of glucose uptake and glucose transporter-1 in macrophages following thermal injury and sepsis in mice. J Leukoc Biol 1996;59(5):639–47.

30. Sorbara LR, Maldarelli F, Chamoun G, et al. Human immunodeficiency virus type 1 infection of H9 cells induces increased glucose transporter expression. J Virol 1996;70(10):7275–9.

31. Ahmed N, Kansara M, Berridge MV. Acute regulation of glucose transport in a monocyte-macrophage cell line: Glut-3 affinity for glucose is enhanced during the respiratory burst. Biochem J 1997;327(Pt 2):369–75.

32. Janus TJ, Kim EE, Tilbury R, et al. Use of [^{18}F]fluorodeoxyglucose positron emission tomography in patients with primary malignant brain tumors. Ann Neurol 1993;33(5):540–8.

33. Spence AM, Muzi M, Mankoff DA, et al. ^{18}F-FDG PET of gliomas at delayed intervals: improved distinction between tumor and normal gray matter. J Nucl Med 2004;45(10):1653–9.

34. Herholz K, Pietrzyk U, Voges J, et al. Correlation of glucose consumption and tumor cell density in astrocytomas. A stereotactic PET study. J Neurosurg 1993;79(6):853–8.

35. Hustinx R, Smith RJ, Benard F, et al. Can the standardized uptake value characterize primary brain tumors on FDG-PET? Eur J Nucl Med 1999;26(11):1501–9.

36. Kubota K. From tumor biology to clinical Pet: a review of positron emission tomography (PET) in oncology. Ann Nucl Med 2001;15(6):471–86.

37. Kim S, Chung JK, Im SH, et al. ^{11}C-methionine PET as a prognostic marker in patients with glioma: comparison with ^{18}F-FDG PET. Eur J Nucl Med Mol Imaging 2005;32(1):52–9.

38. Delbeke D, Meyerowitz C, Lapidus RL, et al. Optimal cutoff levels of F-18 fluorodeoxyglucose uptake in the differentiation of low-grade from high-grade brain tumors with PET. Radiology 1995;195(1):47–52.

39. Kaschten B, Stevenaert A, Sadzot B, et al. Preoperative evaluation of 54 gliomas by PET with fluorine-18-fluorodeoxyglucose and/or carbon-11-methionine. J Nucl Med 1998;39(5):778–85.

40. Ogawa T, Inugami A, Hatazawa J, et al. Clinical positron emission tomography for brain tumors: comparison of fludeoxyglucose F 18 and L-methyl-^{11}C-methionine. AJNR Am J Neuroradiol 1996;17(2):345–53.

41. Tsuchida T, Takeuchi H, Okazawa H, et al. Grading of brain glioma with 1-^{11}C-acetate PET: comparison with ^{18}F-FDG PET. Nucl Med Biol 2008;35(2):171–6.

42. Herholz K, Rudolf J, Heiss WD. FDG transport and phosphorylation in human gliomas measured with dynamic PET. J Neurooncol 1992;12(2):159–65.

43. Fischman AJ, Alpert NM. FDG-PET in oncology: there's more to it than looking at pictures. J Nucl Med 1993;34(1):6–11.

44. Stockhammer F, Thomale UW, Plotkin M, et al. Association between fluorine-18-labeled fluorodeoxyglucose uptake and 1p and 19q loss of heterozygosity in World Health Organization Grade II gliomas. J Neurosurg 2007;106(4):633–7.

45. Di Chiro G. Positron emission tomography using [^{18}F] fluorodeoxyglucose in brain tumors. A powerful diagnostic and prognostic tool. Invest Radiol 1987;22(5):360–71.

46. Alavi JB, Alavi A, Chawluk J, et al. Positron emission tomography in patients with glioma. A predictor of prognosis. Cancer 1988;62(6): 1074–8.

47. Borgwardt L, Højgaard L, Carstensen H, et al. Increased fluorine-18 2-fluoro-2-deoxy-D-glucose (FDG) uptake in childhood CNS tumors is correlated with malignancy grade: a study with FDG positron emission tomography/magnetic resonance imaging coregistration and image fusion. J Clin Oncol 2005;23(13):3030–7.

48. Barker FG 2nd, Chang SM, Valk PE, et al. 18-Fluorodeoxyglucose uptake and survival of patients with suspected recurrent malignant glioma. Cancer 1997;79(1):115–26.

49. Padma MV, Said S, Jacobs M, et al. Prediction of pathology and survival by FDG PET in gliomas. J Neurooncol 2003;64(3):227–37.

50. Patronas NJ, Di Chiro G, Kufta C, et al. Prediction of survival in glioma patients by means of positron emission tomography. J Neurosurg 1985;62(6): 816–22.

51. Tyler JL, Diksic M, Villemure JG, et al. Metabolic and hemodynamic evaluation of gliomas using positron emission tomography. J Nucl Med 1987; 28(7):1123–33.

52. Rozental JM, Cohen JD, Mehta MP, et al. Acute changes in glucose uptake after treatment: the effects of carmustine (BCNU) on human glioblastoma multiforme. J Neurooncol 1993;15(1):57–66.

53. De Souza B, Brunetti A, Fulham MJ, et al. Pituitary microadenoma: a PET study. Radiology 1990;177: 39–44.

54. Kwee SA, Ko JP, Jiang CS, et al. Solitary brain lesions enhancing at MR imaging: Evaluation with fluorine 18-fluorocholine PET. Radiology 2007;244: 557–65.

55. Cremerius U, Striepecke E, Henn W, et al. [[18]FDG-PET in intracranial meningiomas versus grading, proliferation index, cellular density and cytogenetic analysis]. Nuklearmedizin 1994;33(4):144–9.

56. Henry JM, Heffner RR Jr, Dillard SH, et al. Primary malignant lymphomas of the central nervous system. Cancer 1974;34(4):1293–302.

57. Kracht LW, Bauer A, Herholz K, et al. Positron emission tomography in a case of intracranial hemangiopericytoma. J Comput Assist Tomogr 1999; 23(3):365–8.

58. Kim EE, Chung SK, Haynie TP, et al. Differentiation of residual or recurrent tumors from post-treatment changes with F-18 FDG PET. Radiographics 1992; 12(2):269–79.

59. Wurker M, Herholz K, Voges J, et al. Glucose consumption and methionine uptake in low-grade gliomas after iodine-125 brachytherapy. Eur J Nucl Med 1996;23(5):583–6.

60. Brock CS, Young H, O'Reilly SM, et al. Early evaluation of tumour metabolic response using [^{18}F] fluorodeoxyglucose and positron emission tomography: a pilot study following the phase II chemotherapy schedule for temozolomide in recurrent high-grade gliomas. Br J Cancer 2000;82(3): 608–15.

61. Henze M, Mohammed A, Schlemmer HP, et al. PET and SPECT for detection of tumor progression in irradiated low-grade astrocytoma: a receiver-operating-characteristic analysis. J Nucl Med 2004; 45(4):579–86.

62. Ricci PE, Karis JP, Heiserman JE, et al. Differentiating recurrent tumor from radiation necrosis: time for re-evaluation of positron emission tomography? AJNR Am J Neuroradiol 1998;19(3):407–13.

63. Patronas NJ, Di Chiro G, Brooks RA, et al. Work in progress: [^{18}F] fluorodeoxyglucose and positron emission tomography in the evaluation of radiation necrosis of the brain. Radiology 1982;144(4): 885–9.

64. Reinhardt MJ, Kubota K, Yamada S, et al. Assessment of cancer recurrence in residual tumors after fractionated radiotherapy: a comparison of fluorodeoxyglucose, L-methionine and thymidine. J Nucl Med 1997;38(2):280–7.

65. Yamamoto T, Nishizawa S, Maruyama I, et al. Acute effects of stereotactic radiosurgery on the kinetics of glucose metabolism in metastatic brain tumors: FDG PET study. Ann Nucl Med 2001;15(2): 103–9.

66. De Witte O, Levivier M, Violon P, et al. Prognostic value positron emission tomography with [^{18}F]fluoro-2-deoxy-D-glucose in the low-grade glioma. Neurosurgery 1996;39(3):470–6 [discussion: 6–7].

67. Glantz MJ, Hoffman JM, Coleman RE, et al. Identification of early recurrence of primary central nervous system tumors by [^{18}F]fluorodeoxyglucose positron emission tomography. Ann Neurol 1991; 29(4):347–55.

68. Fulham MJ, Brunetti A, Aloj L, et al. Decreased cerebral glucose metabolism in patients with brain tumors: an effect of corticosteroids. J Neurosurg 1995;83(4):657–64.

69. Wong TZ, Turkington TG, Hawk TC, et al. PET and brain tumor image fusion. Cancer J 2004;10(4): 234–42.

70. Kahn D, Follett KA, Bushnell DL, et al. Diagnosis of recurrent brain tumor: value of 201Tl SPECT vs ^{18}F-fluorodeoxyglucose PET. AJR Am J Roentgenol 1994;163(6):1459–65.

71. Ortega-Lopez N, Mendoza-Vasquez RG, Adame-Ocampo G, et al. Validation of MRI and ^{18}F-FDG-PET coregistration in patients with primary brain tumors. Gac Med Mex 2007;143(4):309–16.

72. Wyss M, Hofer S, Bruehlmeier M, et al. Early metabolic responses in temozolomide treated low-grade glioma patients. J Neurooncol 2009 [Epub ahead of print].

73. Pirotte B, Goldman S, Brucher JM, et al. PET in stereotactic conditions increases the diagnostic yield of brain biopsy. Stereotact Funct Neurosurg 1994;63(1-4):144–9.

74. Levivier M, Goldman S, Pirotte B, et al. Diagnostic yield of stereotactic brain biopsy guided by positron emission tomography with [18F]fluorodeoxyglucose. J Neurosurg 1995;82(3):445–52.

75. Goldman S, Levivier M, Pirotte B, et al. Regional methionine and glucose uptake in high-grade gliomas: a comparative study on PET-guided stereotactic biopsy. J Nucl Med 1997;38(9): 1459–62.

76. Massager N, David P, Goldman S, et al. Combined magnetic resonance imaging- and positron emission tomography-guided stereotactic biopsy in brainstem mass lesions: diagnostic yield in a series of 30 patients. J Neurosurg 2000;93(6):951–7.

77. Rosenfeld SS, Hoffman JM, Coleman RE, et al. Studies of primary central nervous system lymphoma with fluorine-18-fluorodeoxyglucose positron emission tomography. J Nucl Med 1992; 33(4):532–6.

78. Hoffman JM, Waskin HA, Schifter T, et al. FDG-PET in differentiating lymphoma from nonmalignant central nervous system lesions in patients with AIDS. J Nucl Med 1993;34(4):567–75.

79. Kim do K, Kim IJ, Hwang S, et al. System L-amino acid transporters are differently expressed in rat astrocyte and C6 glioma cells. Neurosci Res 2004;50:437–46.

80. Isselbacher KJ. Sugar and amino acid transport by cells in culture—differences between normal and malignant cells. N Engl J Med 1972;286(17): 929–33.

81. Jager PL, Vaalburg W, Pruim J, et al. Radiolabeled amino acids: basic aspects and clinical applications in oncology. J Nucl Med 2001;42(3):432–45.

82. Lilja A, Bergstrom K, Hartvig P, et al. Dynamic study of supratentorial gliomas with L-methyl-^{11}C-methionine and positron emission tomography. AJNR Am J Neuroradiol 1985;6(4):505–14.

83. Derlon JM, Bourdet C, Bustany P, et al. [11C]L-methionine uptake in gliomas. Neurosurgery 1989;25(5):720–8.

84. O'Tuama LA, Phillips PC, Strauss LC, et al. Two-phase [11C]L-methionine PET in childhood brain tumors. Pediatr Neurol 1990;6(3):163–70.

85. Ogawa T, Shishido F, Kanno I, et al. Cerebral glioma: evaluation with methionine PET. Radiology 1993;186(1):45–53.

86. Chung JK, Kim YK, Kim SK, et al. Usefulness of ^{11}C-methionine PET in the evaluation of brain lesions that are hypo- or isometabolic on ^{18}F-FDG PET. Eur J Nucl Med Mol Imaging 2002;29(2): 176–82.

87. Herholz K, Holzer T, Bauer B, et al. ^{11}C-methionine PET for differential diagnosis of low-grade gliomas. Neurology 1998;50(5):1316–22.

88. Bergstrom M, Collins VP, Ehrin E, et al. Discrepancies in brain tumor extent as shown by computed tomography and positron emission tomography using [68Ga]EDTA, [11C]glucose, and [11C]methionine. J Comput Assist Tomogr 1983; 7(6):1062–6.

89. Mosskin M, Ericson K, Hindmarsh T, et al. Positron emission tomography compared with magnetic resonance imaging and computed tomography in supratentorial gliomas using multiple stereotactic biopsies as reference. Acta Radiol 1989;30(3): 225–32.

90. Pirotte B, Goldman S, David P, et al. Stereotactic brain biopsy guided by positron emission tomography (PET) with [F-18]fluorodeoxyglucose and [C-11]methionine. Acta Neurochir Suppl 1997;68: 133–8.

91. Kapouleas I, Alavi A, Alves WM, et al. Registration of three-dimensional MR and PET images of the human brain without markers. Radiology 1991; 181(3):731–9.

92. Derlon JM, Petit-Taboue MC, Chapon F, et al. The in vivo metabolic pattern of low-grade brain gliomas: a positron emission tomographic study using ^{18}F-fluorodeoxyglucose and ^{11}C-L-methylmethionine. Neurosurgery 1997;40(2):276–87 [discussion: 87–8].

93. Mosskin M, Bergstrom M, Collins VP, et al. Positron emission tomography with ^{11}C-methionine of intracranial tumours compared with histology of multiple biopsies. Acta Radiol Suppl 1986;369:157–60.

94. Van Laere K, Ceyssens S, Van Calenbergh F, et al. Direct comparison of ^{18}F-FDG and ^{11}C-methionine PET in suspected recurrence of glioma: sensitivity, inter-observer variability and prognostic value. Eur J Nucl Med Mol Imaging 2005;32(1):39–51.

95. De Witte O, Goldberg I, Wikler D, et al. Positron emission tomography with injection of methionine as a prognostic factor in glioma. J Neurosurg 2001;95(5):746–50.

96. Piepmeier J, Christopher S, Spencer D, et al. Variations in the natural history and survival of patients with supratentorial low-grade astrocytomas. Neurosurgery 1996;38(5):872–8 [discussion: 8–9].

97. Lote K, Egeland T, Hager B, et al. Survival, prognostic factors, and therapeutic efficacy in low-grade glioma: a retrospective study in 379 patients. J Clin Oncol 1997;15(9):3129–40.

98. Ribom D, Eriksson A, Hartman M, et al. Positron emission tomography (11)C-methionine and survival in patients with low-grade gliomas. Cancer 2001;92(6):1541–9.

99. Ogawa T, Kanno I, Shishido F, et al. Clinical value of PET with ^{18}F-fluorodeoxyglucose and L-methyl-^{11}C-methionine for diagnosis of recurrent brain tumor and radiation injury. Acta Radiol 1991;32(3): 197–202.

100. Lilja A, Lundqvist H, Olsson Y, et al. Positron emission tomography and computed tomography in differential diagnosis between recurrent or residual glioma and treatment-induced brain lesions. Acta Radiol 1989;30(2):121–8.

101. Sonoda Y, Kumabe T, Takahashi T, et al. Clinical usefulness of ^{11}C-MET PET and ^{201}T1 SPECT for differentiation of recurrent glioma from radiation necrosis. Neurol Med Chir (Tokyo) 1998;38(6): 342–7 [discussion: 7–8].

102. Wienhard K, Herholz K, Coenen HH, et al. Increased amino acid transport into brain tumors measured by PET of L-(2-^{18}F)fluorotyrosine. J Nucl Med 1991;32(7):1338–46.

103. Pruim J, Willemsen AT, Molenaar WM, et al. Brain tumors: L-[1-C-11]tyrosine PET for visualization and quantification of protein synthesis rate. Radiology 1995;197(1):221–6.

104. Weckesser M, Langen KJ, Rickert CH, et al. O-(2-[(18)F]fluoroethyl)-L-tyrosine PET in the clinical evaluation of primary brain tumours. Eur J Nucl Med Mol Imaging 2005;32:422–9.

105. Bader JB, Samnick S, Moringlane JR, et al. Evaluation of I-3-[^{123}I]iodo-alpha-methyltyrosine SPET and [^{18}F]fluorodeoxyglucose PET in the detection and grading of recurrences in patients pretreated for gliomas at follow-up: a comparative study with stereotactic biopsy. Eur J Nucl Med 1999;26(2): 144–51.

106. Biersack HJ, Coenen HH, Stocklin G, et al. Imaging of brain tumors with L-3-[^{123}I]iodo-alpha-methyl tyrosine and SPECT. J Nucl Med 1989;30(1):110–2.

107. Chen W, Silverman DH, Delaloye S, et al. ^{18}F-FDOPA PET imaging of brain tumors: comparison study with ^{18}F-FDG PET and evaluation of diagnostic accuracy. J Nucl Med 2006;47(6):904–11.

108. de Wolde H, Pruim J, Mastik MF, et al. Proliferative activity in human brain tumors: comparison of histopathology and L-[1-(11)C]tyrosine PET. J Nucl Med 1997;38(9):1369–74.

109. Miyagawa T, Oku T, Uehara H, et al. "Facilitated" amino acid transport is upregulated in brain tumors. J Cereb Blood Flow Metab 1998;18:500–9.

110. Weber WA, Wester HJ, Grosu AL, et al. O-(2-[^{18}F]fluoroethyl)-L-tyrosine and L-[methyl-^{11}C]methionine uptake in brain tumours: initial results of a comparative study. Eur J Nucl Med 2000;27(5): 542–9.

111. Floeth FW, Pauleit D, Sabel M, et al. Prognostic value of O-(2-^{18}F-fluoroethyl)-L-tyrosine PET and MRI in low-grade glioma. J Nucl Med 2007;48(4): 519–27.

112. Floeth FW, Sabel M, Stoffels G, et al. Prognostic value of ^{18}F-fluoroethyl-L-tyrosine PET and MRI in small nonspecific incidental brain lesions. J Nucl Med 2008;49(5):730–7.

113. Mehrkens JH, Popperl G, Rachinger W, et al. The positive predictive value of O-(2-[^{18}F]fluoroethyl)-L-tyrosine (FET) PET in the diagnosis of a glioma recurrence after multimodal treatment. J Neurooncol 2008;88(1):27–35.

114. Pauleit D, Floeth F, Hamacher K, et al. O-(2-[^{18}F]fluoroethyl)-L-tyrosine PET combined with MRI improves the diagnostic assessment of cerebral gliomas. Brain 2005;128:678–87.

115. Floeth FW, Pauleit D, Wittsack HJ, et al. Multimodal metabolic imaging of cerebral gliomas: Positron emission tomography with [^{18}F]fluoroethyl L-tyrosine and magnetic resonance spectroscopy. J Neurosurg 2005;102:318–27.

116. Schiepers C, Chen W, Cloughesy T, et al. ^{18}F-FDOPA kinetics in brain tumors. J Nucl Med 2007;48(10): 1651–61.

117. Chen W. Clinical applications of PET in brain tumors. J Nucl Med 2007;48(9):1468–81.

118. Shinoura N, Nishijima M, Hara T, et al. Brain tumors: detection with C-11 choline PET. Radiology 1997; 202(2):497–503.

119. Ohtani T, Kurihara H, Ishiuchi S, et al. Brain tumour imaging with carbon-11 choline: comparison with FDG PET and gadolinium-enhanced MR imaging. Eur J Nucl Med 2001;28(11):1664–70.

120. Hara T, Kosaka N, Shinoura N, et al. PET imaging of brain tumor with [methyl-^{11}C]choline. J Nucl Med 1997;38(6):842–7.

121. Chen W, Cloughesy T, Kamdar N, et al. Imaging proliferation in brain tumors with ^{18}F-FLT PET: comparison with ^{18}F-FDG. J Nucl Med 2005; 46(6):945–52.

122. Choi SJ, Kim JS, Kim JH, et al. [^{18}F]3'-deoxy-3'-fluorothymidine PET for the diagnosis and grading of brain tumors. Eur J Nucl Med Mol Imaging 2005; 32(6):653–9.

123. Saga T, Kawashima H, Araki N, et al. Evaluation of primary brain tumors with FLT-PET: usefulness and limitations. Clin Nucl Med 2006;31(12):774–80.

124. Hatakeyama T, Kawai N, Nishiyama Y, et al. (11)C-methionine (MET) and (18)F-fluorothymidine (FLT) PET in patients with newly diagnosed glioma. Eur J Nucl Med Mol Imaging 2008;35(11):2009–17.

125. Shields AF, Grierson JR, Dohmen BM, et al. Imaging proliferation in vivo with [F-18]FLT and positron emission tomography. Nat Med 1998; 4(11):1334–6.

126. Hengstschlager M, Knofler M, Mullner EW, et al. Different regulation of thymidine kinase during the cell cycle of normal versus DNA tumor virus-transformed cells. J Biol Chem 1994;269(19):13836–42.

127. Brown JM, Giaccia AJ. Tumour hypoxia: the picture has changed in the 1990s. Int J Radiat Biol 1994; 65(1):95–102.

128. Gray LH, Conger AD, Ebert M, et al. The concentration of oxygen dissolved in tissues at the time of irradiation as a factor in radiotherapy. Br J Radiol 1953;26(312):638–48.

129. Janssen HL, Haustermans KM, Balm AJ, et al. Hypoxia in head and neck cancer: how much, how important? Head Neck 2005;27(7):622–38.

130. Hockel M, Schlenger K, Aral B, et al. Association between tumor hypoxia and malignant progression in advanced cancer of the uterine cervix. Cancer Res 1996;56(19):4509–15.

131. Brizel DM, Scully SP, Harrelson JM, et al. Tumor oxygenation predicts for the likelihood of distant metastases in human soft tissue sarcoma. Cancer Res 1996;56(5):941–3.

132. Brizel DM, Sibley GS, Prosnitz LR, et al. Tumor hypoxia adversely affects the prognosis of carcinoma of the head and neck. Int J Radiat Oncol Biol Phys 1997;38(2):285–9.

133. Evans SM, Jenkins WT, Joiner B, et al. 2-Nitroimidazole (EF5) binding predicts radiation resistance in individual 9L s.c. tumors. Cancer Res 1996;56(2):405–11.

134. Ziemer LS, Evans SM, Kachur AV, et al. Noninvasive imaging of tumor hypoxia in rats using the 2-nitroimidazole ^{18}F-EF5. Eur J Nucl Med Mol Imaging 2003;30(2):259–66.

135. Komar G, Seppänen M, Eskola O, et al. ^{18}F-EF5: a new PET tracer for imaging hypoxia in head and neck cancer. J Nucl Med 2008;49(12):1944–51.

136. Koch CJ, Evans SM, Lord EM. Oxygen dependence of cellular uptake of EF5 [2-(2-nitro-1H-imidazol-1-yl)-N-(2,2,3,3,3-pentafluoropropyl)acetamide]: analysis of drug adducts by fluorescent antibodies

vs bound radioactivity. Br J Cancer 1995;72(4):869–74.

137. Chen W, Delaloye S, Silverman DHS, et al. Predicting treatment response of malignant gliomas to bevacizumab and irinotecan by imaging proliferation with ^{18}F fluorothymidine positron emission tomography: a pilot study. J Clin Oncol 2007;25:4714–21.

138. Henze M, Schuhmacher J, Hipp P, et al. PET imaging of SSTR using ^{68}Ga]-DOTA-D Phe1-Tyr3-octreotide (DOTA-TOC): first results in meningioma-patients. J Nucl Med 2001;42:1053–6.

139. Henze M, Dimitrakopoulou-Strauss A, Milker-Zabel S, et al. Characterization of ^{68}Ga-DOTA-D-Phe1-Tyr3-octreotide kinetics in patients with meningiomas. J Nucl Med 2005;46(5):763–9.

140. Levivier M, Wikier D, Goldman S, et al. Integration of the metabolic data of positron emission tomography in the dosimetry planning of radiosurgery with the gamma knife: early experience with brain tumors. Technical note. J Neurosurg 2000; 93(Suppl 3):233–8.

141. Levivier M, Wikler D Jr, Massager N, et al. The integration of metabolic imaging in stereotactic procedures including radiosurgery: a review. J Neurosurg 2002;97(5 Suppl):542–50.

142. Basu S, Zaidi H, Houseni M, et al. Novel quantitative techniques for assessing regional and global function and structure based on modern imaging modalities: implications for normal variation, aging and diseased states. Semin Nucl Med 2007; 37(3):223–39.

143. Vees H, Senthamizhchelvan S, Miralbell R, et al. Assessment of various strategies for (18)F-FET PET-guided delineation of target volumes in high-grade glioma patients. Eur J Nucl Med Mol Imaging 2009;36(2):182–93.

144. Basu S. Selecting the optimal image segmentation strategy in the era of multitracer multimodality imaging: a critical step for image-guided radiation therapy. Eur J Nucl Med Mol Imaging 2009;36(2):180–1.

145. Jacobs A, Voges J, Reszka R, et al. Positron-emission tomography of vector-mediated gene expression in gene therapy for gliomas. Lancet 2001; 358:727–9.

146. Voges J, Weber F, Reszka R, et al. Clinical protocol. Liposomal gene therapy with the herpes simplex thymidine kinase gene/ganciclovir system for the treatment of glioblastoma multiforme. Hum Gene Ther 2002;13:675–85.

147. Larcos G, Maisey MN. FDG-PET screening for cerebral metastases in patients with suspected malignancy. Nucl Med Commun 1996;17(3):197–8.

Therapeutic Advances in Malignant Glioma: Current Status and Future Prospects

H. Ian Robins, MD, PhD[a,b,c], Andrew B. Lassman, MD[d],
Deepak Khuntia, MD[e,*]

KEYWORDS

- Radiation sensitizers • Temozolomide • Glioblastoma
- Pseudoresponse • Pseudoprogression • Targeted agents

Of the approximately 23,000 new cases of malignant central nervous system neoplasms diagnosed annually in the United States, more than half will be categorized as glioblastoma, which is the most aggressive subtype of the malignant gliomas.[1] Despite the application of radiation, chemotherapy, and modern aggressive surgical approaches,[2–4] average survival is approximately 1 year.

However, several strategies are under investigation to improve outcome. The first involves attempts to enhance the benefit from radiation, which is the most powerful nonsurgical tool. Attempts at dose escalation more than 6000 cGy have resulted in increased toxicity without a survival benefit. Therefore, radiation sensitizers have been explored. To improve local control and limit toxicity to normal brain tissue, novel imaging techniques (eg, chemical shift imaging) are being explored to better define radiotherapy fields.[5]

Other confounds to therapy relate to drug resistance or interactions (eg, P450 induction or inhibition) and overcoming the blood–brain barrier with systemic drug therapies. The alkylating agent temozolomide has emerged as a key antineoplastic agent that may also have radiosensitizing effects.[6] Ongoing clinical trials are evaluating temozolomide in combination with other systemic agents (eg, motexafin gadolinium, mammalian target of rapamycin [mTOR] inhibitors, farnesyl-transferase inhibitors, tyrosine kinase inhibitors [TKIs], and antiangiogenesis agents), which have shown promising activity in combination with radiotherapy.

Additionally, the ability to assess progression radiographically has become an ever increasing and daunting task. It has become increasingly apparent that early and late radiotherapy effects can be mistaken for progressive disease with MRI and MR spectroscopy, often called *pseudoprogression*. Pseudoprogression is especially seen with combined modality approaches (eg, temozolomide, radiotherapy), occurring in up to 20% of patients.[7]

[a] Department of Medicine, University of Wisconsin School of Medicine and Public Health, Madison, WI 53792, USA

[b] Department of Neurology, University of Wisconsin School of Medicine and Public Health, Madison, WI 53792, USA

[c] Department of Human Oncology, University of Wisconsin School of Medicine and Public Health, Madison, WI 53792, USA

[d] Department of Neurology and the Brain Tumor Center, Memorial Sloan-Kettering Cancer Center, New York, NY 10065, USA

[e] Department of Human Oncology, University of Wisconsin School of Medicine and Public Health, 600 Highland Avenue, K4-B100, Madison, WI 53792, USA

* Corresponding author.

E-mail address: khuntia@humonc.wisc.edu (D. Khuntia).

Neuroimag Clin N Am 19 (2009) 647–656
doi:10.1016/j.nic.2009.08.015
1052-5149/09/$ – see front matter. Published by Elsevier Inc.

Moreover, the potential for a pseudoresponse in some clinical scenarios is now recognized. The use of vascular endothelial growth factor (VEGF) inhibitors, which affect vascular permeability, can reduce contrast enhancement on MRI and CT scans as a result of diminished penetration of contrast agents. Therefore, scan changes during treatment with VEGF inhibitors may overestimate the extent of response when using traditional imaging criteria.[8] These considerations complicate the care management of individual patients, interpretation of clinical trial data, and development strategies for future clinical investigation.

This article identifies the current status and trends for the treatment of gliomas (focusing on glioblastoma), and describes some of the difficulties and controversies.

NEWLY DIAGNOSED GLIOBLASTOMA: CURRENT STANDARD OF CARE

Until recently, the median overall survival of patients who had glioblastoma generally ranged from 10 to 12 months, with fewer than 10% of patients surviving 2 years.[9] Meta-analyses showed a modest benefit to the use of adjuvant nitrosourea-based chemotherapy,[9,10] and early trials showed that nitrosoureas increased the likelihood of surviving more than 18 months.[11] Strategies for newly diagnosed glioblastoma have varied. Gilbert and colleagues[12] used preradiation temozolomide as an adjunct to treatment. Although preradiation temozolomide resulted in an impressive 41% response rate, response duration was short, and median overall survival was in the typical range of 1 year.

In 2003, the use of carmustine (BCNU)-impregnated wafers (Gliadel) in a phase III placebo-controlled study of patients who had World Health Organization (WHO) grade III and IV gliomas suggested a survival advantage[13]; however, when patients who did not have glioblastomas were removed from the analysis, the study was underpowered to show a statistically significant result.[14] Furthermore, no significant improvement in progression-free survival was seen, which many neurooncologists consider a surrogate marker for overall survival. In addition, wafer implantation may lead to increased difficulty with wound healing and infection, and confound MRI interpretation. Nonetheless, Gliadel wafers are an approved standard of care for newly diagnosed glioblastoma.

A significant therapeutic breakthrough occurred when Stupp and co-workers reported results of the use of daily temozolomide (75 mg/m^2) during radiotherapy (approximately 6 weeks), followed by 6 months of adjuvant therapy at 150 to 200 mg/m^2 on days 1 through 5 for a 28-day cycle.[15] Median survival in this phase II study was 16 months. The rationale for this approach included the possibility of radiosensitization, for which preclinical support now exists.[16]

The concept of daily dosing was also supported by observations showing that extended daily administration of temozolomide depletes the DNA-repair enzyme O-6-methylguanine-DNA methyltransferase (MGMT).[17] MGMT is a proposed resistance mechanism for temozolomide. After MGMT removes a methyl group from DNA (deposited by temozolomide), it is no longer active; hence, MGMT is called a *suicide enzyme*.

This concept was tested in the recurrent setting with encouraging results preliminarily.[18] Use of adjuvant temozolomide starting 1 month postradiotherapy was predicated on the inherent antitumor activity of the drug. This study showed a promising 2-year survival rate of 31% and led to a confirmatory (European/Canadian) phase III trial comparing the phase II regimen with radiotherapy alone. This randomized phase III trial[6] confirmed the earlier phase II study,[15] showing that the experimental regimen (now colloquially known as the *Stupp Regimen*) produces a statistically significant increase in median overall survival of 12.1 versus 14.6 months and, more impressively, an improved 2-year survival of 10% versus 26%. Longer follow-up also shows that the benefit was sustained after 4 and 5 years.[19]

A retrospective analysis of tissue samples from this study also suggested that *MGMT* promoter methylation correlates with improved outcome.[20,21] When the promoter region of the *MGMT* gene is methylated, the gene is silenced (ie, transcriptionally inactive and therefore ultimately not producing MGMT enzyme). Patients who had tumors harboring *MGMT* promoter methylation who were randomized to receive temozolomide had a median survival of 15.3 months and a 2-year survival rate of 46%, compared with 12.7 months and 13.8% for patients who had tumors not exhibiting promoter methylation.

However, several observations suggest the biology may be more complicated. First, patients in the control arm (who received radiotherapy alone at diagnosis and of whom approximately 60% received temozolomide at recurrence), promoter methylation also resulted in clinical benefit (ie, overall survival of 15.3 versus. 11.8 months for patients who had an unmethylated promoter). Other studies have also shown that MGMT promoter methylation correlates with a survival benefit for patients treated with radiotherapy alone.[22]

In addition, immunohistochemistry for MGMT expression does not correlate with survival.[23] Therefore, it is possible that MGMT promoter methylation contributes to prognosis through MGMT inactivation, but may also serve as a marker of as unidentified prognostic factors. Other markers under investigation for prognostic value include epidermal growth factor receptor (EGFR) amplification, tenascin expression, phosphatase and tensin homolog on chromosome 10 (PTEN), loss of chromosome 10, mutation or loss of the *P53* gene, and expression of YKL-40.[24–27] In addition, the finding of MGMT promoter methylation status as a putative marker of response to therapy and outcome has stimulated further laboratory and clinical evaluation of other temozolomide resistance mechanisms, such as the base excision repair pathway. This pathway depends on a group of enzymes in the poly (ADP-ribose) polymerase (PARP) family that provide the energy needed for base excision. PARP-1 inhibitors have been tested preclinically and have moved into phase I and II testing.[28,29]

TARGETED AGENTS IN RECURRENT DISEASE

The marked molecular heterogeneity of glioblastomas provides another opportunity for directed therapy with novel targeted agents based on the recent elucidation of signaling pathways. As single agents, these drugs have shown limited efficacy (Table 1).[30–37,39–45]

However, responses do occur, suggesting that patient subpopulations could be identified that may uniquely benefit from a given drug. For example, the status of the *PTEN* gene, lost or otherwise inactivated in most glioblastomas,[46] is a key regulator of the Akt signal transduction pathway. *PTEN* loss or inactivation leads to Akt activation, which is involved in resistance to apoptosis and acceleration of cell proliferation, and may have implications for prognosis and response to EGFR TKIs.

In a retrospective study, Mellinghoff and colleagues[47] observed that a constitutively activated form of EGFR (ie, the mutant EGFR variant III [*EGFRvIII*]), in association with retained PTEN expression, predicted response to the EGFR TKIs erlotinib and gefitinib. Although some have questioned this result,[48] Haas-Kogan and colleagues[49] also reported that EGFR amplification and low levels of AKT activity (consistent with PTEN retention) predicted response. Prospective trials to accrue patients who have EGFR mutant disease are planned.

Platelet-derived growth factor (PDGF) overexpression has been described in up to 66% of glioblastomas. However, clinical trials performed without regard to molecular prescreening have shown negative results.[40,50,51] Taken collectively, these observations provide the basis for prospective trials involving patients selected based on the molecular characterization of their tumors.

Because results of trials using drugs with one target have been disappointing, current efforts involve combining a single molecularly targeted agent with cytotoxic chemotherapy or radiotherapy.[52–54] Furthermore, the combination of two targeted agents is also an attractive concept

Table 1
Recurrent glioblastoma multiforme remains a challenge

Agent	Class	N	Response Rate	Median OS	Median PFS/TTP	6-Month PFS Rate
TMZ (naïve)[30–32]	Alkylator	382	5%–16%	5–8 mo	2–3 mo	18%–21%
BCNU[33]	Alkylator	40	15%	7.5 mo	3.1 mo	17.5%
Gefitinib[34,35]	EGFR	92	0%	10 mo	2 mo	9%–13%
Erlotinib[36–38]	EGFR	78	0%–8%	10 mo	2–3 mo	0%–17%
Imatinib[39,40]	PDGFR	83	6%	5.9 mo	1.8 mo	3%–16%
CCI-779[41,42]	mTOR	106	<5%	4.4 mo	2.3 mo	2%–8%
Pooled phase II[43]	Various	225	6%	5.7 mo	2 mo	15%
Pooled phase II (no TMZ)[44]	Various, 1998–2002	291	<7%	6.0 mo	1.6 mo	9%

Abbreviations: BCNU, carmustine; EGFR, epithelial growth factor receptor; mTOR, mammalian target of rapamycin; OS, overall survival; PDGFR, platelet-derived growth factor receptor; PFS, progression-free survival; TMZ, temozolomide; TTP, time to progression.

(eg, a receptor tyrosine kinase [eg, EGFR] inhibitor combined with a signal transduction [eg, mTOR] modulator).[53,55,56] Another strategy involves the use of single agents with multiple targets.[57] All of these approaches are being pursued, although some results have been disappointing.[56]

One of the most promising targets in recent studies has been the vascular endothelial growth factor receptor (VEGFR), which is overexpressed in glioblastomas.[58] Bevacizumab is a monoclonal anti-VEGF antibody that has been tested either alone or in combination with chemotherapy or radiotherapy in several phase II trials for patients who had recurrent glioblastomas (Table 2).[59–67]

Drawing from the experience in colon cancer, in which irinotecan (CPT11) has activity, bevacizumab has been combined with CPT11 for recurring glioblastoma, showing responses in up to 56% of patients.[59,60,63,64,67] However, a portion of the biologic rationale for CPT-11/bevacizumab in colon cancer (ie, increased drug penetration and disruption of early blood vessels) may not be entirely applicable to glioblastoma. Whether bevacizumab plus CPT11 has superior efficacy to bevacizumab alone for glioblastoma remains unknown.

Several studies suggest that bevacizumab monotherapy is a reasonable therapeutic approach.[63,67] A phase II study in a pediatric population showed minimal bevacizumab activity, suggesting the possibility of age-related biology.[68,69] Other inhibitors of VEGF/VEGFR are also in active trials, including aflibercept (VEGF-Trap),[66] pazopanib,[70] and cedirinib (AZD2171).[65,70]

RADIOGRAPHIC ASSESSMENT AND THERAPY
Treatment Planning

As reviewed in detail elsewhere,[71] a series of studies showed that involved-field radiotherapy (IFRT) had comparable efficacy to but less toxicity than whole brain radiotherapy. Therefore, IFRT became the standard of care. However, significant limitations exist regarding the delivery radiotherapy for the treatment of glioblastoma. For example, the maximum safe dose of radiotherapy may be increased through concurrent administration of bevacizumab.[64]

In addition, the radiation field defined by conventional imaging underestimates the true volume of tissue infiltrated by tumor. Although CT and MRI have improved the ability to deliver IFRT, these imaging modalities do not define active or microscopic tumor. Standard contrast-enhanced CT and MRI scans also do not distinguish active tumor from radionecrosis. Hence,

innovative imaging techniques are under investigation to better target tumor volumes. For example, magnetic resonance spectroscopy imaging (MRSI), also termed *chemical shift imaging*, can reflect tumor metabolic activity based on levels of cellular metabolites (eg, choline, creatine, N-acetylaspartate, lactate). Thus, detection of alterations in these metabolite levels can potentially predict areas of occult disease and theoretically decrease the rates of local relapse.[72] However, the test requires further perfection before routine incorporation into radiotherapy planning.

In a retrospective study in which the prognostic value of MRSI was explored in patients who had high-grade gliomas treated with radiosurgery, Graves and colleagues[73] showed that the absence of MRSI changes suggesting tumor outside the areas of MRI contrast enhancement was a positive prognostic factor. Pirzkall and colleagues[72] observed metabolically active tumors outside the region of enhancement (≤ 28 mm) on T2-weighted MRIs in 88% of patients (n = 34). They also observed MRIs in general predicted a 50% larger volume of microscopic disease than MRSI, suggesting that targeted radiotherapy based on results of anatomic versus metabolic imaging would likely be of significantly different sizes and locations.[72]

Other modalities under investigation include positron emission tomography (PET) using methyl-11C-L-methionine (MET) and other radiotracers, and 3-iodine-123 (I123)-α-methyl-tyrosine single-photon emission tomography (IMT-SPECT).[74,75] Experience using IMT-SPECT in 30 patients who had unresected gliomas found that the IMT region of abnormality was 69% greater than the region of enhancement on T1-weighted contrast MRI.[76]

The aforementioned represent a sampling of novel imaging techniques under consideration. Clearly, continued study is needed to evolve an improved standard diagnostic approach in the evaluation and treatment of glioblastoma.

Pseudoprogression

Many neurooncologists over the past decade recognized that brain MRI scans performed immediately after radiotherapy showed increased contrast enhancement that improved spontaneously. Some investigators speculated that this imaging artifact was related to treatment-induced BBB disruption. Therefore, delaying a patient's first MRI until 4 to 6 weeks postradiation became standard. Fig. 1 presents an example from the authors' experience.

Table 2
Efficacy and safety of vascular endothelial growth factor/vascular endothelial growth factor receptor inhibitors

Agent(s)	Study Type	N	Response Rate	Median OS	Median PFS	6-month PFS Rate	Notable Major Toxicity
Bevacizumab + irinotecan[59,60]	Phase II	35	56	9.7 mo	5.5 mo	46%	1 CNS bleed, 4 PE/DVT, 4 severe fatigue
Bevacizumab + irinotecan/other[61]	Retrospective	23	34%	8.2 mo	5.5 mo	42%	2 CNS bleeds (asymptomatic), 4 PE, 1 SMV thrombosis 1 colon perforation
Bevacizumab[62]	Phase II	85	28%	9.2 mo	Not described	43%	2.4% fatal AE
Bevacizumab[63]	Phase II	48	35%	7.3 mo	3.7 mo	29%	Thromboembolism (12.5%), hypertension (12.5%), hypophosphatemia (6%), thrombocytopenia (6%), bowel perforation (2%); 0 CNS bleeds
Bevacizumab + irinotecan[62]	Phase II	82	38%	8.7 mo	Not described	50%	1.3% fatal AE
Bevacizumab + re-radiation[64]	Pilot	20 GBM	50%	12.5 mo	7.3 mo	65%	1 each: CNS bleed, bowel perforation, gastrointestinal bleed, wound dehiscence; no radionecrosis
Cediranib (AZD2171)[65]	Phase II	31	56%	7.3 mo	3.8 mo	26%	Hypertension, headache
Aflibercept[66]	Phase II	32	30%	Not described	Not described	Not described	1 CNS ischemia, 1 systemic hemorrhage, others

Abbreviations: AE, adverse event; CNS, central nervous system; DVT, deep vein thrombosis; GBM, glioblastoma; OS, overall survival; PE, pulmonary embolism; PFS, progression-free survival; SMV, superior mesenteric vein.

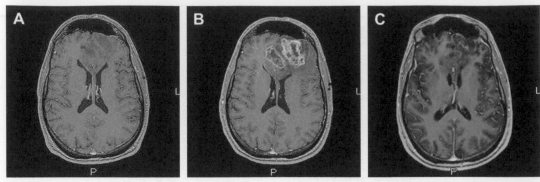

Fig. 1. Patient who has a grade 2 astrocytoma (with non-enhancing disease) initially treated with surgery followed by 18 cycles of temozolomide on a clinical trial who developed a recurrence based on T2/FLAIR images. The patient was then treated with radiotherapy to 54 Gy at 1.8 Gy per fraction and subsequently developed enhancing changes consistent with progression or radiation changes. The enhancing resolved spontaneously without further therapy, representing a pseudoprogression induced by radiotherapy alone. (A) Preradiotherapy T1-contrast MRI just before radiotherapy. (B) T1-contrast MRI 4 months after radiotherapy, representing pseudoprogression. (C) After 9 months, resolution of pseudoprogression on T1-contrast MRI.

This pseudoprogression[77] was recently revisited, showing that spontaneous stabilization or improvement occurred in approximately one third of patients, some of whom experienced the initial worsening a few months after the end of radiotherapy rather than immediately after.[78]

In 2006, Chamberlain and colleagues[79] characterized this phenomenon pathologically in patients treated with radiation and concurrent temozolomide. All symptomatic patients who were believed to have a progressive disease underwent re-resection, and nearly one half showed treatment injury rather than active tumor histologically. In this series, the rate of pseudoprogression was 58% within the first 3 months of completing radiotherapy and concurrent temozolomide. These authors also commented that this finding might underestimate the problem, because their patients represented a subgroup that were candidates for surgery.

Others have also suggested the rate of pseudoprogression may be as high as 64%.[80] The implications are profound within the context of clinical trials. For example, improvement of pseudoprogression could be interpreted falsely as a response to an experimental therapy. Others have reported the pseudoprogression as high as 75% if patients who have equivocal imaging results are included.[80–82] In addition, Brandes and colleagues[80] noted that MGMT promoter methylation may correlate with pseudoprogression.

Despite a plethora of available imaging techniques (eg, proton MRSI,[81,83,84] perfusion MRI,[14,81] fluoro-deoxyglucose-PET,[80,81] and diffusion-weighted MRI[83]), distinguishing progressive disease from pseudoprogression radiographically remains more art than science, with definitive diagnosis dependent on histology. Preliminary work using ferumoxytol for dynamic perfusion imaging has shown some promise but requires further study.[85] This area clearly requires further study and delineation.

Vascular Endothelial Growth Factor Receptor Inhibitors and Implications for Disease Assessment and Management

The effects of VEGFR inhibition confound interpretation of contrast-enhanced brain MRI. VEGF/VEGFR-targeted therapy appears to benefit many patients. However, measuring that benefit using radiographic response rate is difficult, and progression-free survival is also dependent on scan interpretation. Although phase II studies suggest a survival advantage and long-term control in a small subset of patients, no phase III study has been conducted. Therefore, caution is suggested in interpreting response as a true antineoplastic effect because it could instead represent a pseudoresponse.

VEGFR inhibitors may affect capillary permeability, resulting in contrast-enhancing tumors becoming nonenhancing in a subset of patients. This effect was observed in some cases within 96 hours of treatment,[63] and cannot be regarded as a true response as traditionally viewed. This effect often occurs simultaneously with worsening T2/FLAIR abnormality that is not steroid-responsive, arguing against increased edema as the explanation, and rather for progression of disease. **Fig. 2** shows this phenomenon. Additionally,

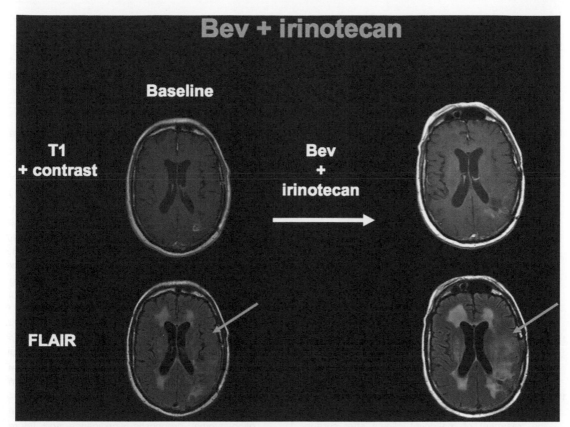

Fig. 2. A patient's MRI showing progressive glioblastoma treated with bevacizumab and irinotecan. The patient experienced clinical deterioration. T1-contrast MRI improved, whereas FLAIR images show progression of disease, consistent with pseudoresponse.

studies have clearly shown that this class of drugs reduces peritumoral edema and associated corticosteroids use.[61,65]

Finally, after VEGF/VEGFR-directed therapy, diffuse infiltrative disease occurs,[61,86] occasionally spreading on subependymal surfaces. This finding suggests that this therapy may change the natural history of the disease to a more infiltrative phenotype in a subset of patients. Therefore, randomized clinical trials with appropriate correlative studies are needed to gain insight into the biologic effects of this new class of agents.

SUMMARY

Numerous strategies are under investigation for treating malignant gliomas. Major recent developments include the survival benefit from temozolomide, exploration of resistance mechanisms, the concept of radiosensitization, and the application of antiangiogenesis agents. Identification of genomic markers that correlate with response may also allow enrichment of patients in the

conduct of clinical trials. This approach, coupled with improved evaluation of patients using radiographic imaging technology, should result in the ability to tailor therapy to individual patients.

REFERENCES

1. 2007–2008 primary brain tumors in the United States statistical report 2000–2004 years of data collected. In: Kruchko C, editor. Central brain tumor registry of the United States. Hinsdale (IL), 2008. Available at: http://www.cbtrus.org/reports//2007 2008/2007report.pdf.

2. Stummer W, Pichlmeier U, Meinel T, et al. Fluorescence-guided surgery with 5-aminolevulinic acid for resection of malignant glioma: a randomised controlled multicentre phase III trial. Lancet Oncol 2006;7:392.

3. Stummer W, Reulen HJ, Meinel T, et al. Extent of resection and survival in glioblastoma multiforme: identification of and adjustment for bias. Neurosurgery 2008;62:564.

4. Van den Bent M, Stupp R, Hildebrand J, et al. Impact of extent of resection and outcome to

adjuvant chemotherapy: a meta-analysis of three EORTIC studies. Neuro Oncol 2008;10:822.

5. Nelson DF, Diener-West M, Horton J, et al. Combined modality approach to treatment of malignant gliomas—re-evaluation of RTOG 7401/ECOG 1374 with long-term follow-up: a joint study of the Radiation Therapy Oncology Group and the Eastern Cooperative Oncology Group. NCI Monogr 1988;6:279–84.

6. Stupp R, Mason WP, van den Bent MJ, et al. Radiotherapy plus concomitant and adjuvant temozolomide for glioblastoma. N Engl J Med 2005;352:987.

7. Brandsma D, Stalpers L, Taal W, et al. Clinical features, mechanisms, and management of pseudoprogression in malignant gliomas. Lancet Oncol 2008;9:453.

8. Macdonald DR, Cascino TL, Schold SC Jr, et al. Response criteria for phase II studies of supratentorial malignant glioma. J Clin Oncol 1990;8:1277.

9. Stewart LA. Chemotherapy in adult high-grade glioma: a systematic review and meta-analysis of individual patient data from 12 randomised trials. Lancet 2002;359:1011.

10. Fine HA, Dear KBG, Loeffler JS, et al. Meta-analysis of radiation therapy with and without adjuvant chemotherapy for malignant gliomas in adults. Cancer 1993;71:2585.

11. Walker MD, Green SB, Byar DP, et al. Randomized comparisons of radiotherapy and nitrosoureas for the treatment of malignant glioma after surgery. N Engl J Med 1980;303:1323.

12. Gilbert MR, Friedman HS, Kuttesch JF, et al. A phase II study of temozolomide in patients with newly diagnosed supratentorial malignant glioma before radiation therapy. Neuro Oncol 2002;4:261.

13. Westphal M, Hilt DC, Bortey E, et al. A phase 3 trial of local chemotherapy with biodegradable carmustine (BCNU) wafers (Gliadel wafers) in patients with primary malignant glioma. Neuro Oncol 2003; 5:79.

14. Catalaa I, Henry R, Dillon WP, et al. Perfusion, diffusion and spectroscopy values in newly diagnosed cerebral gliomas. NMR Biomed 2006;19:463.

15. Stupp R, Dietrich PY, Ostermann Kraljevic S, et al. Promising survival for patients with newly diagnosed glioblastoma multiforme treated with concomitant radiation plus temozolomide followed by adjuvant temozolomide. J Clin Oncol 2002;20:1375.

16. Chakravarti A, Erkkinen MG, Nestler U, et al. Temozolomide-mediated radiation enhancement in glioblastoma: a report on underlying mechanisms. Clin Cancer Res 2006;12:4738.

17. Tolcher AW, Gerson SL, Denis L, et al. Marked inactivation of O6-alkylguanine-DNA alkyltransferase activity with protracted temozolomide schedules. Br J Cancer 2003;88:1004.

18. Perry JR, Rizek P, Cashman R, et al. Temozolomide rechallenge in recurrent malignant glioma by using a continuous temozolomide schedule: the "rescue" approach. Cancer 2008;113:2152.

19. Stupp R, Hegi ME, Mason WP, et al. Effects of radiotherapy with concomitant and adjuvant temozolomide versus radiotherapy alone on survival in glioblastoma in a randomised phase III study: 5-year analysis of the EORTC-NCIC trial. Lancet Oncol 2009;10(5):459–66.

20. Hegi ME, Diserens AC, Gorlia T, et al. MGMT gene silencing and benefit from temozolomide in glioblastoma. N Engl J Med 2005;352:997.

21. Hegi ME, Liu L, Herman JG, et al. Correlation of O6-methylguanine methyltransferase (MGMT) promoter methylation with clinical outcomes in glioblastoma and clinical strategies to modulate MGMT activity. J Clin Oncol 2008;26:4189.

22. Pelloski CE, Rivera AL, De La Cruz Guerrero C, et al. MGMT promoter methylation is an independent prognostic factor in the absence of alkylating chemotherapy in glioblastoma. Int J Radiat Oncol Biol Phys 2008;72(Suppl 1):S9.

23. Preusser M, Janzer RC, Felsberg J, et al. Anti-O6-methylguanine-methyltransferase (MGMT) immunohistochemistry in glioblastoma multiforme: observer variability and lack of association with patient survival impede its use as clinical biomarker. Brain Pathol 2008;18:520.

24. Hill C, Hunter SB, Brat DJ. Genetic markers in glioblastoma: prognostic significance and future therapeutic implications. Adv Anat Pathol 2003;10: 212.

25. Sansal I, Sellers WR. The biology and clinical relevance of the PTEN tumor suppressor pathway. J Clin Oncol 2004;22:2954.

26. Smith JS, Tachibana I, Passe SM, et al. PTEN mutation, EGFR amplification, and outcome in patients with anaplastic astrocytoma and glioblastoma multiforme. J Natl Cancer Inst 2001; 93:1246.

27. Tanwar MK, Gilbert MR, Holland EC. Gene expression microarray analysis reveals YKL-40 to be a potential serum marker for malignant character in human glioma. Cancer Res 2002;62:4364.

28. Tentori L, Graziani G. Chemopotentiation by PARP inhibitors in cancer therapy. Pharmacol Res 2005; 52:25.

29. Tentori L, Leonetti C, Scarsella M, et al. Brain distribution and efficacy as chemosensitizer of an oral formulation of PARP-1 inhibitor GPI 15427 in experimental models of CNS tumors. Int J Oncol 2005;26:415.

30. Brada M, Hoang-Xuan K, Rampling R, et al. Multicenter phase II trial of temozolomide in patients with glioblastoma multiforme at first relapse. Ann Oncol 2001;12:259.

31. Chang SM, Theodosopoulos P, Lamborn K, et al. Temozolomide in the treatment of recurrent malignant glioma. Cancer 2004;100:605.

32. Yung WK, Albright RE, Olson J, et al. A phase II study of temozolomide vs. procarbazine in patients with glioblastoma multiforme at first relapse. Br J Cancer 2000;83:588.

33. Brandes AA, Tosoni A, Amista P, et al. How effective is BCNU in recurrent glioblastoma in the modern era? A phase II trial. Neurology 2004;63:1281.

34. Lieberman FS, Cloughesy T, Malkin M, et al. Phase I-II study of ZD-1839 for recurrent malignant gliomas and meningiomas progressing after radiation therapy [abstract 421]. J Clin Oncol 2003;22:105.

35. Rich JN, Reardon DA, Peery T, et al. Phase II trial of gefitinib in recurrent glioblastoma. J Clin Oncol 2004;22:133.

36. Raizer JJ, Abrey LE, Wen P, et al. A phase II trial of erlotinib (OSI-774) in patients with recurrent malignant gliomas not on EIAEDs [abstract]. J Clin Oncol 2004;22:1502.

37. Vogelbaum MA, Peerboom G, Stevens G, et al. Phase II trial of the EGFR tyrosine kinase inhibitor erlotinib for single agent therapy of recurrent glioblastoma multiforme: interim results [abstract]. J Clin Oncol 2004;22:1558.

38. Yung A, Vredenburgh J, Cloughesy T, et al. Erlotinib HCL for glioblastoma multiforme in first relapse, a phase II trial [abstract]. J Clin Oncol 2004;22:15554.

39. Raymond E, Brandes A, van Oosterom A, et al. Multicentre phase II study of imatinib mesylate in patients with recurrent glioblastoma: an EORTC: NDDG/BTG Intergroup study [abstract]. J Clin Oncol 2004;22:1501.

40. Wen PY, Yung WK, Lamborn KR, et al. Phase I/II study of imatinib mesylate for recurrent malignant gliomas: North American Brain Tumor Consortium Study 99–08. Clin Cancer Res 2006;12:4899.

41. Chang SM, Wen P, Cloughesy T, et al. Phase II study of CCI-779 in patients with recurrent glioblastoma multiforme. Invest New Drugs 2005;23:357.

42. Galanis E, Buckner JC, Maurer MJ, et al. Phase II trial of temsirolimus (CCI-779) in recurrent glioblastoma multiforme: a North Central Cancer Treatment Group study. J Clin Oncol 2005;23:5294.

43. Wong ET, Hess KR, Gleason MJ, et al. Outcomes and prognostic factors in recurrent glioma patients enrolled onto phase II clinical trials. J Clin Oncol 1999;17:2572.

44. Lamborn KR, Yung WK, Chang SM, et al. Progression-free survival: an important end point in evaluating therapy for recurrent high-grade gliomas. Neuro Oncol 2008;10:162.

45. Lassman AB, Rossi MR, Raizer JJ, et al. Molecular study of malignant gliomas treated with epidermal growth factor receptor inhibitors: tissue analysis from North American Brain Tumor Consortium Trials 01-03 and 00-01. Clin Cancer Res 2005;11:7841.

46. Lassman AB. Molecular biology of gliomas. Curr Neurol Neurosci Rep 2004;4:228.

47. Mellinghoff IK, Wang MY, Vivanco I, et al. Molecular determinants of the response of glioblastomas to EGFR kinase inhibitors. N Engl J Med 2005;353:2012.

48. Brandes AA, Franceschi E, Tosoni A, et al. Epidermal growth factor receptor inhibitors in neuro-oncology: hopes and disappointments. Clin Cancer Res 2008;14:957.

49. Haas-Kogan DA, Prados MD, Tihan T, et al. Epidermal growth factor receptor, protein kinase B/Akt, and glioma response to erlotinib. J Natl Cancer Inst 2005;97:880.

50. Dresemann G. Imatinib and hydroxyurea in pretreated progressive glioblastoma multiforme: a patient series. Ann Oncol 2005;16:1702.

51. Guha A, Dashner K, Black PM, et al. Expression of PDGF and PDGF receptors in human astrocytoma operation specimens supports the existence of an autocrine loop. Int J Cancer 1995;60:168.

52. Chakravarti A, Chakladar A, Delaney MA, et al. The epidermal growth factor receptor pathway mediates resistance to sequential administration of radiation and chemotherapy in primary human glioblastoma cells in a RAS-dependent manner. Cancer Res 2002;62:4307.

53. Fan QW, Specht KM, Zhang C, et al. Combinatorial efficacy achieved through two-point blockade within a signaling pathway-a chemical genetic approach. Cancer Res 2003;63:8930.

54. Nagane M, Narita Y, Mishima K, et al. Human glioblastoma xenografts overexpressing a tumor-specific mutant epidermal growth factor receptor sensitized to cisplatin by the AG1478 tyrosine kinase inhibitor. J Neurosurg 2001;95:472.

55. Goudar RK, Shi Q, Hjelmeland MD, et al. Combination therapy of inhibitors of epidermal growth factor receptor/vascular endothelial growth factor receptor 2 (AEE788) and the mammalian target of rapamycin (RAD001) offers improved glioblastoma tumor growth inhibition. Mol Cancer Ther 2005;4:101.

56. Kreisl TN, Lassman AB, Mischel PS, et al. A pilot study of everolimus and gefitinib in the treatment of recurrent glioblastoma (GBM). J Neurooncol 2009;92:99.

57. Lassman AB, Wang W, Gilbert MR, et al. Phase II trial of dasatinib for recurrent glioblastoma (RTOG 0627). Neuro Oncol 2008;10:824.

58. Stupp R, Hegi ME, van den Bent MJ, et al. Changing paradigms an update on the multidisciplinary management of malignant glioma. Oncologist 2006;11:165.

59. Vredenburgh JJ, Desjardins A, Herndon JE 2nd, et al. Phase II trial of bevacizumab and irinotecan in recurrent malignant glioma. Clin Cancer Res 2007;13:1253.

60. Vredenburgh JJ, Desjardins A, Herndon JE 2nd, et al. Bevacizumab plus irinotecan in recurrent glioblastoma multiforme. J Clin Oncol 2007;25:4722.

61. Norden AD, Young GS, Setayesh K, et al. Bevacizumab for recurrent malignant gliomas: efficacy,

toxicity, and patterns of recurrence. Neurology 2008; 70:779.

62. Cloughesy TF, Prados MD, Wen PY, et al. A phase II, randomized, non-comparative clinical trial of the effect of bevacizumab (BV) alone or in combination with irinotecan (CPT) on 6-month progression free survival (PFS6) in recurrent, treatment-refractory glioblastoma (GBM) [abstract 2010b, oral presentation update] [abstract]. J Clin Oncol 2008;26:2010b.

63. Kreisl TN, Kim L, Moore K, et al. Phase II trial of single-agent bevacizumab followed by bevacizumab plus irinotecan at tumor progression in recurrent glioblastoma. J Clin Oncol 2009;27:740.

64. Gutin PH, Iwamoto FM, Beal K, et al. Safety and efficacy of bevacizumab with hypofractionated stereotactic irradiation for recurrent malignant gliomas. Int J Radiat Oncol Biol Phys 2009;75(1):156–63.

65. Batchelor TT, Sorensen AG, di Tomaso E, et al. AZD2171, a pan-VEGF receptor tyrosine kinase inhibitor, normalizes tumor vasculature and alleviates edema in glioblastoma patients. Cancer Cell 2007;11:83.

66. de Groot JF, Wen PY, Lamborn K, et al. Phase II single arm trial of aflibercept in patients with recurrent temozolomide-resistant glioblastoma: NABTC 0601 [abstract 2020]. J Clin Oncol 2008;26:2020.

67. Cloughesy TF, Prados MD, Wen PY, et al. A phase II, randomized, non-comparative clinical trial of the effect of bevacizumab (BV) alone or in combination with irinotecan (CPT) on 6-month progression free survival (PFS6) in recurrent, treatment-refractory glioblastoma (GBM) [abstract]. J Clin Oncol 2008;26:2010b.

68. Gururangan S, Chi S, Onar A, et al. Phase II study of bevacizumab plus irinotecan in children with recurrent malignant glioma and diffuse brainstem glioma— a Pediatric Brain Tumor Consortium study (PBTC-022). Neuro Oncol 2008;10:833.

69. Hurwitz H, Dowlati A, Savage S, et al. Safety, tolerability and pharmacokinetics of oral administration of GW786034 in pts with solid tumors [abstract]. J Clin Oncol 2005;23:3012.

70. Wedge SR, Kendrew J, Hennequin LF, et al. AZD2171: a highly potent, orally bioavailable, vascular endothelial growth factor receptor-2 tyrosine kinase inhibitor for the treatment of cancer. Cancer Res 2005;65:4389.

71. Chang JE, Khuntia D, Robins HI, et al. Radiotherapy and radiosensitizers in the treatment of glioblastoma multiforme. Clin Adv Hematol Oncol 2007;5:894.

72. Pirzkall A, McKnight TR, Graves EE, et al. MR-spectroscopy guided target delineation for high-grade gliomas. Int J Radiat Oncol Biol Phys 2001; 50:915.

73. Graves EE, Nelson SJ, Vigneron DB, et al. A preliminary study of the prognostic value of proton magnetic resonance spectroscopic imaging in gamma knife radiosurgery of recurrent malignant gliomas. Neurosurgery 2000;46:319.

74. Mosskin M, Ericson K, Hindmarsh T, et al. Positron emission tomography compared with magnetic resonance imaging and computed tomography in supratentorial gliomas using multiple stereotactic biopsies as reference. Acta Radiol 1989;30:225.

75. Ogawa T, Shishido F, Kanno I, et al. Cerebral glioma: evaluation with methionine PET. Radiology 1993; 186:45.

76. Grosu AL, Weber W, Feldmann HJ, et al. First experience with I-123-alpha-methyl-tyrosine p in the 3-D radiation treatment planning of brain gliomas. Int J Radiat Oncol Biol Phys 2000;47:517.

77. Hoffman WF, Levin VA, Wilson CB. Evaluation of malignant glioma patients during the postirradiation period. J Neurosurg 1979;50:624.

78. de Wit MC, de Bruin HG, Eijkenboom W, et al. Immediate post-radiotherapy changes in malignant glioma can mimic tumor progression. Neurology 2004;63:535.

79. Chamberlain MC, Glantz MJ, Chalmers L, et al. Early necrosis following concurrent Temodar and radiotherapy in patients with glioblastoma. J Neurooncol 2007;82:81.

80. Brandes AA, Franceschi E, Tosoni A, et al. MGMT promoter methylation status can predict the incidence and outcome of pseudoprogression after concomitant radiochemotherapy in newly diagnosed glioblastoma patients. J Clin Oncol 2008;26:2192.

81. Clarke JL, Abrey LE, Karimi S, et al. Pseudoprogression (PsPr) after concurrent radiotherapy (RT) and temozolomide (TMZ) for newly diagnosed glioblastoma multiforme (GBM) [abstract]. J Clin Oncol 2008;26:2025.

82. Taal W, Brandsma D, de Bruin HG, et al. Incidence of early pseudo-progression in a cohort of malignant glioma patients treated with chemoirradiation with temozolomide. Cancer 2008;113:405.

83. Schlemmer HP, Bachert P, Henze M, et al. Differentiation of radiation necrosis from tumor progression using proton magnetic resonance spectroscopy. Neuroradiology 2002;44:216.

84. Schlemmer HP, Bachert P, Herfarth KK, et al. Proton MR spectroscopic evaluation of suspicious brain lesions after stereotactic radiotherapy. AJNR Am J Neuroradiol 2001;22:1316.

85. Neuwelt E, Raslan A, Gahramanov S, et al. DSC-MRI using ferumoxytol may help differentiate pseudoprogression from true progression in patients with glioblastoma. A preliminary report. Neuro Oncol 2008;10:894.

86. Lassman AB, Iwamoto FM, Gutin PH, et al. Patterns of relapse and prognosis after bevacizumab (BEV) failure in recurrent glioblastoma (GBM) [abstract]. J Clin Oncol 2008;26:2028.

Brain Irradiation: Effects on Normal Brain Parenchyma and Radiation Injury

Pia C. Sundgren, MD, PhD[a,c,*], Yue Cao, PhD[b]

KEYWORDS

- Irradiation • Radiation injury • Neurotoxicity
- Diffusion tensor imaging • MR imaging • MR spectroscopy

Radiation therapy (RT) is a major treatment modality for malignant and benign brain tumors. Concerns of radiation effects on the brain tissue and neurocognitive function and quality of life increase, however, because survival of the patients treated for brain tumors is improving. Radiation effects on the brain manifest as late neurologic sequelae and neurocognitive dysfunction with or without gross tissue necrosis.[1–4] Late neurocognitive dysfunction presents as diminishing mental capacity for working memory, learning ability, executive function, and attention. Recent multicenter studies of patients with low-grade gliomas who are without clinical signs of tumor recurrence after radiation treatment show that both a high total dose and a high dose per fraction are associated with neurocognitive deterioration, especially memory functions.[4,5] Radiation-induced functional, metabolic, and molecular changes in the brain structures and neural networks, which can be assessed by in vivo imaging, could be responsible for neurocognitive function changes.

This article discusses clinical and neurobehavioral symptoms and signs of radiation-induced brain injury; possible histopathology; and the potential of functional, metabolic, and molecular imaging as a biomarker for assessment and prediction of neurotoxicity after brain irradiation and imaging findings in radiation necrosis.

CLINICAL, RADIOLOGIC, AND NEUROBEHAVIORAL SYMPTOMS AND SIGNS
Clinical Symptoms and Signs

Classically, clinical complications after brain therapeutic irradiation have been described as acute (days to weeks after irradiation); subacute or early delayed (2–6 months after the completion of RT); and late effects (6 months to years after the completion of RT).[1,6,7]

The acute reaction to conventional fractionated brain irradiation is usually mild, characterized by headache, nausea, drowsiness, and sometimes worsening of neurologic symptoms. Corticosteroids are usually successful in relieving acute complications.

Reports on early delayed reactions increase with frequency following contemporary cranial irradiation techniques. General neurologic deterioration during this interval (2–6 months after RT) is believed to be secondary to transient, diffuse demyelination. Many focal neurologic signs following radiation treatment of intracranial tumor have been attributed to intralesional reactions, probably indicative of tumor response or perilesional reactions (ie, edema or demyelination). Periventricular white matter (WM) lesions start to appear on conventional MR imaging or CT during this interval, however, even with standard fractionated partial brain RT.[8,9] Following high-dose,

a Diagnostic Centre for Imaging and Functional Medicine, Malmö University Hospital, University of Lund, SE-205 02 Malmö, Sweden
b Department of Radiation Oncology and Radiology, University of Michigan, Ann Arbor, MI 48109–0010, USA
c Department of Radiology, University of Michigan, Ann Arbor, MI 48109-0030, USA
* Corresponding author. Diagnostic Centre for Imaging and Functional Medicine, Malmö University Hospital, University of Lund, SE-205 02 Malmö, Sweden.
E-mail address: pia.sundgren@med.lu.se (P.C. Sundgren).

Neuroimag Clin N Am 19 (2009) 657–668
doi:10.1016/j.nic.2009.08.014
1052-5149/09/$ – see front matter © 2009 Elsevier Inc. All rights reserved.

volume-limited stereotactic radiosurgery (SRS), transient WM alterations are often apparent on conventional MR imaging, generally beginning 6 or more months after treatment.[10,11] Following high-dose, large brain-volume treatment and concurrent chemotherapy, necrosis, particularly in WM, starts to develop in this interval, and the location of necrosis is often near the site of the original tumor.[12,13]

The classical late effect following brain irradiation is either localized or multifocal necrosis, often associated with high-dose and large brain-volume treatment.[7,12–14] Complications include worsening neurologic signs and symptoms, seizures, and increased intracranial pressure. Nevertheless, WM abnormality is a much more common late effect, and is often noted extending peripherally beyond the high-dose volume following partial brain irradiation.[8,9] WM abnormality and necrosis are progressive[8–11] and the imaging findings are discussed later.

Neurologic symptoms and neurocognitive impairments related to WM injury range from mild personality change to progressive memory loss, and to marked, incapacitating dementia.[15]

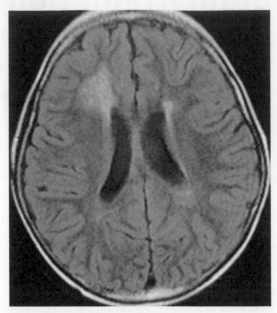

Fig. 1. Axial fluid attenuation inversion recovery image demonstrates the increased signal in predominately right frontal lobe in a patient with radiation injury secondary to irradiation.

Radiologic Signs

The radiologic signatures of WM alterations have been categorized as (1) periventricular changes, (2) focal extension of intense signal into WM, (3) diffuse extension into WM, and (4) diffuse coalescence of white and gray matter into intense signal region, loss of architecture, cortical atrophy, and hydrocephalus.[8]

Following focal or whole-brain irradiation asymptomatic focal edema is a commonly seen finding both on CT and MR imaging, typically presenting as increased signal on T2-weighted and fluid attenuation inversion recovery images in the WM on MR imaging (**Fig. 1**) and as decreased attenuation in the WM on CT.

Radiation necrosis is often difficult to differentiate from recurrent tumor because the imaging pattern is very similar and they have many shared characteristics, such as an origin that often is at or in the vicinity of the original tumor, and they often demonstrate heterogeneous contrast enhancement. Commonly, radiation necrosis presents as a single focal enhancing lesion but it can be multifocal, or even in the contralateral size. The side may vary and range from small nodular enhancement to large areas of necrosis and heterogeneous enhancement.[16] Most lesions consist of an enhancing mass with a central area of necrosis often in a so-called "soap-bubble" or "Swiss-cheese pattern" (**Fig. 2**).[13] On T2-weighted

images, the solid portion of the radiation-induced necrotic mass has low signal intensity, and the central necrotic component shows increased signal intensity.[13]

In the milder forms of radiation-induced injury the pattern of enhancement can be nodular, linear, or curvilinear and present as single or multiple

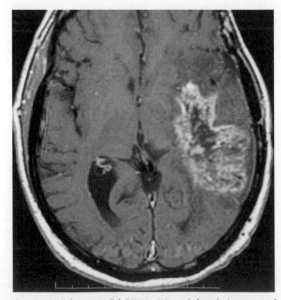

Fig. 2. Axial post–Gd-DTPA T1-weighted image of Swiss-cheese appearance of contrast enhancement in a case of surgically proved radiation necrosis.

lesions of varying sizes. Commonly, the lesion growth over time demonstrates surrounding edema, and causes mass effect. Typical locations for radiation necrosis are in the postsurgical tumor bed, in the periventricular WM especially corpus callosum and centrum semiovale (on top of the ventricles) because the periventricular WM is very susceptible to radiation. Radiation injury and radiation necrosis can occur outside the high-dose radiation dose field (**Fig. 3**).[16]

Neurobehavioral Symptoms and Signs

In recent years, many efforts have been focused on late neurocognitive dysfunction and quality of life of patients with brain tumors who had been treated by RT with or without concurrent chemotherapy. Although a few studies find that the deterioration of neurocognitive function is an indicator of tumor progression,[17,18] a recent multicenter study of patients with low-grade gliomas who had no clinical signs of tumor recurrence at least 1 year after treatment showed that a high total dose correlated with a decline in working memory and that a high dose per fraction interfered with long-term memory storage and retrieval.[4] Also, in a randomized trial of low- (50.4 Gy) versus high-dose (64.8 Gy) RT in patients with supratentorial low-grade glioma, significant cognitive deterioration from baseline was found in those without tumor progression, with rates of 8.2%, 4.6%, and 5.3% at years of 1, 2, and 5, respectively, as assessed by the relatively insensitive Folstein Mini-Mental State Examination.[5] Moreover, the rate of cognitive impairment is even higher using a battery of neuropsychologic tests, which are much more sensitive to cognitive functions than the Mini-Mental State Examination.[4,15,19,20] Also, neurocognitive dysfunction is observed without radiation necrosis,[15] consistent with the findings in an animal study.[21]

The cognitive domains of these dysfunctions present primarily in memory function, learning ability, and executive function, and to a lesser extent in fine motor skills and attention.

The potential effect of RT on neurocognitive outcomes is an important factor in the determination of the risks versus benefits of treatment,[22] which should be an integral part of clinical decision-making. Given the late nature of neurocognitive dysfunction, it is important to identify in vivo imaging biomarkers for early assessment and prediction of late neurotoxicity.

HISTOPATHOLOGY IN RADIATION-INDUCED BRAIN INJURY

Radiation-induced injury in cerebral tissue is a highly complex and interactive process involving multiple tissue elements.[2,23,24] Cerebral vascular injury has long been recognized to occur acutely and precedes subacute demyelination and reactive astrocytic and microglial responses.[25–28] Histopathologic studies reveal that lifting of endothelium from the basement membrane, dilation and thickening of blood vessels, endothelial cell nuclear enlargement, and hypertrophy of perivascular astrocytes are among the first effects after irradiation.[29–31] Early endothelial cell death and apoptosis after irradiation have been

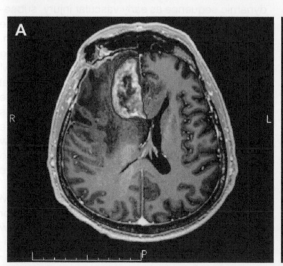
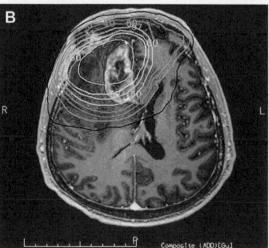

Fig. 3. Axial post–Gd-DTPA T1-weighted image demonstrates a focal heterogeneously enhancing lesion in the right frontal lobe. (*A*) The lesion that was histopathology-proved radiation necrosis is outlined in red. (*B*) The lesions is so-called "in-field" of the radiation dosage volume but only parts of the lesion are in the high 60-Gy field, whereas other parts are outside the high dose.

detected.[26,27,32] Possible mechanisms of endothelial apoptosis include generation of intracellular ceramide by acidic sphingomyelinase and adhering leukocytes by tumor necrosis factor-α.[27,32,33] The initial injury of vessels is followed by the formation of platelet matrix and thrombus, which eventually results in occlusion and thrombosis in microvessels within weeks to months.[23,34] Furthermore, cerebral vascular injury is followed by degenerative structural changes in WM.[29–31,35] The lag time between vascular injury and WM degeneration depends on the severity of the injury. Together, these observations strongly support the concept that cerebral vascular injury is of crucial importance for the development of WM injury following irradiation.

In addition to vascular abnormalities, demyelination is another typical histopathological of radiation-induced brain tissue injury. It has been shown that irradiation results in the loss of reproductive capacity of the oligodendrocyte type 2 astrocyte (O-2A) progenitor cells in both brain and spinal cord of adult rats.[36–38] Presumably, radiation-induced loss of O-2A progenitor cells results in failure to replace normal turned-over oligodendrocytes, with the eventual consequence of demyelination. The kinetics of oligodendrocyte loss is inconsistent, however, with the late onset of necrosis.

The brain is a highly integrated system, comprising a number of disparate phenotypes of cells. Brain irradiation could affect not only vasculature and O-2A progenitors, but also astrocytes, microglia, neurons, and recently identified neural stem cells.[39] As suggested, the response of neural tissue to irradiation also involves oxygen stress, inflammatory response, secondary reactive processes, and enhanced cytokine gene expression.[2,23,24] To date, the understanding of histopathology and molecular biology after brain response to irradiation is limited.

RADIATION NECROSIS AND PSEUDOPROGRESSION

The differentiation of recurrent tumor or progressive tumor from radiation injury after radiotherapy is often a radiologic dilemma regardless of the technique used (CT or MR imaging). Most of these brain neoplasms have been subjected to radiation or chemotherapy and many of the tumors do not have specific imaging characteristics that enable the neuroradiologist to discriminate tumor recurrence from the inflammatory or necrotic change that can result from treatment with radiation or chemotherapy. Both entities typically demonstrate contrast enhancement. It is often the clinical course, a brain biopsy, or imaging over a lengthy follow-up interval that enable the distinction of recurrent tumor from a treatment-related lesion and not the specific imaging itself.[13]

Although the difficulties in differentiation between radiation necrosis and a recurrent tumor often occur several months after the initial therapy, recent studies have described transient increases in contrast enhancement immediately after chemoradiation, which mimics tumor progression and has been termed pseudoprogression.[40–44]

The incidence of pseudoprogression following concurrent chemoradiation has been reported to occur in approximately 15% to 30% of patients.[40–44] Most patients remained clinically stable despite imaging changes suggestive of tumor progression. Radiation-induced vascular changes leading to focal transient increase in gadolinium enhancement following irradiation have been considered a possible mechanism.[40] The combination of chemotherapy and RT may increase the incidence of pseudoprogression, possibly because of the increased radiosensitive effect of temozolomide on adjacent normal tissue.[41–44] Pseudoprogression is further discussed elsewhere in this issue.

IMAGING AS A BIOMARKER FOR RADIATION-INDUCED NEUROTOXICITY AND RADIATION NECROSIS

Today, a large body of converging evidence from histopathology, molecular biology, animal models, and clinical observations suggests that radiation-induced neurotoxicity follows an interactive and dynamic sequence as early vascular injury, subsequent focal and diffuse demyelination, late tissue degeneration, and neurocognitive dysfunction. Although limited, functional and metabolic imaging have been used to investigate vascular injury, WM demyelination, and metabolic change in cerebral tissue after irradiation without apparent tissue necrosis. The functional and metabolic changes have been associated with radiation dose, dose volume, and fraction size. Furthermore, a few studies have attempted to link the functional and metabolic changes in the brain to neurocognitive function changes.

The following sections review the studies of WM injury and radiation necrosis using diffusion tensor imaging (DTI), and changes in cerebral blood flow (CBF), cerebral blood volume (CBV), and metabolism using functional MR imaging, proton spectroscopy, and positron emission tomography. Changes in CBF and CBV in the work-up to distinguish radiation necrosis from recurrent brain tumor are discussed elsewhere in this issue.

Diffusion Tensor Imaging

DTI is the most sensitive technique to assess WM integrity and histopathologic changes before structural changes are visible on any other imaging modalit. DTI is able to assess water diffusion and anisotropic diffusion in the tissue structures.[45-47] In WM, the tight myelin sheaths surrounding the axon substantially restrict water diffusion in the direction perpendicular to the axon axis ($\lambda_\perp$) compared with water diffusion in the direction along the axon axis ($\lambda_{||}$). Anisotropic water diffusion can be used to characterize tissue types (eg, grey and white matter), and to provide information on the density and orientation of WM fiber tracts. Furthermore, the quantitative indices obtained from DTI can aid in distinguishing between myelin loss and axonal injury. For example, an increase in $\lambda_\perp$ with or without a change in $\lambda_{||}$ has been confirmed to be an in vivo biomarker for demyelination with pathology in myelin-deficient rats.[48] In a recent study of radiation-induced WM damage in a rodent model, an early delayed increase in $\lambda_\perp$ after irradiation was correlated with demyelination histologically, whereas a decrease in $\lambda_{||}$ was correlated with reactive astrogliosis without necrosis.[49] Either $\lambda_\perp$ increase or $\lambda_{||}$ decrease can lead to fractional anisotropy (FA) decreases.

DTI has been used to assess WM injury in pediatric and adult patients treated with brain radiation. In a recent study of children with medulloblastoma treated with craniospinal irradiation, decreased FA in WM after radiation was found to be correlated inversely with the age at treatment and positively with craniospinal dose.[50] In a cross-sectional study of survivors of childhood medulloblastoma and acute lymphoblastic leukemia treated with craniospinal irradiation, differences of WM FA in the patients and in age-matched control group had a significant effect on intelligence quotient scores after adjusting effects of age at treatment, craniospinal dose, and time interval since treatment.[51] In another study of the survivors of acute lymphoblastic leukemia 17 to 37 years after craniospinal irradiation, FA was analyzed in the temporal lobe, hippocampus, and thalamus, and found to be reduced compared with aged-matched control.[52] Because neurocognitive functions in these patients were not evaluated, however, neurobehavioral consequences of degradation of these functional structures are unknown. Although findings from these cross-sectional studies identify several interesting factors that might contribute to radiation-induced neurocognitive injury in the pediatric population, future prospective studies are required to test hypotheses generated from these preliminary investigations.

In the adult patients who undergo partial or whole-brain RT, several prospective studies showed changes in DTI indices of normal-appearing WM.[53,54] In a study of 25 patients who had high-grade glioma, low-grade glioma, or benign tumors and underwent partial brain RT, progressive decreases in FA from the start of RT to 45 weeks after were observed in large WM fibers of the genu and splenium of corpus callosum.[53] Also, the decrease in FA was dose-dependent. Further analysis showed progressive increases in $\lambda_\perp$ but little change in $\lambda_{||}$, suggesting demyelination predominantly after WM irradiation. In another study of 26 patients who underwent prophylactic cranial irradiation, decreases in FA of several WM anatomic sites, including frontal WM, corona radiata, and cerebellum, were observed at the end of RT, and 6 weeks after RT, the extent of which seems to depend on risk factors of vascular diseases.[54] Whether the radiation-induced WM injury is structural selective is a question that remains to be answered. Also, how these observed WM changes are associated with neurocognitive function changes remains to be tested.

Recent studies using diffusion weighted imaging to differentiate recurrent tumor from radiation injury[55] have shown that the apparent diffusion coefficient (ADC) ratio in the contrast-enhancing lesion is lower in recurrent tumor than in radiation-induced injury[55]; however, other investigators using DTI[56] demonstrated significantly higher ADC values in the contrast-enhancing part of the lesion in patients with tumor recurrence than in the contrast-enhancing lesion in patients with radiation injury. That study also showed that the ADC ratios in the WM tracts in the perilesion edema were significantly higher in radiation-injury patients compared with those with recurrent tumor and also that the FA ratios were significantly higher in normal-appearing WM tracts adjacent to the edema in patients diagnosed with radiation injury compared with those with recurrent tumours.[56] Both $\lambda_\perp$ and $\lambda_{||}$ values were significantly higher in contrast-enhancing lesions in patients with recurrent tumor than in those with radiation injury ($P = .02$) and in the perilesional edema for both patient groups compared with normal-appearing WM. It can be anticipated that higher ADC values found in areas of tumor recurrence could be caused by increased extracellular space and micronecrosis, as commonly found in brain tumors, although a high-cell-density tumor exhibits low ADC. Lower ADC value in radiation injury could be a result of gliosis, fibrosis, macrophage invasion, vascular changes, and demyelination. These radiation-induced effects restrict water mobility (lower ADC) relative to simple noncellular or cystic necrosis, which elevates ADC. Contradictory are results from another study that demonstrated higher ADC values in treatment-related changes and radiation necrosis than in solid tumors, suggesting that solid tumors may have more densely packed cells than necrotic tissues, resulting in a lower ADC for recurrent tumor.[57] It has been suggested and supported by data both from animal and human studies that diffusion imaging may be sensitive for evaluating early tumor response to therapy,[36,58,59] suggesting that early increase in ADC values during therapy may relate to therapy-induced cell necrosis. The subsequent drop in tumor ADC to pretreatment levels could be an indicator of tumor regrowth.[58,59]

Proton Spectroscopy

MR spectroscopy is a noninvasive technique for measurement of chemical substances (metabolites) in the brain and may serve as a sensitive imaging tool to noninvasively detect neurochemical changes as evidence of neurotoxicity in the irradiated brain.[60–68] The technique has been used to differentiate recurrent tumor from radiation necrosis,[69–71] whereas only a few prospective studies evaluating interval changes in metabolic activity in normal-appearing brain parenchyma during and following cranial RT for primary brain neoplasm have been published.[63–68,72]

The most common technique has been single-voxel 1H MR spectroscopy technique with only a limited part of the brain evaluated and only at one or two time points during and after irradiation.[63–65,72] Less frequently, two-dimensional multivoxel spectroscopy[66,68] or three-dimensional spectroscopic imaging[67] have been used for interval follow-up during or after RT.

It has been hypothesized that structural degradation in cerebral tissue after RT would be predicted by early changes in metabolic activity detectable by MR spectroscopy before the development of neurocognitive symptoms or anatomic changes seen on conventional MR imaging. This hypothesis is supported by the findings in a recent study of 11 adult patients with either low-grade glioma or benign tumors without previous cranial irradiation.[68] That study demonstrated that significant alterations in brain metabolites occurred in normal-appearing human brain parenchyma early during radiation treatment and that interval progression of some of these changes occurred over at least a 6-month period.[68] This was especially evident by the interval decrease in

N-acetylaspartate/creatine (NAA/Cr) and choline/creatine (Cho/Cr) ratios from the pretreatment values at 3 weeks of radiation treatment and the progressive decline seen in the ratios at 6 months after the completion of radiation treatment (Fig. 4).[68] The conclusion from that study was that the decrease in the NAA/Cr ratio is most likely caused by neuronal damage, neuronal cell death caused by apoptosis, and neuronal dysfunction secondary to the irradiation. The metabolite NAA is predominantly present in neurons and believed to represent a marker of neuronal density and function, and creatine is a marker of energy metabolism and is considered to be fairly stable under most conditions. The presumption that NAA decreases following radiation is also supported by other previous studies demonstrating a decrease in whole-brain NAA and in the NAA concentration of irradiated brain.[62–64,72] Observations of decreases in both choline and choline compounds, and the decreased Cho/Cr ratio, have also been reported after irradiation.[60,67,68,73] The choline compound is correlated with cell membrane biosynthesis and metabolic turnover in proliferative tissue and it has been suggested that the decrease in Cho seen in normal-appearing brain tissue after irradiation might be caused by membrane damage in the myelin or the myelin-producing oligodendrocytes, accompanied by impaired tissue perfusion.[74] One of the few previous reports of metabolic changes after prophylactic irradiation, in patients with acute lymphoblastic leukemia,[60] found that the lower NAA/Cr and Cho/Cr ratio was associated with the presence of hemosiderin but not with imaging findings of leukoencephalopathy.

Also, recent animal studies have demonstrated significant differences in brain metabolite concentrations in irradiated rat brain,[75] accompanied by worsening on behavioral tests in the irradiated rats compared with sham-irradiated rats 54 weeks after radiation treatment.[76]

Specific spectroscopic changes that occur in radiation necrosis have been reported and include slight depression of NAA and variable changes in Cho and Cr.[71,77–79] In addition, radiation necrosis may show a broad peak between 0 and 2 ppm, probably reflecting cellular debris containing fatty acids, lactate, and amino acids (Fig. 5).[80] Also, other metabolites have been suggested to be present in radiation necrosis. For example, in one study monitoring the progression of severe cerebral radiation injuries in the temporal lobes in patients previously treated for nasopharyngeal carcinoma an unknown resonance named Px in the 2.37 to 2.40 ppm region was found in affected temporal lobes. The authors speculated if Px could be associated with anaerobic glycolysis producing

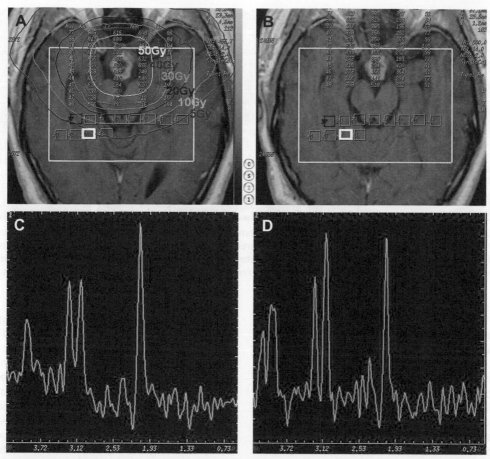

Fig. 4. (*A–D*) Post–Gd-DTPA T1-weighted images before RT (*top left*) and 6 months after the completion of RT (*top right*). The large white boxes represent the volume of interest for MR spectroscopy acquisition, and small white boxes depict the individual volume of interest for spectral analysis. The two representative spectra before radiation treatment (*bottom left*) and 6 months after radiation treatment (*bottom right*) were from the corresponding bright white boxes in top panels. Color contours denote isodose lines of radiation.

pyruvate (2.37 ppm) or succinate (2.40 ppm), as can be seen in brain abscess formations.[81]

Overall, it looks like higher Cho/NAA and Cho/Cr ratios are to be expected in areas of recurrent tumor compared with areas of radiation injury and with normal adjacent brain tissue as reported by several studies. Different MR spectroscopy studies using different spectroscopy technique have reported an 80% to 97% success rate to retrospectively differentiate recurrent tumor from radiation injury with significantly increased Cho/NAA and Cho/Cr ratios.[69,70,79]

Different so-called "metabolic cut-off values" have been suggested to differentiate recurrent tumor from radiation injury.[69] A previous study using two-dimensional CSI reported that when cut-off values of 1.8 for either Cho/NAA or Cho/Cr were used (ie, values above 1.8 being diagnostic for tumor recurrence) 27 out of 28 patients were retrospectively correctly diagnosed.[69] Values

that are in agreement with those in a previous study using multivoxel 1H-MRSI and correlation with histologic specimens[70] in which the investigators claim that a Cho/Cr ratio over 1.79 or lipid or lactate (Lip-lac)/Cho ratio less than 0.75 has a sevenfold increased odds of being pure tumor compared with pure necrosis and the odds of the biopsy's being pure necrosis and having either the Cho/nCr values less than 0.89 or a Cho/nCho value less than 0.66 are six times the odds of the biopsy's being pure tumor.[70] Another study using receiver operating characteristic analysis reported the sensitivity, specificity, and diagnostic accuracy of three-dimensional 1H-MR spectroscopy to be 94.1%, 100%, and 96.2%, respectively, based on the cut-off values of 1.71 for Cho/Cr or 1.71 for Cho/NAA or both as tumor criterion.[82] The Cho/Lip or Lac is another ratio that has been used to diagnose radiation necrosis. In another study the authors reported positive predictive

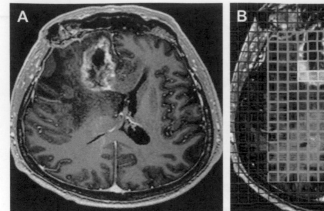
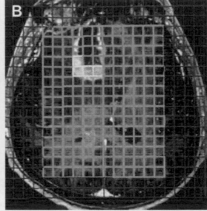
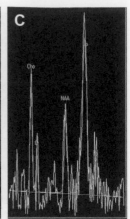

Fig. 5. (*A–C*) Axial post–Gd-DTPA T1-weighted image demonstrates a focal heterogeneously enhancing lesion in the right frontal lobe. The volume of interest of the three-dimensional chemical shift imaging MR spectroscopy (*B*) and corresponding spectra with significantly elevated lipid peak, slight decrease in NAA peak, and slight increase in the choline peak. The lesion was surgically removed and was proved to be radiation necrosis.

values of a Cho/Lip or Lac ratio less than 0.3 and the positive predictive values of a Cho/Cr ratio less than 2.48 for diagnosing radiation necrosis were 100% and 71.4%, respectively.[83]

Many of these newly occurring lesions do not only consist of large areas of pure tumor or radiation injury and necrosis but rather are a mixture of tumor cells and tissue with radiation injury present. This assumption is supported by a prior study of multivoxel MR spectroscopy that found that "spectral patterns do allow reliable differential diagnostic statements to be made when the tissues are composed of either pure tumor or pure necrosis, but the spectral patterns are less definitive when tissues composed of varying degrees of mixed tumor and necrosis are examined."[84]

Positron Emission Tomography

Previous positron emission tomography studies have shown that areas of radiation injury have lower glucose metabolism than normal brain tissue because they have lower cellular density.[85] A previous positron emission tomography review reports the sensitivity of positron emission tomography to be 80% to 90% and the specificity to be 50% to 90% in differentiating late-delayed radiation injury from recurrent high-grade glioma.[86] Another study of 15 patients with histopathologically confirmed diagnosis reported that fluorodeoxyglucose (FDG) positron emission tomography was only 43% sensitive in distinguishing recurrent tumor from radiation effect, and was least accurate when the lesion volume was less than 6 mL.[87] False-positive FDG positron emission

tomography and Tl-201 single-photon emission CT have been reported with biopsy-proved radiation necrosis.[88]

FDG positron emission tomography and ^{15}O positron emission tomography (CBF) have been used to relate dose-dependent radiologic defined changes in normal brain tissue to neurocognitive dysfunction. In that recent study a dose-dependent response of central nervous system tissue was detected using FDG positron emission tomography and the decrease in central nervous system metabolism correlated with decreased performance on neuropsychologic tests.[89] They also demonstrated transient changes in CBF with ^{15}O; increased relative CBF with increasing dose measured by an increase in ^{15}O changes at 3 weeks after treatment in areas receiving greater then 30 Gy by significantly lower levels at 6 months after treatment.[89]

^{11}C-Methonine (Met) positron emission tomography has in a few recent studies demonstrated the possibility to accurately distinguish recurrent brain tumor from radiation necrosis. In a recent MET positron emission tomography study of 21 patients previously treated for primary or secondary neoplasm presenting with a total of 27 lesions the authors report intense MET uptake in patients with recurrent tumor (mean 1.79 ± 0.32 vs 1.05 ± 0.11, $P<0.0001$), whereas no significant MET uptake was seen in patients with radiation necrosis with 100% sensitivity, specificity, and accuracy of visual interpretation of the MET uptake.[90]

More about the use of positron emission tomography imaging to differentiate radiation necrosis from recurrent tumor is discussed elsewhere in this issue.

Vascular Imaging

There are limited reports about the CBF and CBV changes in normal brain that has been irradiated. The limited existing reports indicate that there are changes in the CBF and CBV after irradiation and that these changes might be dose-dependent.[89,91–94]

In a prospective study of DCE MR imaging of prediction of radiation-induced neurocognitive dysfunction Cao and coworkers[92] found that vascular volumes and blood-brain barrier (BBB) permeability increased significantly in the high-dose regions during RT, followed by a decrease after RT. Changes in both vascular volume and BBB permeability correlated with the doses accumulated at the time of scans at weeks 3 and 6 during RT and 1 month after RT. The effect of the dose-volume on the vascular volume was also observed. Finally, changes in verbal learning scores 6 months after RT were significantly correlated with changes in vascular volumes of left temporal and frontal lobes and changes in BBB permeability of left frontal lobes during RT. Similar correlation was found between recall scores and BBB permeability. These data suggest that the early changes in cerebral vasculature may predict delayed alterations in verbal learning and total recall, which are important components of neuro-cognitive function.

Mean and regional CBF was measured at before, 2 weeks, and 3 months after SRS in a 99mTc-HMPAO to elucidate the radiation effect on the normal brain after SRS.[92] They found significant reductions in mean CBF (by 7%) and regional CBF in the peritarget areas (by 5%–7%) and out-of-field areas (by 6%–22%) were recognized at 2 weeks and 3 months after SRS.[93]

Another study using dynamic-susceptibility contrast perfusion MR imaging demonstrated lower relative CBV in normal-appearing brain tissue 2 months after radiotherapy suggesting a dose-dependent decline in vessel density and increase in vascular permeability or tortuosity in irradiated normal-appearing brain tissue.[91]

A recent study using perfusion CT demonstrated higher nCBV and nCBF and lower nMTT compared with radiation necrosis.[94] More about the use of perfusion imaging both with MR imaging and CT to differentiate radiation necrosis from recurrent tumor is discussed elsewhere in this issue.

SUMMARY

Several different imaging techniques point in the same direction that occult injury to the normal brain occurs during radiation treatment. In the future these different imaging biomakers might be able to compare the effects of different radiation treatment regimens and to evaluate neuroprotective therapies with the potential to minimize the neurotoxicity of brain radiation treatment.

The differentiation of recurrent tumor from radiation injury remains a challenge and the combination of conventional MR imaging and more than one of the other more advanced imaging modalities, such as MR spectroscopy and positron emission tomography, are often needed to come to a conclusion.

REFERENCES

1. Schultheiss TE, Kun LE, Ang KK, et al. Radiation response of the central nervous system. Int J Radiat Oncol Biol Phys 1995;31:1093–112.
2. Tofilon PJ, Fike JR. The radioresponse of the central nervous system: a dynamic process. Radiat Res 2000;153:357–70.
3. Khuntia D, Brown P, Li J, et al. Whole-brain radiotherapy in the management of brain metastasis. J Clin Oncol 2006;24:1295–304.
4. Klein M, Heimans JJ, Aaronson NK, et al. Effect of radiotherapy and other treatment related factors on mid-term to long-term cognitive sequelae in low-grade gliomas: a comparative study. Lancet 2002; 360:1361–8.
5. Brown PD, Buckner JC, O'Fallon JR, et al. Effects of radiotherapy on cognitive function in patients with low-grade glioma measured by the Folstein mini-mental state examination. J Clin Oncol 2003;21: 2519–24.
6. Hopewell JW, Wright EA. The nature of latent cerebral irradiation damage and its modification by hypertension. Br J Radiol 1970;43:161–7.
7. Sheline GE, Wara WM, Smith V. Therapeutic irradiation and brain injury. Int J Radiat Oncol Biol Phys 1980;6:1215–28.
8. Constine LS, Konski A, Ekholm S, et al. Adverse effects of brain irradiation correlated with MR and CT imaging. Int J Radiat Oncol Biol Phys 1988;15: 319–30.
9. Isuruda JS, Kortman KE, Bradley WG, et al. Radiation effects on cerebral white matter: MR evaluation. AJR Am J Roentgenol 1987;49:165–71.
10. Flickinger JC, Lunsford LD, Kondziolka D, et al. Radiosurgery and brain tolerance: an analysis of neurodiagnostic imaging changes after gamma knife radiosurgery for arteriovenous malformations. Int J Radiat Oncol Biol Phys 1992;23:19–26.
11. Loeffler JS, Siddon RL, Wen PY, et al. Stereotactic radiosurgery of the brain using a standard linear accelerator: a study of early and late effects. Radiother Oncol 1990;17:311–21.

12. Van Tassel P, Bruner JM, Maor MH, et al. MR of toxic effects of accelerated fractionation radiation therapy and carboplatin chemotherapy for malignant gliomas. AJNR Am J Neuroradiol 1995;16: 715–26.

13. Kumar AJ, Leeds NE, Fuller GN, et al. Malignant gliomas: MR imaging spectrum of radiation therapy- and chemotherapy-induced necrosis of the brain after treatment. Radiology 2000;217:377–84.

14. Kramer S. Radiation effect and tolerance of the central nervous system. Front Radiat Ther Oncol. 1972;6:332–45.

15. Postma TJ, Klein M, Verstappen CC, et al. Radiotherapy-induced cerebral abnormalities in patients with low-grade glioma. Neurology 2002;59:121–3.

16. Sundgren PC, Elias A, Rogers L, et al. Correlation of MR imaging morphologic abnormalities, MR spectroscopy, and radiation treatment dose volumes in histologically proved cerebral radiation necrosis. In: Programs and abstracts of the 47th Annual Meeting of the American Society of Neuroradiology. Vancouver (Canada), May 16–21, 2009. p. 219–20.

17. Mehta MP, Shapiro WR, Glantz MJ, et al. Lead-in phase to randomized trial of motexafin gadolinium and whole-brain radiation for patients with brain metastases: centralized assessment of magnetic resonance imaging, neurocognitive, and neurologic end points. J Clin Oncol 2002;20:3445–53.

18. Meyers CA, Brown PD. Role and relevance of neurocognitive assessment in clinical trials of patients with CNS tumors. J Clin Oncol 2006;24:1305–9.

19. Roman DD, Sperduto PW. Neuropsychological effects of cranial radiation: current knowledge and future directions. Int J Radiat Oncol Biol Phys 1995;31:983–98.

20. Crossen JR, Garwood D, Glatstein E, et al. Neurobehavioral sequelae of cranial irradiation in adults: a review of radiation-induced encephalopathy. J Clin Oncol 1994;12:627–42.

21. Hodges H, Katzung N, Sowinski P, et al. Late behavioural and neuropathological effects of local brain irradiation in the rat. Behav Brain Res 1998;91: 99–114.

22. Mulhern RK, Palmer SL, Merchant TE, et al. Neurocognitive consequences of risk-adapted therapy for childhood medulloblastoma. J Clin Oncol 2005; 23:5511–9.

23. Belka C, Budach W, Kortmann RD, et al. Radiation induced CNS toxicity: molecular and cellular mechanisms. Br J Cancer 2001;85:1233–9.

24. Wong CS, Van der Kogel AJ. Mechanisms of radiation injury to the central nervous system: implications for neuroprotection. Mol Interv 2004;4:273–84.

25. Price RE, Langford LA, Jackson EF, et al. Radiation-induced morphologic changes in the rhesus monkey (Macaca mulatta) brain. J Med Primatol 2001;30: 81–7.

26. Ljubimova NV, Levitman MK, Plotnikova ED, et al. Endothelial cell population dynamics in rat brain after local irradiation. Br J Radiol 1991;64:934–40.

27. Pena LA, Fuks Z, Kolesnick R. Radiation-induced apoptosis of endothelial cells in the murine central nervous system: protection by fibroblast growth factor and sphingomyelinase deficiency. Cancer Res 2000;60:321–7.

28. Li YQ, Chen P, Haimovitz-Friedman A, et al. Endothelial apoptosis initiates acute blood-brain barrier disruption after ionizing radiation. Cancer Res 2003;63:5950–6.

29. Calvo W, Hopewell JW, Reinhold HS, et al. Time- and dose-related changes in the white matter of the rat brain after single doses of X rays. Br J Radiol 1988;1:1043–52.

30. Reinhold HS, Calvo W, Hopewell JW, et al. Development of blood vessel-related radiation damage in the fimbria of the central nervous system. Int J Radiat Oncol Biol Phys 1990;8:37–42.

31. Okeda R, Okada S, Kawano A, et al. Neuropathology of delayed encephalopathy in cats induced by heavy-ion irradiation. J Radiat Res (Tokyo) 2003; 44:345–52.

32. Santana P, Pena LA, Haimovitz-Friedman A, et al. Acid sphingomyelinase-deficient human lymphoblasts and mice are defective in radiation-induced apoptosis. Cell 1996;86:189–99.

33. Eissner G, Kohlhuber F, Grell M, et al. Critical involvement of transmembrane tumor necrosis factor-alpha in endothelial programmed cell death mediated by ionizing radiation and bacterial endotoxin. Blood 1995;86:4184–93.

34. Verheij M, Dewit LG, Boomgaard MN, et al. Ionizing radiation enhances platelet adhesion to the extracellular matrix of human endothelial cells by an increase in the release of von Willebrand factor. Radiat Res 1994;137:202–7.

35. Fike JR, Sheline GE, Cann CE, et al. Radiation necrosis. Prog Exp Tumor Res 1984;28:136–51.

36. van der Maazen RW, Kleiboer BJ, Verhagen I, et al. Irradiation in vitro discriminates between different O-2A progenitor cell subpopulations in the perinatal central nervous system of rats. Radiat Res 1991; 128:64–72.

37. van der Maazen RW, Kleiboer BJ, Verhagen I, et al. Repair capacity of adult rat glial progenitor cells determined by an in vitro clonogenic assay after in vitro or in vivo fractionated irradiation. Int J Radiat Biol 1993;63:661–6.

38. van der Maazen RW, Verhagen I, Kleiboer BJ, et al. Radiosensitivity of glial progenitor cells of the perinatal and adult rat optic nerve studied by an in vitro clonogenic assay. Radiother Oncol 1991;20:258–64.

39. Monje ML, Mizumatsu S, Fike JR, et al. Irradiation induces neural precursor-cell dysfunction. Nat Med 2002;8:955–62.

40. DeWit MC, de Bruin HG, Eijkenboom W, et al. Immediate post-radiotherapy changes in malignant glioma can mimic tumor progression. Neurology 2004;63(3):535–7.

41. Brandsma D, Stalphers L, Taal W, et al. Clinical features, mechanisms, and management of pseudo-progression in malignant gliomas. Lancet Oncol 2008;9(5):453–61.

42. Taal W, Brandsma D, de Bruin H, et al. Incidence of early pseudo-progression in a cohort of malignant glioma patients treated with chemoirradiation with temozolomide. Cancer 2008;113(2):405–10.

43. Brandes AA, Franceschi E, Tosoni A, et al. MGMT promoter methylation status can predict the incidence and outcome of pseudoprogression after concomitant radiochemotherapy in newly diagnosed glioblastoma patients. J Clin Oncol 2008; 26(13):2192–7.

44. Gerstner ER, McNamara MB, Norden AD, et al. Effect of adding temozolomide to radiation therapy on the incidence of pseudo-progression. J Neuro-oncol 2009;94:97–101 [epub Feb, 17].

45. Basser PJ, Pierpaoli C. Microstructural and physiological features of tissues elucidated by quantitative-diffusion-tensor MRI. J Magn Reson B 1996; 111:209–19.

46. Basser PJ, Pierpaoli C. A simplified method to measure the diffusion tensor from seven MR images. Magn Reson Med 1998;39:928–34.

47. Pierpaoli C, Jezzard P, Basser PJ, et al. Diffusion tensor MR imaging of the human brain. Radiology 1996;201:637–48.

48. Song SK, Sun SW, Ramsbottom MJ, et al. Dysmyelination revealed through MRI as increased radial (but unchanged axial) diffusion of water. Neuroimage 2002;17:1429–36.

49. Wang S, Wu EX, Qiu D, et al. Longitudinal diffusion tensor magnetic resonance imaging study of radiation-induced white matter damage in a rat model. Cancer Res 2009;69:1190–8.

50. Khong PL, Leung LH, Chan GC, et al. White matter anisotropy in childhood medulloblastoma survivors: association with neurotoxicity risk factors. Radiology 2005;236:647–52.

51. Khong PL, Leung I H, Fung AS, et al. White matter anisotropy in post-treatment childhood cancer survivors: preliminary evidence of association with neurocognitive function. J Clin Oncol 2006;24:884–90.

52. Dellani PR, Eder S, Gawehn J, et al. Late structural alterations of cerebral white matter in long-term survivors of childhood leukemia. J Magn Reson Imaging 2008;27:1250–5.

53. Nagesh V, Tsien CI, Chenevert TL, et al. Radiation-induced changes in normal-appearing white matter in patients with cerebral tumors: a diffusion tensor imaging study. Int J Radiat Oncol Biol Phys 2008; 70:1002–10.

54. Welzel T, Niethammer A, Mende U, et al. Diffusion tensor imaging screening of radiation-induced changes in the white matter after prophylactic cranial irradiation of patients with small cell lung cancer: first results of a prospective study. AJNR Am J Neuroradiol 2008;29:379–83.

55. Hein PA, Eskey CJ, Dunn JF, et al. Diffusion-weighted imaging in the follow-up of treated high-grade gliomas: tumor recurrence versus radiation injury. AJNR Am J Neuroradiol 2004;25:201–9.

56. Sundgren PC, Fan XY, Weybright P, et al. Differentiation of recurrent brain tumor versus radiation injury using diffusion tensor imaging in patients with new contrast enhancing lesions. Magn Reson Imaging 2006;44:1131–42.

57. Zhou XJ, Leeds NE, Kumar AJ, et al. Differentiation of tumor recurrence from treatment-induced necrosis using quantitative diffusion MRI. In: Proceedings for the 9th Annual meeting of the International Society of Magnetic Resonance in Medicine. Glasgow (Scotland), April 21–27, 2001. p. 726.

58. Chenevert T, McKeever P, Ross B. Monitoring early response of experimental brain tumors to therapy using diffusion magnetic resonance imaging. Clin Cancer Res 1997;3:1457–66.

59. Chenevert T, Stegman L, Taylor JM, et al. Diffusion magnetic resonance imaging: an early surrogate marker of therapeutic efficacy in brain tumors. J Natl Cancer Inst. 2000;92:2029–36.

60. Chan YL, Roebuck DJ, Yuen MP, et al. Long-term cerebral metabolite changes on proton magnetic resonance spectroscopy inpatients cured of acute lymphoblastic leukemia with previous intrathecal methotrexate and cranial irradiation prophylaxis. Int J Radiat Oncol Biol Phys 2001;50(3):759–63.

61. Davidson A, Tait DM, Payne GS, et al. Magnetic resonance spectroscopy in the evaluation of neurotoxicity following cranial irradiation for childhood cancer. Br J Radiol 2000;73(868):421–4.

62. Chan YL, Yeung DKW, Leung SF, et al. Proton magnetic resonance spectroscopy of late delayed radiation-induced injury of the brain. J Magn Reson Imaging 1999;10:130–7.

63. Usenius T, Usenius JP, Tenhunen M, et al. Radiation-induced changes in human brain metabolites as studied by 1H nuclear magnetic resonance spectroscopy in vivo. Int J Radiat Oncol Biol Phys 1995; 33(3):719–24.

64. Kaminaga T, Shirai K. Radiation-induced brain metabolic changes in the acute and early delayed phase detected with quantitative proton magnetic resonance spectroscopy. J Comput Assist Tomogr. 2005;29(3):293–7.

65. Walecki J, Sokól M, Pieniázek P, et al. Role of short Te 1H-MR spectroscopy in monitoring of post-operation irradiated patients. Eur J Radiol 1999;30: 154–61.

66. Estève F, Rubin C, Grand S, et al. Transient metabolic changes observed with proton MR spectroscopy in normal human brain after radiation therapy. Int J Radiat Oncol Biol Phys 1998;40:279–86.

67. Lee MC, Pirzkall A, McKnight TR, et al. ^{1}H-MRS of radiation effects in normal-appearing white matter: dose-dependence and impact on automated spectral classification. J Magn Reson Imaging 2004;19:379–88.

68. Sundgren PC, Nagesh V, Elias A, et al. Metabolic alterations; a biomarker for radiation-induced injury of normal brain. An spectroscopy study. J Magn Reson Imaging 2009;29(2):291–7.

69. Weybright P, Sundgren PC, Gomez-Hassan D, et al. Differentiation of tumor recurrence from treatment related changes using 2D-CSI MR spectroscopy. AJR Am J Roentgenol 2005;185:1471–6.

70. Rock JP, Hearshen D, Scarpace L, et al. Correlations between magnetic resonance spectroscopy and image-guided histopathology, with special attention to radiation necrosis. Neurosurgery 2002;51:912–9.

71. Schlemmer JP, Bachert P, Henze M, et al. Differentiation of radiation necrosis from tumor progression using proton magnetic resonance spectroscopy. Neuroradiology 2002;44:216–22.

72. Movsas B, Li BSY, Babb JS, et al. Quantifying radiation therapy-induced brain injury with whole brain proton MR spectroscopy: initial observations. Radiology 2001;221:327–31.

73. Isobe T, Matsumura A, Anno I, et al. Changes in 1H-MRSin glioma patients before and after irradiation: the significance of quantitative analysis of choline-containing compounds. No Shinkei Geka 2003;31(2): 167–72 [abstract in English, article in Japanese].

74. Virta A, Patronas N, Raman R, et al. Spectroscopic imaging of radiation-induced effects in the white matter of glioma patients. J Magn Reson Imaging 2000;18:851–7.

75. Atwood T, Robbins ME, Zhu J-M. Quantitative in vivo proton MR spectroscopic evaluation of the irradiated rat brain. J Magn Reson Imaging 2007;26(6):1590–6.

76. Atwood T, Payne VS, Zhao W, et al. Quantitative magnetic resonance spectroscopy reveals a potential relationship between radiation-induced changes in rat brain metabolites and cognitive impairment. Radiat Res 2007;168(5):574–81.

77. Chong VF, Rumpel H, Fan YF, et al. Temporal lobe changes following radiation therapy: imaging and proton MR spectroscopic findings. Eur Radiol 2001;11:317–24.

78. Chong VF, Rumpel H, Aw YS, et al. Temporal lobe necrosis following radiation therapy for nasopharyngeal carcinoma: 1H MR spectroscopic findings. Int J Radiat Oncol Biol Phys 1999;45:699–705.

79. Schlemmer HP, Bachert P, Herfarth K, et al. Proton MR spectroscopic evaluation of suspicious brain lesions after stereotactic radiotherapy. ANJR Am J Neuroradiol 2001;22:1316–24.

80. Castillo M, Kwock L, Mukherji SK. Clinical applications of proton MR spectroscopy. AJNR Am J Neuroradiol 1996;17:1–15.

81. Yeung DK, Chan Y, Leung S, et al. Detection of an intense resonance at 2.4 ppm in 1H MR spectra of patients with severe late-delayed, radiation-induced brain injuries. Magn Reson Med 2001;45:994–1000.

82. Zeng QS, Li CF, Zhang K, et al. Multivoxel 3D proton MR spectroscopy in the distinction of recurrent glioma from radiation injury. J Neurooncol 2007;84:63–9.

83. Kimura T, Sako K, Gotoh T, et al. In vivo single voxel proton MR spectroscopy in brain lesions with ring-like enhancement. NMR Biomed 2001;14:339–49.

84. Rock JP, Scarpace L, Hearshen D, et al. Associations among magnetic resonance spectroscopy, apparent diffusion coefficients and image-guided histopathology with special attention to radiation necrosis. Neurosurgery 2004;54:1111–9.

85. Di Chiro G, Oldfield E, Wright DC. Cerebral necrosis after radiotherapy and/or intraarterial chemotherapy for brain tumors. PET and neuropathologic studies. AJR Am J Roentgenol 1988;150:189–97.

86. Langleben DD, Segall GM. PET in differentiation of recurrent brain tumor from radiation injury. J Nucl Med 2000;41:1861–7.

87. Thompson TP, Lunsford LD, Kondziolka D. Distinguishing recurrent tumor and radiation necrosis with positron emission tomography versus stereotactic biopsy. Stereotact Funct Neurosurg 1999;73:9–14.

88. Matheja P, Rickert C, Weckesser M, et al. Scintigraphic pitfall: delayed radionecrosis: case illustration. J Neurosurg 2000;92:732.

89. Hahn CA, Zhou SM, Raynor R, et al. Dose-dependent effects of radiation therapy on cerebral blood flow, metabolism, and neurocognitive dysfunction. Int J Radiat Oncol Biol Phys 2009;73(4):1082–7.

90. Katoh N, Nakada K, Takei T, et al. Methionine PET in differentiating recurrent brain tumor from radiation necrosis following cranial radiation. Int Congr Ser 2004;1264:217–21.

91. Lee MC, Cha S, Chang SM, et al. Dynamic susceptibility contrast perfusion imaging of radiation effects in normal-appearing brain tissue: changes in the first-pass and recirculation phases. J Magn Reson Imaging 2005;21(6):683–93.

92. Cao Y, Tsien CI, Sundgren P, et al. DCE MRI as a biomarker for prediction of radiation-induced neurocognitive dysfunction. Clinical Cancer Research 2009;15(5):1747–54.

93. Taki S, Higashi K, Oguchi M, et al. Changes in regional cerebral blood flow in irradiated regions and normal brain after stereotactic radiosurgery. Ann Nucl Med 2002;16(4):273–7.

94. Jain R, Scarpace L, Ellika S, et al. First-pass perfusion computed tomography: initial experience in differentiating recurrent brain tumors from radiation effects and radiation necrosis. Neurosurgery 2007;61:778–86.

Imaging of the Central Skull Base

KEYWORDS

- Central skull base • CT • MR imaging
- Skull base pathology • Skull base tumors
- Sellar and parasellar lesions

The central skull base (CSB), the ultimate frontier between the intracranial compartment and the extracranial head and neck, can be affected by intrinsic lesions originating from the bony-cartilaginous structures of the skull base proper or by lesions originating from the neighboring structures from the intracranial compartment above or from the extracranial head and neck below. Because clinical assessment of the CSB is limited, cross-sectional imaging has become the mainstay for the diagnosis, treatment planning, and follow-up of patients with skull base lesions.[1–3] Developments in cross-sectional imaging and in surgical and targeted radiation therapy techniques have largely contributed to improve the prognosis of patients with skull base tumors and to decrease the surgical-related morbidity and mortality.[2–6] Multidisciplinary skull base teams, including ear, nose, and throat (ENT) surgeons; neurosurgeons; radiation therapists; radiologists; and oncologists, have been created to provide a comprehensive approach to patients with skull base lesions with the aim of maximizing the chances for long-term survival with the minimum amount of dysfunction and disfigurement possible.[3,6,7]

Cross-sectional imaging can narrow down the differential diagnoses according to the site of origin, pattern of growth, and imaging features of a given lesion; can accurately delineate tumor margins; and can determine the precise relations between the lesion and important surrounding structures.[3,8,9]

This review focuses on the contribution of imaging to patient management, providing a systematic approach to CSB lesions based on an anatomic division of the CSB and on the tissue constituents present in each division. Detailed knowledge of skull base anatomy is required for correct imaging diagnosis and for accurate delineation of lesions.

ANATOMY

Viewed from above, the skull base shows three naturally contoured regions that grossly correspond to the anterior skull base, CSB, and posterior skull base. The CSB makes up the floor of the middle cranial fossa and is mainly composed of the sphenoid and temporal bone anterior to the petrous ridge (Fig. 1). It is separated from the anterior skull base by a line that follows the tuberculum sella, the anterior clinoid processes, the posterior margin of the lesser sphenoid wings, and the anterior and superior rim of the greater sphenoid wings and is separated from the posterior skull base by a line following the spheno-occipital synchondrosis medially and the petroclival synchondrosis and superior ridge of the petrous and mastoid bones posteriorly and laterally.[3,4,8–10]

IMAGING APPROACH TO PATHOLOGIC FINDINGS

For diagnostic imaging purposes, it is useful to subdivide the CSB further into midline sagittal, off-midline parasagittal, and lateral compartments by drawing vertical lines passing medially to the petroclival fissure and just lateral to the foramen ovale, respectively (Fig. 2).[8,9,10] The midline sagittal compartment includes the body of the sphenoid and the portion of the clivus anterior to the spheno-occipital synchondrosis (basisphenoid),

The reprint of this artical from August 2009 provides readers corrected images for Figures 4E-F, 6A-B, 15C-D, 22A, 25B-F, and 27C-D.

Radiology Departement, Instituto Português de Oncologia de Francisco Gentil- Centro de Lisboa Rua Prof. Lima Basto, 1093, Lisboa, Portugal
E-mail address: borgalexandra@gmail.com

Neuroimag Clin N Am 19 (2009) 669–696
doi:10.1016/j.nic.2009.11.001
1052-5149/09/$ – see front matter © 2009 Published by Elsevier Inc.

neuroimaging.theclinics.com

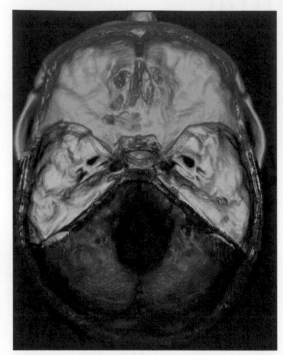

Fig. 1. Three-dimensional CT reconstruction represents the skull base division into anterior (*green*), central (*light orange*), and posterior (*blue*) compartments.

contains the sphenoid sinus, and is bordered superiorly by the sella turcica and inferiorly by the roof and posterior wall of the nasopharynx (**Fig. 3**). It is pierced by the intracranial opening of the orbital apex, giving passage to the optic nerves (**Fig. 4**A). The parasagittal compartment includes the petroclival synchondrosis, foramen

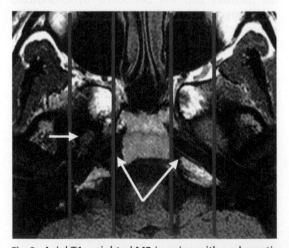

Fig. 2. Axial T1-weighted MR imaging with a schematic representation of the CSB subdivision into sagittal, parasagittal, and lateral compartments. The medial red lines pass in the medial aspect of the petroclival synchondrosis (*long white arrows*). The lateral red lines pass immediately lateral to the foramen ovale (*short white arrow*).

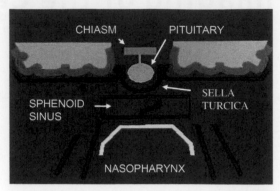

Fig. 3. Schematic representation of the central sagittal skull base with the body of the sphenoid and sphenoid sinus medially, the sella turcica and pituitary gland above, and the nasopharyngeal mucosal space below.

lacerum, and medial aspect of the greater sphenoid wing. It is bordered superiorly and medially by the parasellar region containing the cavernous sinus, superiorly and laterally by the basal temporal lobes, and inferiorly by the parapharyngeal and masticator spaces of the suprahyoid neck. Most of the neurovascular foramina of the CSB lay in this compartment, including the intracranial opening of the superior orbital fissure traversed by cranial nerves III, IV, V1, and VI and the superior ophthalmic vein on their way from the cavernous sinus to the orbit; the foramen rotundum giving passage to V2 on its way from the cavernous sinus to the pterygopalatine fossa; the vidian canal containing the vidian nerve and artery extending from the foramen lacerum to the high pterygopalatine fossa; the foramen ovale traversed by V3 on its way to the masticator space; and the foramen spinosum crossed by the middle meningeal artery. The cavernous sinus, the most important component of the parasagittal CSB, contains, from superior to inferior, cranial nerves III, IV, V1, and V2 enclosed within a dural leaflet of its lateral wall and the cavernous carotid artery and cranial nerve VI within the sinus itself. Finally, the lateral division of the CSB comprises the lateral aspect of the greater sphenoid wing, including the sphenoid triangle, temporal squamosa, and the glenoid cavity of the temporomandibular joint (TMJ).[3,8,9]

In addition to location, knowing the major tissue constituents of the CSB can help in establishing further possible differential diagnoses for a skull base lesion. Although some tissues are common to all subdivisions of the CSB, including bone and the pachymeninges investing the intracranial aspect of the skull base, others are site specific.[8,9] The surgical approach to CSB lesions also varies according to lesion location in each of these compartments (transsphenoidal, transmastoid, temporopteryonal, and frontotemporal approaches).[7,8]

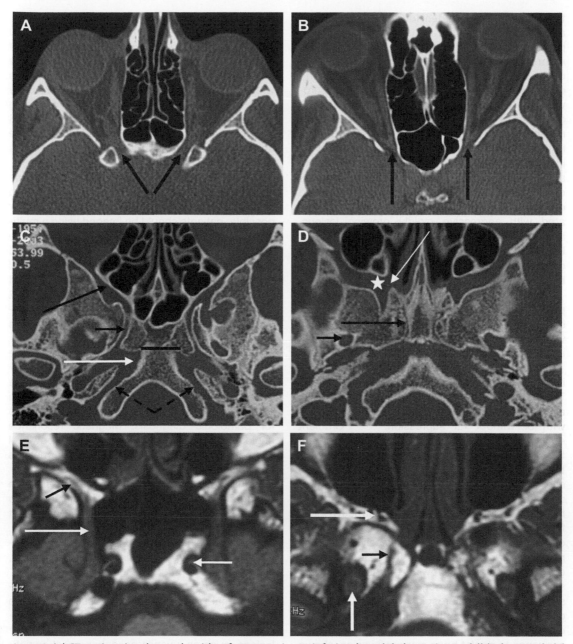

Fig. 4. Axial CT sections in a bone algorithm from superior to inferior show (A) the optic canal (*black arrows*); (B) the superior orbital fissure (*black arrows*); (C) the inferior orbital fissure (*long black arrow*), foramen rotundum (*short black arrow*), foramen lacerum (*white arrow*), the petroclival (*dashed black arrows*) and spheno-occipital (*black line*) synchondroses; (D) the high pterygopalatine fossa (*white star*), the sphenopalatine foramen (*long white arrow*); the vidian canal (*long black arrow*) and foramen ovale (*short black arrow*). Axial sensitivity encoding (SENSE) T1W MR images shows (E) V2 within foramen rotundum (*white arrow*), the inferior orbital branch within the inferior orbital fissure (*black arrow*) and (F) V3 within foramen ovale (*white arrow*), the vidian nerve (*short black arrow*) and the sphenopalatine ganglion in the high pterygopalatine fossa (*long black arrow*).

IMAGING MODALITIES AND IMAGING TECHNIQUE

In assessing the CSB, CT and MR imaging have a complementary role and are often used together to establish the presumptive diagnosis and to depict the full extent of a lesion.[8] MR imaging is preferred to assess the soft tissue component and to determine its relations with adjacent structures. It is the modality with the highest accuracy to depict intracranial extent (dural, leptomeningeal, and brain parenchyma invasion), perineural and perivascular spread, and bone marrow involvement.[8,11,12] CT remains the technique of choice to define the bony anatomy of the skull base and to depict the thin cortical margins of skull base neurovascular foramina.[3,8,12,13] It is quite specific in the diagnosis of primary bone lesions (neoplastic and non-neoplastic), is more sensitive than MR imaging in the depiction of calcifications, and can provide information regarding the rate of growth and aggressiveness of a lesion by showing its effect on adjacent bone.[8,13] Whereas permeative and erosive patterns of bone involvement are associated with aggressive rapidly growing lesions, malignant neoplasms, or infectious processes, bone expansion and remodeling with smooth cortical thinning are usually associated with more benign slow-growing processes.[8,9,13]

Therefore, in most institutions with multidisciplinary skull base teams, imaging evaluation of skull base lesions includes a full MR imaging study with gadolinium and a high-resolution CT scan using a bone algorithm during the same visit.[7]

The magnetic resonance protocol should include images in the three orthogonal planes using T1 and T2 weighting, short-tau inversion recovery (STIR), and gadolinium-enhanced T1-weighted images with or without fat supression.[8,11–13] Gradient echo T2* images may be useful to demonstrate the presence of susceptibility artifacts related to the presence of paramagnetic substances, such as calcifications, blood degradation products, or melanin within a lesion.[11,14,15] High-resolution highly T2-weighted sequences (constructive interference in the steady state or driven equilibrium radiofrequency reset pulse) can nicely depict the relation between a lesion and the cisternal course of cranial nerves by showing the nerves as dark structures traveling through the high signal intensity of the cerebrospinal fluid (CSF)–filled cisterns.[12,13] A conventional spin echo or fast spin echo T1-weighted sequence is the single best sequence to depict bone marrow invasion, shown as replacement of the hyperintense fatty marrow by hypointense material.[11–16] Intravenous administration of gadolinium is mandatory to depict meningeal invasion and perineural spread and usually maximizes tumor contrast against adjacent structures that do not enhance to the same degree.[11–15] The use of fat suppression, particularly employing techniques based on frequency-selective fat-suppression pulses, is not consensual. Although it can potentially increase the conspicuity of an enhancing lesion against a fat-containing background, failure of fat suppression attributable to the numerous interfaces seen at the CSB (where

bone, air-containing sphenoid sinus, soft tissues, and fat lay close together) is often a problem and may lead to false-positive results.[8,13,17] The use of STIR, which is not based on frequency-selective pulses, or contrast-enhanced T1-weighted images with appropriate windowing is preferred by some.[8,17] High-resolution sensitivity encoding (SENSE) parallel imaging and high-field 3-T MR imaging are being increasingly used to depict fine anatomic detail, particularly to study cranial nerves and the walls of the cavernous sinus.[13,18]

CT studies of the skull base must include images in at least two orthogonal planes with a slice thickness less than 3 mm. Whenever possible, patients should be imaged using a multidetector helical or volumetric scanner, with a single acquisition in the axial plane further reconstructed in different planes as needed without additional radiation to the patient.[8,11] When CT is obtained as an adjunct to a prior contrast-enhanced MR imaging study, orthogonal images in a high-resolution bone algorithm should suffice.[4,7,8] When CT is used as a single examination, a full contrast-enhanced study should be obtained in soft tissue and bone algorithms.[8,16]

CT and open-field MR imaging scanners can be used for image guidance of fine-needle aspiration cytology or core biopsy to obtain a tissue sample for pathologic diagnosis. Magnetic resonance angiography and CT angiography can be powerful adjuncts in the depiction of vascular malformations and in assessing hypervascular lesions.[3,4,8,12]

[18]F-fluorodeoxyglucose positron emission tomography is essentially used in the follow-up of skull base tumors to differentiate post-treatment changes from persistent or recurrent neoplasm. No routine role has been found in the primary evaluation of patients presenting with CSB lesions, however.[8]

Conventional angiography is mainly used for interventional procedures and to assess the circle of Willis when a carotid artery needs to be sacrificed. Preoperative embolization of hypervascular lesions, such as juvenile nasopharyngeal angiofibromas (JNAs), paragangliomas, a few meningiomas, hemangiopericytomas, and hypervascular metastasis, has greatly reduced surgical mortality and morbidity related to bleeding.[3,4,8–13]

MAJOR IMAGING ISSUES AND DIAGNOSTIC DILEMMAS: HOW TO REPORT A CENTRAL SKULL BASE IMAGING STUDY

To issue a useful imaging report, the radiologist should be aware of the main factors that influence treatment options and may have an impact on the surgical approach.[8] To plan treatment, the surgeon needs to know the exact location and extent of a skull base lesion to decide whether it can be excised with acceptable morbidity and to choose the best surgical approach and the best route to obtain a biopsy specimen.[3,4,7,8]

Specific contraindications for surgical resection of skull base lesions vary from one institution to another and often among different surgeons.[3,4,7] Usually, they comprise invasion of the lateral or superior walls of the sphenoid sinus, invasion of the cavernous sinus, bilateral optic nerve or optic chiasm involvement, and invasion of the nasopharynx or prevertebral fascia.[3–8]

On every imaging study of the skull base, the radiologist should always report on the amount of bony skull base involvement; on the presence and extent of intracranial and orbital invasion; and on the relation of the lesion to the cavernous sinus, cranial nerves, and vessels, all of which have important implications on treatment planning and prognosis.[3,4,8,12]

Dural invasion is the single most important prognostic factor in skull base tumors.[19–21] Whereas an extradural lesion can be resected by means of an inferior ENT approach, a lesion that has transgressed the dura requires a combined craniofacial approach and is associated with a significant decrease in the 5-year survival rate and the specific disease-free interval.[8,19–21] Contrast-enhanced MR imaging is the best imaging modality to depict dural invasion.[8,12,13] Imaging signs of dural invasion in decreasing order of positive predictive value include contrast enhancement or edema of the brain parenchyma adjacent to tumor, leptomeningeal enhancement, nodular dural enhancement, and linear dural enhancement thicker than 5 mm.[8,19–21] Dural enhancement less than 5 mm is the most sensitive but least specific of all imaging signs because it can result from fibrovascular changes and does not necessarily indicate dural invasion.[8,13]

Orbital involvement is another important issue in surgical planning. The most common site of orbital invasion by CSB lesions is by way of the orbital fissures or orbital apex (Fig. 5D). Loss of fat and abnormal enhancement within these neural foramina indicate invasion.[8,11,12,22] Because of the close relation between the periorbita and the dural sheath of the optic nerve, involvement of the orbital apex by a skull base lesion usually requires orbital exenteration with sacrifice of the optic nerve.[8,9]

Invasion of the cavernous sinus usually precludes complete resection of a lesion. Imaging signs of cavernous sinus invasion include compression, encasement, stenosis, or irregularity of the cavernous carotid artery; loss of contrast enhancement of the cavernous sinus, which is best depicted on a dynamic coronal MR imaging study; and bulging of the lateral sinus wall, which is concave under normal conditions (see Fig. 5E, F).[8,9,11–13,18] When subtle, cavernous sinus invasion may be hard to depict, even using optimal technique. Because the dural leaflets are not clearly visible, it is often difficult to differentiate a bulge of the sinus walls because of compression by an extrinsic lesion from actual dural transgression. The use of 3-T MR imaging scanners seems promising in solving this issue. It should also be kept in mind that the cavernous sinus may be affected by interdural lesions laying within the dural leaflets of the lateral wall or by true intracavernous lesions. Whereas the former tend to displace the cavernous carotid artery without encasement or stenosis, the latter tend to encase and narrow its lumen.[3,4,12,18]

PATHOLOGIC FINDINGS

Most patients with CSB problems present with headache, cranial nerve deficits, proptosis, Eustachian tube dysfunction, or other symptoms related to the nasopharyngeal airway.[8,11–15] Because clinical examination of the CSB is limited, surgeons often have to rely on imaging studies to reach a diagnosis and plan subsequent treatment.

The following description of CSB lesions is based on a radiologist's friendly approach and on the frequency and propensity for certain disease processes to occur at specific sites. Lesions that are not site specific, originating from the bony skull base, such as fibro-osseous conditions and primary and secondary bone tumors, are discussed at the end of this article.

Midline Sagittal Central Skull Base Lesions

Midline sagittal CSB lesions comprise lesions arising from the sphenoid body, sphenoid sinus, and clivus; from the sella turcica immediately above; and from the nasopharynx immediately below (see Fig. 3). Whereas lesions arising within the sella turcica tend to displace the sellar floor inferiorly, intrinsic lesions of the clivus and those arising from the nasopharynx tend to push the sellar floor and pituitary gland superiorly.[2,4,9,12]

Lesions of the sphenoid sinus can be inflammatory and neoplastic. Chronic obliteration of sinus drainage may lead to mucocele formation. Sphenoid mucoceles, as is the case with those seen elsewhere, present as expansile lesions thinning and remodeling the sinus walls and eventually leading to cortical bone dehiscence.[9,10] This tumor, made of retained secretions, may show variable density and signal intensity on imaging studies depending on the degree of hydration, protein concentration,

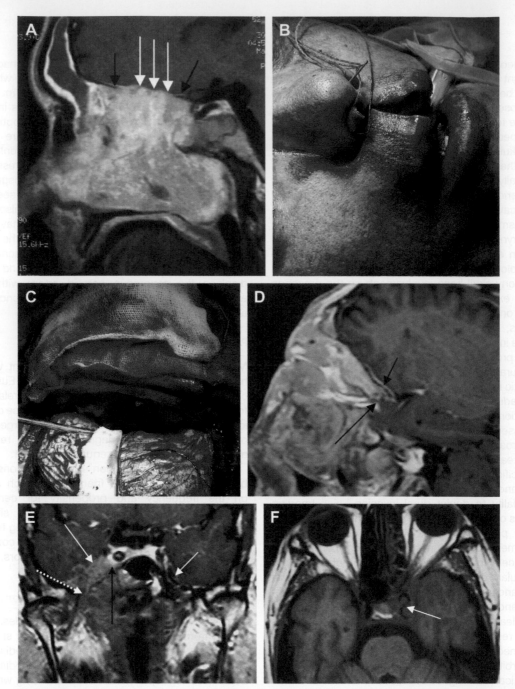

Fig. 5. (*A*) Gadolinium-enhanced sagittal T1-weighted MR imaging shows a large enhancing sinonasal neoplasm transgressing the skull base at the level of the planum sphenoidale. Note the discontinuity of the thin enhancing line corresponding to the dura (*black arrows*) with small areas of tumoral enhancement effacing the adjacent subarachnoid space (*white arrows*), reflecting transdural growth (pathologically proved). No brain edema or enhancement is seen to suggest invasion of the parenchyma. Images of a combined craniofacial resection: paranasal ear, nose, and throat approach (*B*) and bifrontal neurosurgical approach (*C*). (*D*) Gadolinium-enhanced sagittal T1-weighted image shows another sinonasal mass with orbital invasion and posterior extension into the orbital apex (*long black arrow*). Also note the smooth linear dural enhancement along the floor of the anterior cranial fossa (*short black arrow*), suggesting reactive fibrovascular changes. (*E*) Gadolinium-enhanced coronal T1-weighted image demonstrates a nasopharyngeal mass with infiltrative borders transgressing the CSB. Note the partial obliteration of the left cavernous sinus enhancement (*long black arrow*) and outward bulging of its lateral wall (*long white arrow*). Also, note tumor growth along V3, back to the foramen ovale (*dashed white arrow*), with complete obliteration of Meckel's cave (note the Meckel's cave on the normal side; *short white arrow*). (*F*) Axial T1-weighted image shows irregularity and stenosis of the right cavernous carotid artery (*white arrow*) attributable to a mass lesion invading the cavernous sinus and orbital apex.

and presence of calcification or fungal colonization (mycetoma) and does not enhance after intravenous administration of contrast material, except for a thin peripheral rim corresponding to the sinus mucosa (**Fig. 6**). The imaging appearance is that of a benign slow-growing lesion, and the diagnosis is usually straightforward in the absence of complications.[9,10,14,15]

Primary neoplasms of the sphenoid sinus are quite rare, because the sphenoid is most often secondarily invaded by tumors originating elsewhere.[3,4,10] Tumor histologic findings are similar to those seen in other paranasal sinuses, with squamous cell carcinoma being the most common.[3,10]

Clivus lesions include hematogenous bone metastasis, plasmacytoma or multiple myeloma, primary bone tumors, chordoma, and chondrosarcoma.

Clival chordoma is a benign locally invasive neoplasm originating from embryonic remnants of notochord that become entrapped within the basisphenoid, accounting for its typical midline sagittal location.[14,15,23,24] Seldom can it be seen in the nasopharynx or in the intracranial compartment.[23,24] Chordomas present as expansile lytic lesions, often with an aggressive pattern of bone destruction. MR imaging can nicely depict the replacement of the fatty marrow of the clivus by a hypointense tissue mass on plain sagittal T1-weighted images. Density and signal intensity are variable because of the presence of hemorrhage, cystic or myxoid components, calcification, and fragments of trabecular bone that become engulfed within the tumor mass.[9,23,24] After contrast, a lobulated pattern of enhancement is usually described (**Fig. 7**).[9,14,15,23,24]

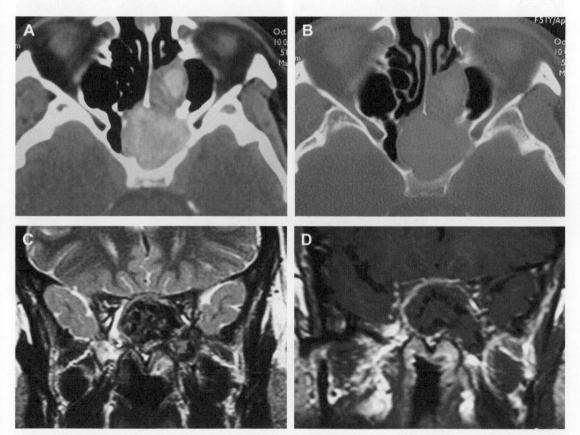

Fig. 6. Axial CT scan in soft tissue (*A*) and a bone algorithm (*B*) shows a heterogeneous but mostly spontaneous hyperdense mass filling in and expanding the right sphenoid sinus and posterior ethmoid cells. Note the thinning and remodeling of the bony walls of the sphenoid sinus without elements of frank destruction, suggestive of a slow-growing process. Corresponding MR imaging, coronal T2-weighted image (*C*) and gadolinium-enhanced coronal T1-weighted image (*D*), show that the material filling in the sinus is markedly heterogeneous, predominantly of low signal intensity on T2-weighted images, with serpiginous areas of signal void. Only peripheral enhancement is noted after gadolinium administration (sphenoid sinus mucocele superinfected by fungal hypha-mycetoma).

Sellar lesions that may invade the CSB include mainly macroadenomas and, in a far distant second place, craniopharyngiomas.[3,4,9] Pituitary macroadenomas tend to fill and expand the sella; may remodel the sellar floor and dorsum sella; extend superiorly into the suprasellar cistern through the diaphragm sella; and expand laterally into the cavernous sinus, wherein they can displace or encase the cavernous carotid artery without narrowing its lumen.[3,4,8] Invasive macroadenomas can breach the sellar floor and clivus and may extend into the sphenoid sinus.[3,4,9] Occasionally, pituitary macroadenomas are completely intraosseous and may cause a diagnostic dilemma. Sagittal and coronal MR imaging is particularly helpful in making the diagnosis. Diagnostic clues include the presence of an empty sella; off-midline deviation of the pituitary stalk; and the presence of an intact sellar floor, often displaced inferiorly, differentiating pituitary macroadenomas from lesions arising primarily from the clivus or from the sphenoid sinus (Fig. 8).[9,12]

Craniopharyngiomas are histologically benign lesions originating from embryonic remnants of the pharyngohypophyseal canal or Rathke's pouch.[3,4,9] They can be seen anywhere from the nasopharynx to the hypothalamus, with the most common location being suprasellar.[3,4,11,12] When completely intraosseous within the sphenoid, they may be hard to diagnose. Typically, craniopharyngiomas are largely cystic or mixed tumors, often showing calcifications.[3,4,11,12] The solid component enhances after intravenous contrast administration (Fig. 9).

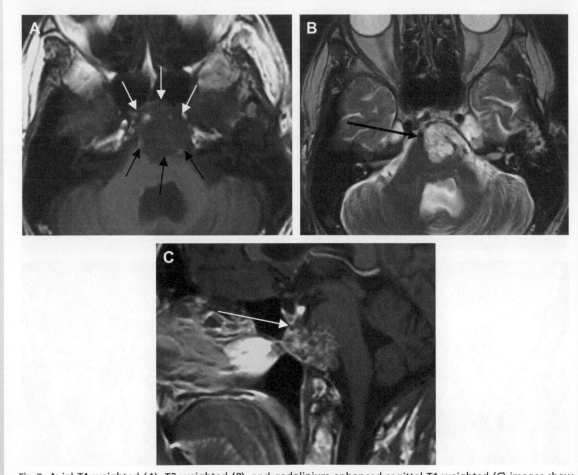

Fig. 7. Axial T1-weighted (*A*), T2-weighted (*B*), and gadolinium-enhanced sagittal T1-weighted (*C*) images show a mass lesion expanding and replacing the fatty marrow of the clivus, with frank destruction of the superior cortical margin. The lesion extends into the posterior cranial fossa, obliterates the prepontine cistern, displaces the basilar artery to the right (*long black arrow in B*), and compresses the ventral pons (*short black arrows in A*). Anteriorly, it bulges into the sphenoid sinus (*small white arrows in A*), and, superiorly, it stops at the sellar floor (*long white arrow in C*). The lesion is of intermediate signal intensity on T1-weighted imaging and hyperintense on T2-weighted imaging, with a faint trabecular pattern, and shows lobulated honeycombed-like enhancement (clival chordoma).

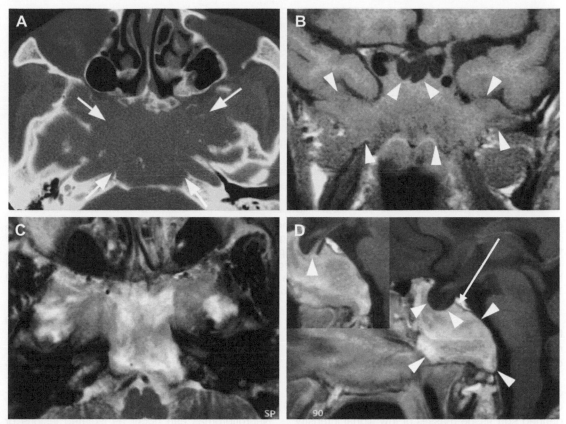

Fig. 8. Axial CT scan in a bone algorithm shows a large destructive lesion almost entirely replacing the sphenoid bone (*A*), retaining its original shape and with small bony fragments engulfed within the lesion (*white arrowheads in B*). Coronal T1-weighted (*B*) and contrast-enhanced sagittal T1-weighted (*D*) MR images show to advantage the soft tissue mass delineating the sphenoid (*white arrowheads*). Note the presence of an empty sella (*black arrowheads*), the inferior displacement of the sellar floor, and the rightward deviation of the pituitary stalk. The high signal intensity of the neurohypophysis can be seen in a normal anatomic location (*long white arrow in D*). (*C*) On T2-weighted imaging, the lesion is heterogeneous in signal intensity but predominantly hyperintense (intra-osseous pituitary adenoma).

Meningiomas of the sellar and parasellar regions account for 20% to 25% of all meningiomas.[3,4,7] The most common sites of origin include the planum sphenoidale, tuberculum sella, clinoid processes, and sellar diaphragm.[3,4,7] They present as broad dural-based masses and are isointense to gray matter, enhancing vividly and homogeneously after contrast administration, often showing a dural tail.[3,4,10–12] Sellar meningiomas tend to push and compress the pituitary gland against the sellar floor (**Fig. 10**). Associated hyperostosis with upward blistering of the planum sphenoidale and tuberculum sella and pneumosinus dilatans are typical features that can be nicely depicted on CT and MR imaging scans.[3,4,9–12]

Nasopharyngeal lesions, infectious and neoplastic, may affect the CSB from below. Because of the tough buccopharyngeal and pharyngobasilar fascias, tumor spread is usually directed superiorly against the clivus and foramen lacerum (**Fig. 11**).[22,25] It should be kept in mind that nasopharyngeal cancers can occasionally be completely submucosal, presenting with extensive CSB destruction and only a slight bulge in the nasopharyngeal mucosal space with normal overlying mucosa.[9,22,25] In this case, deep transnasal biopsies are required to make the diagnosis.

Parasagittal Central Skull Base Lesions

Parasagittal CSB lesions originate from the greater sphenoid wing, cavernous sinus, cranial nerves traversing the neurovascular foramina, and petroclival synchondrosis. Developmental lesions, such as basal transsphenoidal cephaloceles, may also be seen.

Cavernous sinus lesions include primary and secondary cranial nerve tumors; vascular malformations; meningiomas; and inflammatory conditions, such as neuritis and Tolosa-Hunt syndrome.

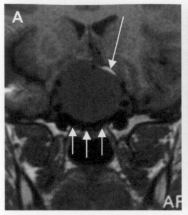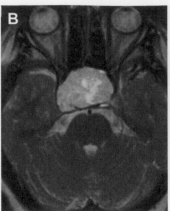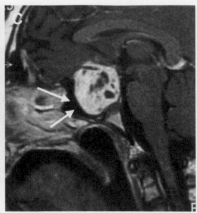

Fig. 9. Coronal T1-weighted (A), axial T2-weighted (B) and gadolinium-enhanced sagittal T1-weighted (C) images show a rounded well-marginated mass lesion, expanding the sella and growing into the suprasellar cistern. Note the inferior displacement of the sellar floor, almost collapsing the sphenoid sinus (*small white arrows in A and C*). The lesion is of intermediate signal intensity on T1-weighted and T2-weighted images with small T2-weighted hyperintense and nonenhancing cystic areas. Also, note a thin spontaneously hyper-intense rim on the coronal T1-weighted image suggesting marginal calcification (*long white arrow in A*) (craniopharyngioma).

Peripheral nerve sheath tumors (PNSTs) tend to follow the axis of the nerve of origin, and the diagnosis is straightforward once the anatomic course of the nerve is recognized.

Schwannomas and neurofibromas are the most common lesions and can affect virtually any cranial nerve. Schwannomas present as well-defined soft tissue masses of low signal intensity on T1-weighted MR imaging and have intermediate to high signal on T2-weighted MR imaging, moderately enhancing after gadolinium administration.[9,12,14,15,26,27] Large tumors tend to show cystic or necrotic areas, and peripheral CSF cysts can also be seen.[14,15,26,27] Fatty degeneration can occur in long-standing neurofibromas, accounting for low density on CT and T1-weighted hyperintensity on MR imaging.[14,15,26,27] These benign slow-growing neoplasms tend to remodel rather then erode adjacent bone, and when extending peripherally, they produce smooth enlargement of the exiting skull base neural foramina (**Fig. 12**).[14,15,25–27] Neurofibromas can occur as isolated lesions or as part of neurofibromatosis type I.[14,15,26,27] Malignant PNSTs, however, are most commonly associated with neurofibromatosis type 1.[9,15,27] These are more aggressive infiltrative lesions that spread diffusely along peripheral branches and show ill-defined borders.[26,27]

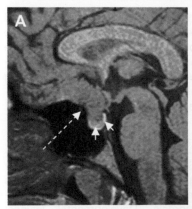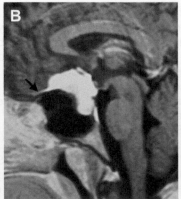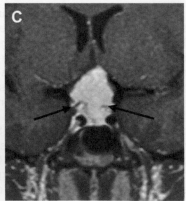

Fig. 10. Sagittal T1-weighted image (A) and gadolinium-enhanced sagittal (B) and coronal (C) T1-weighted images show a dural-based lesion along the posterior aspect of the planum, transgressing the diaphragm and growing into the sella, compressing the pituitary gland against the sellar floor (*small white arrows in A*). Note the hourglass shape of the lesion, which is best appreciated on the coronal plane, with a stricture at the sellar diaphragm (*black arrows in C*). The lesion is isointense with gray matter and enhances homogeneously, showing a thin dural tail along the planum (*small black arrow in B*). Bone sclerosis, with blistering of the sphenoid roof (*dashed white arrow in A*) and pneumosinus dilatans, can also be seen (sphenosellar meningioma).

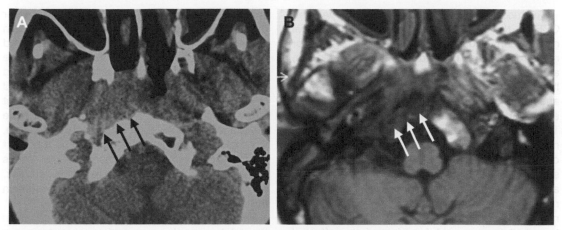

Fig. 11. Plain axial CT scan (*A*) and axial T1-weighted MR image (*B*) show a mass lesion in the posterolateral wall of the nasopharynx obliterating the fossa of Rosenmüller, effacing the parapharyngeal fat, and growing posteriorly into the jugular foramen. Note the sclerosis and slight irregularity of the cortical margin of the right lateral aspect of the clivus on the CT image (*black arrows*) corresponding to replacement of the fatty marrow, which is best appreciated on MR imaging (*white arrows*).

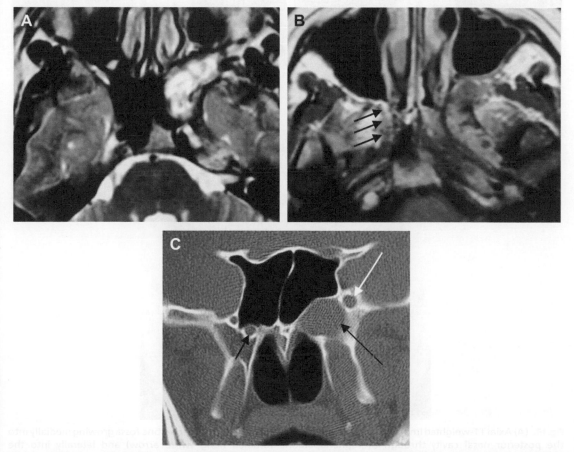

Fig. 12. Axial T2-weighted (*A*) and gadolinium-enhanced T1-weighted (*B*) images show a sausage-shaped lesion extending from the foramen lacerum posteriorly into the high pterygopalatine fossa anteriorly, following the course of the vidian nerve. (*C*) Coronal CT image in the bone algorithm shows the smooth enlargement of the vidian canal (*long black arrow*) and superior displacement of the foramen rotundum (*white arrow*). Note the vidian nerve on contralateral side (*short black arrows* on *B* and *C*).

The most commonly affected cranial nerve in the CSB is the trigeminal nerve. [26–28] The cranial nerves can also be affected by anterograde or retrograde spread of head and neck malignancies, a phenomenon known as perineural spread. [22,26,29] It manifests as focal or segmental enlargement and abnormal enhancement along the course of a cranial nerve, often with skip areas. [14,15,26,29] This type of spread is most often seen with squamous cell carcinoma, the most frequent neoplasm of the head and neck, but can also be seen with salivary gland malignancies (mainly adenoid cystic and mucoepidermoid carcinomas), hematologic malignancies, and melanoma. [26,29] On CT, perineural spread can be depicted by enlargement of the skull base neural foramina of the affected nerve, by effacement of the foraminal fat, or indirectly through denervation atrophy of the muscles supplied by a particular nerve. [14,15,26,29] MR

imaging is more sensitive, allowing earlier detection of this type of spread. [9,12,26,29] Plain T1-weighted images and fat-suppressed contrast-enhanced T1-weighted images are particularly well suited to detect perineural spread through effacement of neuroforaminal fat and areas of focal or segmental enhancement (**Fig. 13**). [26,28,29] Cranial nerve neuritis can have the exact same appearance on imaging; therefore, the clinical setting is crucial to achieve a correct diagnosis (**Fig. 14**). In most cases, neuritis results from viral infection secondary to herpes simplex, herpes zoster, cytomegalovirus, or HIV, to mention the most common infections. [14,15,26,29]

Pyogenic and fungal infections originating from the orbit, nasopharynx, and paranasal sinuses may access the cavernous sinus, spreading along neurovascular structures. Skull base osteomyelitis, abscess formation and cavernous sinus, and

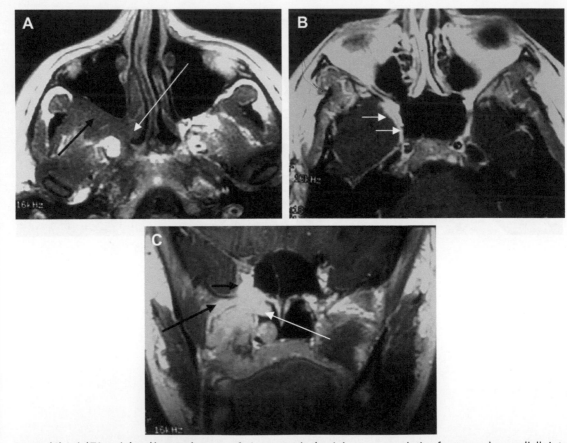

Fig. 13. (A) Axial T1-weighted image shows a soft tissue mass in the right pterygopalatine fossa growing medially into the posterior nasal cavity through the sphenopalatine foramen (*long white arrow*) and laterally into the infratemporal fossa and retroantral fat through the pterygomaxillary fissure (*long black arrow*). Postgadolinium axial (B) and coronal (C) T1-weighted images demonstrate abnormal enhancement of V2 along the foramen rotundum back to the cavernous sinus (*short white arrows in B*). Also, note the enlargement of the inferior cavernous sinus (*short black arrow in C*), tumor growth into the posterior nasal cavity through the sphenopalatine foramen (*long white arrow*) and laterally, into the infratemporal fossa via the pterygomaxillary fissure (*long black arrow*).

superior ophthalmic vein thrombosis are potential complications best demonstrated by magnetic resonance imaging.[3,4,9,12]

Inflammatory pseudotumor of the cavernous sinus and orbital apex, Tolosa-Hunt syndrome, is a diagnosis of exclusion after all infectious and specific inflammatory conditions, particularly sarcoidosis, have been ruled out.[26,28] It is characterized by painful ophthalmoplegia with deficits of cranial nerves III, IV, V1, and VI and a prompt response to steroid therapy.[3,15,26] MR imaging is the modality of choice, showing abnormal enhancing soft tissue within the cavernous sinus and orbital apex, often extending along the floor of the middle cranial fossa, and, occasionally, irregular narrowing of the cavernous carotid artery.[15,26] This tissue tends to be isointense to muscle on T1-weighted images and of low to intermediate signal intensity on T2-weighted images (**Fig. 15**).[12,15,26]

Cavernous sinus vascular malformations, including aneurysms, carotid-cavernous fistulas, and hemangiomas, are all associated with focal or diffuse enlargement of the cavernous sinus with outward bulging of its lateral wall; when long standing, they can also lead to remodeling of the inner wall of the sphenoid sinus.[3,4,9,26] These are imaging diagnoses that should be ruled out before any attempts to obtain tissue diagnosis are made.

Giant cavernous carotid aneurysms present as expansile lesions of the cavernous sinus with variable signal characteristics.[3,4,9,12] When the aneurysm lumen is completely patent, a fusiform or saccular flow void on MR imaging is the rule. When a varying amount of thrombosis is present, signal intensity is heterogeneous, reflecting the presence of blood products in different stages of degradation, calcifications, and flowing blood (**Fig. 16**).[9,11,12] The presence of flow-related

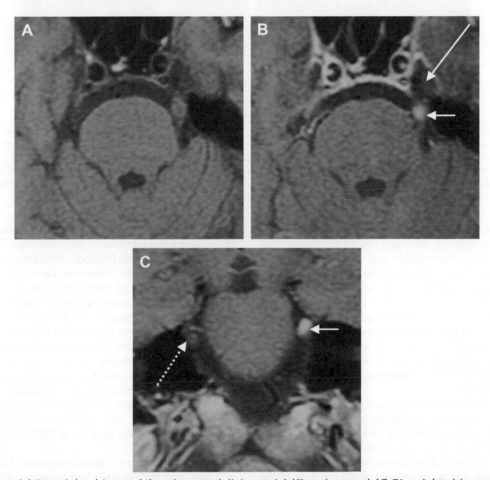

Fig. 14. Axial T1-weighted image (*A*) and postgadolinium axial (*B*) and coronal (*C*) T1-weighted images show a small focus of enhancement and slight enlargement of the cisternal segment of the left trigeminal nerve (*short white arrows*), which does not extend into Meckel's cave (*long white arrow in B*). Note the cisternal segment of the right trigeminal nerve (*dashed white arrow in C*). (This focal enhancement disappeared on follow-up scans, and a presumptive diagnosis of neuronitis was made).

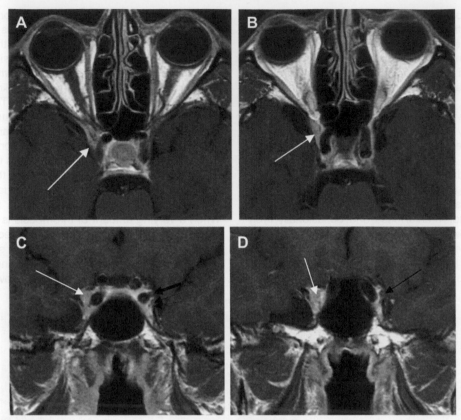

Fig. 15. Post-gadolinium (*A and B*) and coronal (*B and C*) T1W MR images demonstrate soft tissue thickening and abnormal enhancement in the lateral wall of the right cavernous sinus, superior orbital fissure and optic canal (*long white arrows in A–C*). In (*C*) note cranial nerves III (*thick black arrow*), IV (*thin black arrow*), and V1 (*dashed black arrow*) in the lateral wall of the cavernous sinus on the left side, from superior to inferior. (*D*) On the affected side the nerves are enhancing and can hardly be recognized within the enhancing sinus (enhancing oculomotor nerve- *short white arrow*) (Tolosa-Hunt syndrome).

artifacts on the phase-encoding axis may be a clue to the diagnosis. Whereas recent thrombus containing deoxihemoglobin and intracellular methemoglobin layers close to the patent lumen, old thrombus containing extracellular metahemoglobin and hemosiderin tends to layer at the periphery.[9,11,12] On CT, a potential pitfall is to mistake a largely patent aneurysm for a cavernous sinus meningioma when a CT angiogram is not performed. Angio-CT or angio-MR imaging should be used to confirm the diagnosis and clearly delineate the aneurysm.[9,12]

Sphenocavernous and petroclival meningiomas are the most common neoplasms affecting the parasagittal CSB, originating from the intracranial compartment (**Fig. 17**). Cavernous meningiomas lead to bulging of the lateral wall of the cavernous sinus and can grow laterally along the floor of the middle cranial fossa, anteriorly into the superior orbital fissure and orbital apex, medially into the sphenoid sinus and sella, posteriorly into Meckel's cave and posterior cranial fossa, and inferolaterally

into the masticator space along the foramen ovale (mimicking a trigeminal nerve schwannoma).[9,12,14,15] Intradiploic growth into the body of the sphenoid and clivus is not infrequent. These lesions tend to follow the signal intensity of gray matter in all imaging sequences and to enhance vividly and homogeneously after administration of gadolinium.

Cephaloceles of the parasagittal CSB are of rare occurrence and consist of herniation of the intracranial contents (meninges or brain parenchyma) through a skull base defect in the greater sphenoid wing into the masticator space immediately below (**Fig. 18**).[3,4,9,12] Coronal and sagittal imaging is helpful in establishing this imaging diagnosis. An unaware biopsy may lead to a CSF fistula and meningitis.

Chondroid tumors, chondromyxoid fibroma, and low- and high-grade chondrosarcomas originate from cartilaginous remnants of the skull base synchondroses, most commonly from the petroclival synchondrosis, accounting for the off-midline parasagittal location of these

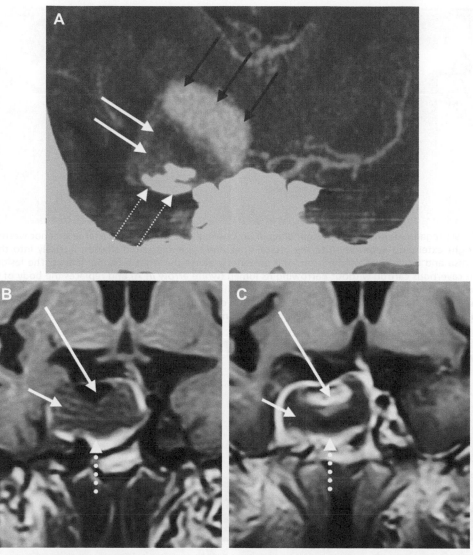

Fig. 16. Coronal CT reconstruction from a CT angiogram (*A*) demonstrates a giant cavernous carotid aneurysm shown as a complex lesion in the right cavernous sinus and supraclinoid region, with an area of early enhancement which corresponds to the patent lumen (*black arrows*) and a non-enhancing hypodense area suggesting thrombus (*white arrows*). Also noted are extensive, layered atheromatous calcifications (*white dashed arrows*). Coronal pre-gadolinium (*B*) and post-gadolinium (*C*) T1W MR images (on another patient) show a complex lesion in the right cavernous sinus at the expected location of the cavernous carotid artery. The lesion has an eccentric flow void enhancing after gadolinium, corresponding to the patent arterial lumen (*long white arrows in C–D*), hypointense material consistent with early clot (*short white arrows*) and, at the periphery, spontaneous T1 hyperintensity, suggesting the presence of metahemoglobin (*white dashed arrows*). (Cavernous carotid artery aneurysm).

neoplasms.[9,14,15,30–32] Chondroid type calcifications are typical for these tumors and are best appreciated on CT.[9,30–32] On MR imaging, high signal intensity on T2-weighted images, often higher than that of CSF, is also a distinctive feature.[9,15,30–32] The signal intensity of calcifications is variable depending on the size and composition of calcium crystals.[15,30–32] Cranial nerve VI palsy is a common clinical presentation

because of involvement of Dorello's canal (**Fig. 19**).[9,15,30–32] Nasopharyngeal cancer can also affect the parasagittal skull base through the foramen lacerum and by means of V3 perineural extension along the foramen ovale.[22]

JNA is a vascular neoplasm occurring exclusively in adolescent boys. It originates in the posterior nasal fossa in the region of the sphenopalatine foramen, extending into the pterygopalatine fossa and, from

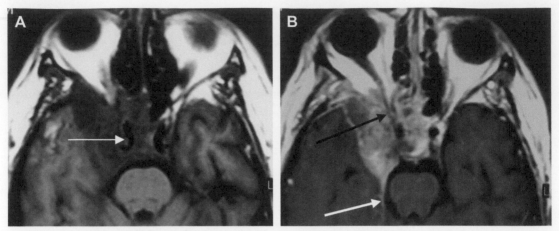

Fig. 17. Axial pregadolinium (*A*) and postgadolinium (*B*) T1-weighted images show a large sphenocavernous lesion on the right extending anteriorly into the orbital apex and sphenoethmoid sinuses, laterally into the middle cranial fossa and lateral wall of the orbit, and posteriorly along the right tentorial leaflet. The lesion encases the right cavernous carotid without narrowing its lumen (*white arrow in A*) and replaces the body of the sphenoid, clivus, and greater sphenoid wing. Postcontrast enhancement is slightly heterogeneous, and a dural tail is noted along the tentorium (*white arrow in B*). Note the encasement and compression of the optic nerve at the optic canal (*black arrow in B*) and secondary proptosis (intradiploic sphenocavernous meningioma).

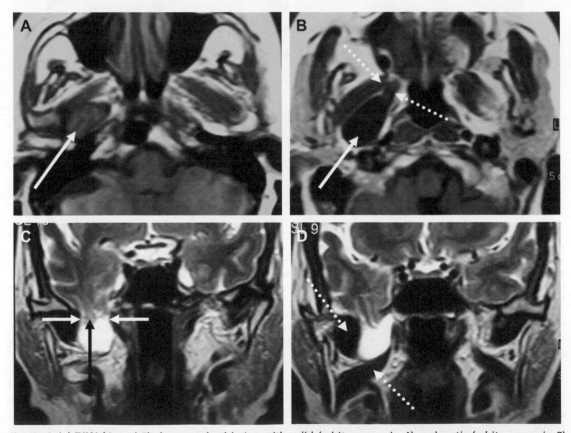

Fig. 18. Axial T1W (*A and B*) show a mixed lesion with solid (*white arrow in A*) and cystic (*white arrow in B*) components on the right parasagittal central skull base centred on foramen ovale and extending into the masticator space in between the medial and lateral pterygoid muscles (*dashed white arrows in B and D*). Coronal T2W images (*C and D*) clearly demonstrate a bony defect at the greater sphenoid wing involving the region of foramen ovale (*white arrows*) with herniation of the intracranial contents, both meninges and the inferior temporal gyrus (*black arrow*), into the masticator space (basal transphenoidal meningoencephalocele).

there, into the parasagittal skull base by way of the foramen rotundum or the vidian canal.[3,4,9,11,12] These highly vascular tumors demonstrate intense contrast enhancement in an early arterial phase and may show a "salt and pepper" pattern on MR imaging, with the salt corresponding to the tumor stroma or hemorrhage and the pepper corresponding to vascular flow voids (**Fig. 20**).[9,11,12] Recurrent epistaxis is the rule. Clinical setting, location, and imaging features are pathognomonic.

Lateral Central Skull Base Lesions

The lateral CSB includes the far lateral aspect of the greater sphenoid wings, the lateral aspect of the temporal bone, and the TMJ. On axial imaging, the anterior-lateral aspect of the greater sphenoid wing has a grossly triangular shape, usually referred to as the sphenoid triangle (**Fig. 21**A white arrows). This anatomic region constitutes a crossroad between the orbit, the middle cranial fossa, and the temporal fossa (suprazygomatic masticator space) and can be affected by any lesion originating from these compartments.[3,4,8]

Globular, and particularly intradiploic (en plaque), meningiomas are of common occurrence in this region, seen on CT as extensive bone sclerosis, often with an irregular contour mimicking osteoblastic metastases or osteosarcoma.[9,11–15] On MR imaging, they show low signal intensity

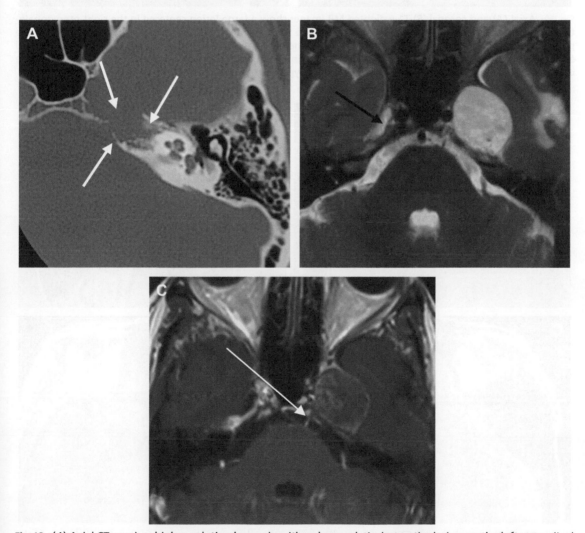

Fig. 19. (*A*) Axial CT scan in a high-resolution bone algorithm shows a lytic destructive lesion on the left petroclival region (*white arrows*). (*B*) Axial T2-weighted and (*C*) postgadolinium axial T1-weighted images show an expansile lesion in the left petroclival region. The lesion is of high signal intensity on T2-weighted images, similar to CSF, and shows only slight to moderate enhancement after administration of gadolinium. It involves cranial nerve IV (*white arrow in C*) at Dorello's canal and obliterates Meckel's cave (note the normal cave on the contralateral side; *black arrow in B*). No gross calcifications are noted within the lesion (petroclival chondrosarcoma).

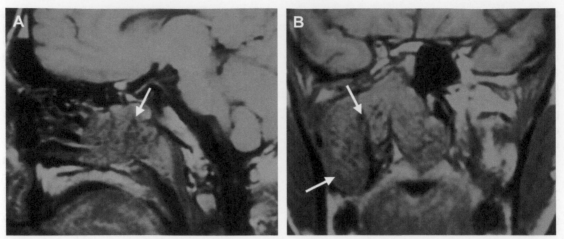

Fig. 20. Axial (*A*) and coronal (*B*) T1-weighted MR images show a large lesion centered in the right pterygopalatine fossa, extending laterally into the masticator space through the pterygomaxillary fissure, medially into the posterior nasal cavity through the sphenopalatine foramen, and posteriorly and superiorly along the vidian canal and foramen rotundum. The lesion is slightly lobulated in contour but is well marginated. Also, note the presence of serpentine flow voids (*white arrows*) reflecting its hypervascular nature (JNA).

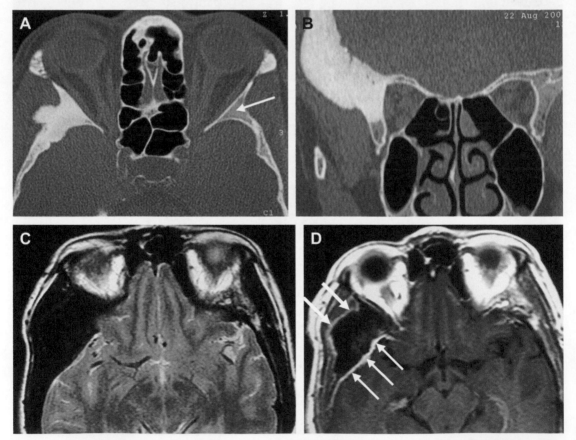

Fig. 21. (*A, B*) Axial and coronal CT images in a bone algorithm demonstrate an expansile sclerotic lesion in the lateral CSB involving the sphenoid triangle and lateral orbital wall, bulging medially into the middle cranial fossa and laterally into the suprazygomatic masticator space (note the sphenoid triangle on the normal side- *white arrow*). On the axial T2-weighted image (*C*), the lesion follows the signal intensity of compact bone (signal void), and on the postgadolinium axial T1-weighted image (*D*), it shows only peripheral enhancement (*white arrows*) (intradiploic meningioma).

on T1- and T2-weighted images and on gadolinium enhancement, with a dural tail along the middle cranial fossa (see **Fig. 21**).[9,15]

Lesions arising from the TMJ are site specific and include a variety of tumors and tumor-like conditions and infectious-inflammatory processes that may spread into the middle cranial fossa. Synovial chondromatosis and benign and malignant synovial tumors can all arise in this synovial joint.[9,33,34]

Pigmented villonodular synovitis can occasionally extend into the middle cranial fossa along the greater sphenoid wing. The hallmark of this lesion is the presence of frond-like hyperplastic synovium; blood degradation products attributable to repeated hemorrhage; and giant foam cells containing hemosiderin, which are responsible for the heterogeneous signal intensity on MR imaging and relative hyperdensity on plain CT studies.[9,33,34] Frond-like enhancement is the rule.[9,33,34] Pressure erosion on the articular surfaces leads to expansion of the joint space and remodeling of adjacent bone.[9,33,34]

Chondroblastoma or chondromatous giant cell tumor is an exclusively epiphyseal neoplasm that is exceedingly rare in the skull base. It may occasionally originate in the mandibular condyle, affect the TMJ, and grow into the lateral CSB.[35,36] Around 90% of cases are diagnosed before the age of 30 years. On CT, it presents as an expansile, eccentric, lytic lesion with geographic margins and a lobulated contour. Calcifications, punctate or irregularly shaped, are seen in approximately half of the cases, and joint involvement, often with effusion, may occur.[35,36] MR imaging tends to overestimate tumor aggressiveness. The tumor matrix is of intermediate to low signal intensity on T1- and T2-weighted images, except when associated with an aneurysmal bone cyst (highly hyperintense on T2-weighted images, often with fluid-fluid levels).[35,36] Peripheral enhancement is the rule (**Fig. 22**).

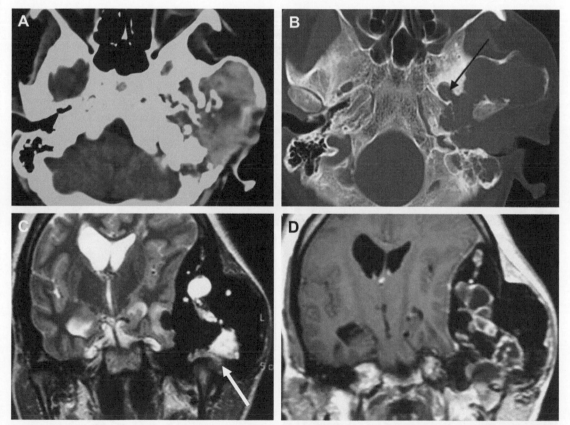

Fig. 22. Axial CT images in soft tissue (*A*) and a bone window (*B*) show a large lytic lesion expanding the lateral aspect of the greater sphenoid wing, temporal bone, and glenoid cavity and involving the left TMJ. Extensive bone remodeling and thinning, with some areas of bony dehiscence and fine bony septa, are also shown. Note the bony dehiscence on the lateral margin of the foramen ovale (*black arrow*). Coronal T2-weighted (*C*) and postgadolinium T1-weighted (*D*) images show to advantage the craniocaudad extent of the lesion, the presence of multiple cysts, and joint effusion (*white arrow in C*). Also, note the dramatic mass effect upon the intracranial structures (chondroblastoma).

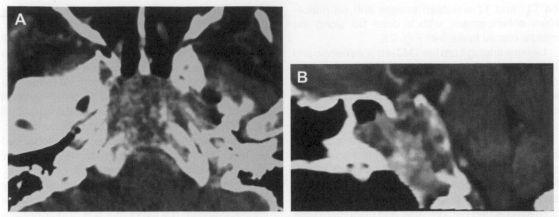

Fig. 23. Contrast-enhanced axial (*A*) and sagittal (*B*) CT reconstruction on a soft tissue window show a destructive lytic lesion centered on the clivus and eroding its cortical margins, with an associated soft tissue mass enhancing heterogeneously in a man with a prior history of colonic adenocarcinoma (clival metastasis).

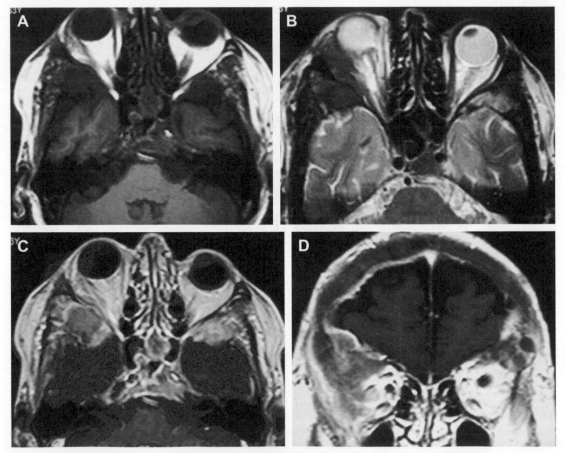

Fig. 24. Axial T1-weighted image (*A*), T2-weighted image (*B*), and contrast-enhanced axial (*C*) and coronal (*D*) T1-weighted images show multiple predominantly sclerotic lesions (hypointense on T1-weighted and T2-weighted images) in the lateral aspect of the greater sphenoid wing, sphenoid triangle, and lateral orbital wall, which enhance vividly on the postgadolinium images. Except for the enhancement, the imaging features are similar to those shown in **Fig. 21** (bone metastases from prostate cancer).

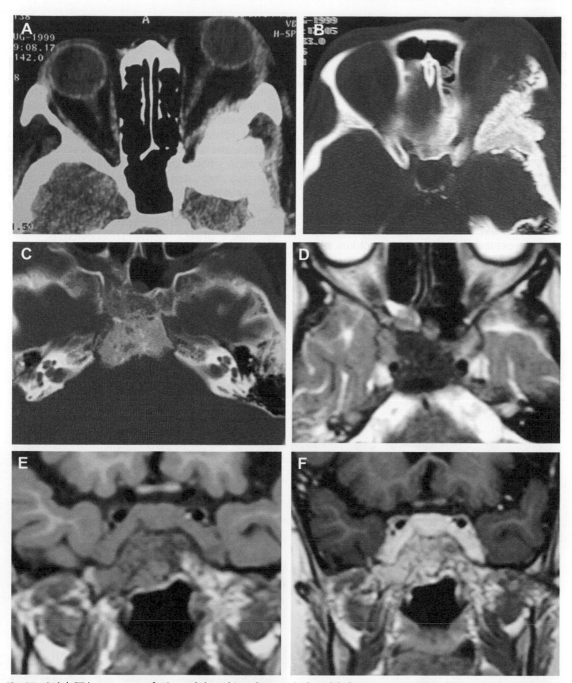

Fig. 25. Axial CT images on soft tissue (*A*) and in a bone window (*B*) show an expansile sclerotic lesion in the left sphenoid triangle and lateral orbital wall with an aggressive sunburst pattern of periosteal reaction leading to proptosis (osteogenic osteosarcoma). (*C*) Axial CT image in a bone window in another patient shows a permeative lesion involving the clivus that is predominantly sclerotic but has small ill-defined lytic areas. Axial T2-weighted image (*D*) and coronal precontrast (*E*) and postcontrast (*F*) T1-weighted images in the same patient show that the lesion is markedly hypointense on T2-weighted imaging, is of intermediate signal intensity on T1-weighted imaging, and enhances vividly after gadolinium administration. The lesion bulges inferiorly in the left nasopharyngeal roof (osteosarcoma secondary to prior irradiation of a posterior fossa medulloblastoma).

Intrinsic Non–Site-Specific Central Skull Base Lesions

Primary and secondary bone neoplasms, fibro-osseous conditions, a variety of systemic bone diseases, and infection can occur in any of the subdivisions of the CSB.

Metastasis is the most common neoplasm affecting the skull base in an adult patient; therefore, it should be included in the differential diagnosis of any intrinsic skull base lesion.[3,4,9,11–15] Because bone metastases are mostly attributable to hematogenous spread, they tend to occur in bones with higher marrow content, such as the clivus, petrous apex, sphenoid triangle, and diploe of the calvarium.[9,11–15] Lesions are primarily centered in the bony structures of the skull base and can be lytic, sclerotic, or mixed (**Figs. 23** and **24**). The lung, breast, prostate, and kidney are the most common primaries to metastasize to the skull base.[4,9,12] Occasionally, a skull base metastasis can be the presenting feature of a neoplasm elsewhere, although malignant disease is already known in most cases. Osteoblastic metastasis can mimic an intradiploic meningioma or an osteosarcoma.[9,14,15] When diffuse, bone metastases can be mistaken for Paget's disease or other fibro-osseous conditions (**Fig. 24**). Hypervascular metastases, such as those from the kidney, thyroid, melanoma, carcinoid, or choriocarcinoma, can potentially be confused with other hypervascular lesions, such as paragangliomas, JNAs, hemangiopericytomas, and meningiomas.[9,11,12]

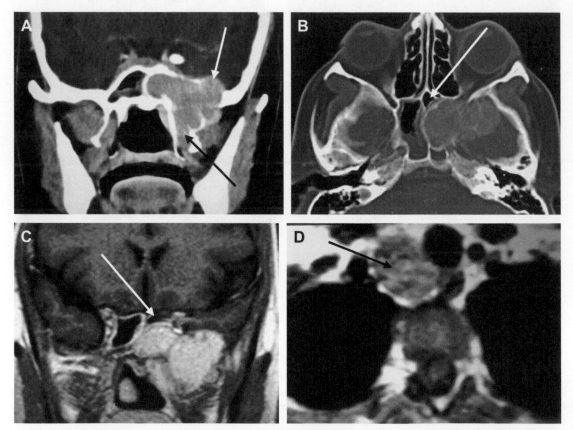

Fig. 26. Contrast-enhanced coronal CT image on soft tissue (*A*), axial CT image on a bone algorithm (*B*), and coronal postgadolinium MR imaging (*C*) demonstrate a well-defined expansile lesion centered in the greater sphenoid wing, bulging medially into the sphenoid sinus (partially obliterated by the lesion) (*white arrows in B and C*), bulging superiorly into the middle cranial fossa (*white arrow in A*), and bulging inferiorly into the pterygoid plates (*black arrow in A*). Note the bone remodeling and thinning without frank bone erosion, suggesting a slow-growing benign process. Also note the vivid enhancement of the lesion. (*D*) Axial T1-weighted image through the lower neck shows a rounded mass lesion on the right tracheoesophageal groove immediately below the inferior pole of the right thyroid lobe (*black arrow in D*) (brown tumor attributable to primary hyperparathyroidism).

Plasmacytoma and multiple myeloma can occur in the skull base, presenting as an expansile destructive lytic lesion with a soft tissue component spontaneously hyperdense on CT scans and showing intermediate signal intensity on T1- and T2-weighted MR imaging.[9,14,15] These imaging features are typical for hypercellular, small, round-cell tumors with a high nucleo-cytoplasmic ratio, which is also a hallmark of lymphoma and leukemic infiltrates (chloromas/granulocytic sarcomas).

In the skull base the most common primary malignant bone tumor is osteosarcoma. This are of rare occurrence in the skull base, often secondary to prior radiation therapy or Paget's disease. Osteosarcomas are characterized by new bone formation and by an aggressive pattern of periosteal reaction, with a spiculated hair-on-end or sunburst appearance, which is best depicted on CT scans (**Fig. 25**).[9,12,14,15]

Any benign bone tumor can potentially occur in the skull base and share the same imaging features as elsewhere. Giant cell tumors, such as osteoclastoma, aneurysmal bone cyst, and brown tumor, are remarkable for the presence of multinucleated giant cells and hemosiderin-laden macrophages secondary to intratumoral hemorrhage and may not be differentiated from each other on the basis of pathologic findings alone.[9,37] The presence of iron, in the form of hemosiderin and ferritin, accounts for tumor hyperdensity on plain CT scans and low signal intensity on T2-weighted MR imaging, with a blooming effect on T2* sequences attributable to susceptibility artifact.[37] These are usually benign-appearing, slow-growing, expansile lytic lesions that remodel and thin cortical bone (**Fig. 26**).[9,37] The diagnosis of brown tumors is supported by laboratory findings of hyperparathyroidism.[9,37] These are highly vascularized

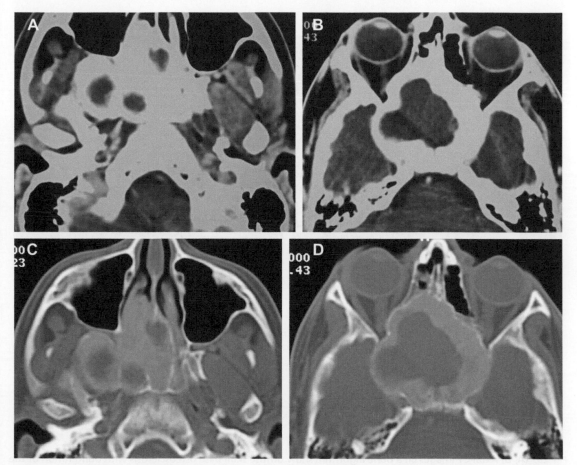

Fig. 27. Axial CT images on soft tissue (*A* and *B*) and bone window (*C* and *D*), show an expansile lesion centered in the sphenoid body, which obliterates the sphenoid sinus extends inferiorly into the pterygoid plates and anteriorly into the posterior nasal septum and nasal turbinates. The lesion is homogeneously hypodense, surrounded by a thick rim of sclerotic bone with a ground-glass pattern excluding sphenoid mucocele as a possible diagnosis (ossifying fibroma).

lesions demonstrating vivid enhancement after contrast administration.[9,37]

Osteoblastoma can seldom be seen in the skull base. It is a benign bone-forming neoplasm of children and young adults, usually presenting before the age of 30 years.[3,4,9] Imaging shows a sharply circumscribed, expansile, predominantly lytic or mixed lytic-sclerotic lesion depending on the degree of mineralization of the tumor matrix, often in the form of bony septa.[9,15] A peripheral sclerotic rim resembling an eggshell is the rule.

Fibro-osseous conditions, such as fibrous dysplasia, ossifying fibroma, and Paget's disease, can affect the skull base. Overall, CT is more specific in the diagnosis, although MR imaging can provide additional information regarding disease activity.

Fibrous dysplasia is primarily a disease of the medullary cavity, sparing cortical bone, which is an important distinctive feature from Paget's disease.[3,4,9,38,39] Woven bone is replaced by myxofibrous tissue with different degrees of mineralization depending on the phase of disease activity. Initially, cystic spaces, more or less coalescent, predominate; a mixed-sclerotic pattern with a ground-glass appearance then ensues; and, finally, intense mineralization results in a sclerotic pattern.[9,38,39] Bone expansion is the rule, which may lead to stenosis of skull base neurovascular foramina and to secondary neurologic deficits.[9,38,39] Affected bones tend to merge imperceptibly with normal-appearing bones.[38,39] A periosteal reaction, when present, indicates pathologic fracture or malignant degeneration, most often into osteosarcoma.[9,14,15,38,39] Contrast-enhanced MR imaging can be used to determine whether the disease is active (showing moderate to intense enhancement) or quiescent (non-enhancing).[15,38,39]

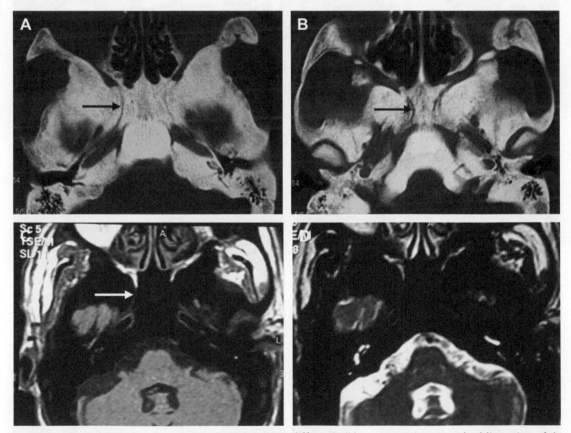

Fig. 28. (A, B) Axial CT images on a bone algorithm show diffuse skull base osteosclerosis with obliteration of the normal trabecular pattern by dense, amorphous, and structureless bone. Note the involvement of the temporal bone including the otic capsule. Axial T1-weighted (C) and T2-weighted (D) images show extensive signal void of the entire skull base reflecting the replacement of the bone marrow by dense compact bone. There is slight bone expansion leading to stenosis of the neurovascular foramina of the skull base. Note the stenotic foramen rotundum compressing V2 (*black arrows in A and C*) and the vidian canal (*white arrow in B*).

Ossifying fibroma is a monostotic form of fibrous dysplasia with a more aggressive behavior. It often leads to marked bone expansion and compressive signs and symptoms (**Fig. 27**).[9,38,39]

Whereas fibrous dysplasia is a disease of children and young adults, Paget's disease tends to occur beyond the fifth decade of life. It thickens cortical bone, and although lytic, mixed, and sclerotic stages are also recognized, the hallmark of the disease is bone expansion and sclerosis with coarse bony trabecula. As opposed to fibrous dysplasia, it may affect the otic capsule.[3,4,9,38,39]

Osteopetrosis is a rare hereditary disorder, leading to defective osteoclast function and loss of normal bone resorption and remodelling.[4] Bones become thick and sclerotic with an increased propensity to fracture. Bone expansion in the skull base may lead to compressive neurovascular symptoms and signs (**Fig. 28**).[4,9,11,12]

Eosinophilic granuloma is part of the spectrum of Langerhans' cell histiocytosis, a pathologic condition characterized by the presence of a histiocytic-like cell. It is seen in the pediatric age group and manifests as a punched-out lytic lesion without marginal sclerosis and with bevelled edges.[9,11,12] Spontaneous hyperdensity on CT and intermediate to low signal intensity on T2-weighted MR imaging are the rule, imposing the differential diagnosis with other small round-cell tumors (**Fig. 29**).[9,11]

Skull base osteomyelitis can result from the spread of infection, usually from the sinonasal region or middle ear cavity, often caused by aggressive bacterial or invasive fungal infections in immunocompromised hosts.[9,12] Invasive forms of *Aspergillus* and *Mucor* species and *Pseudomonas aeruginosa* infections in the form of malignant or necrotizing otitis externa are most commonly seen. Invasive funguses are remarkable for their angiocentric growth, leading to vessel irregularity, stenosis, and occlusion.[9,12,14,15] On

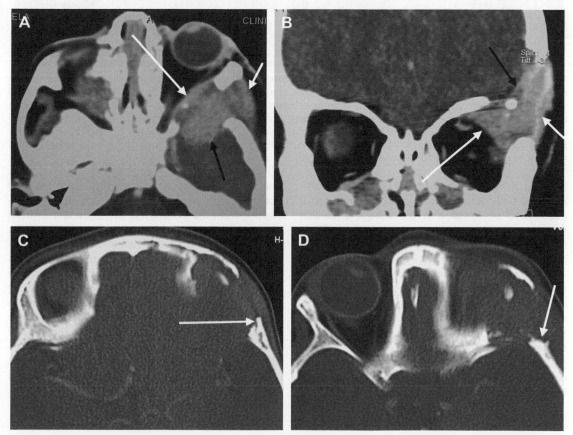

Fig. 29. Contrast-enhanced axial (*A*) and coronal (*B*) CT images in soft tissue window show a vividly enhancing mass lesion on the left sphenoid triangle bulging medially into the orbit (*long white arrows*), laterally into the suprazygomatic masticator space (*short white arrows*) and posteriorly into the middle cranial fossa (*black arrows*). Axial images on a bone algorithm (*C and D*) show a lytic expansile lesion with bevelled edges (*white arrows*) in a 9 month old child (Langerhans cell histyocitosis).

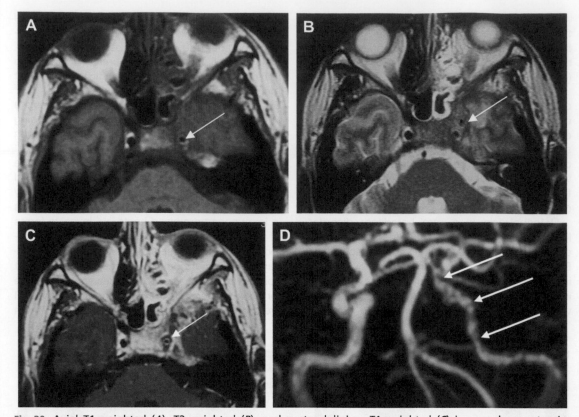

Fig. 30. Axial T1-weighted (*A*), T2-weighted (*B*), and postgadolinium T1-weighted (*C*) images show extensive replacement of the central bony skull base by a soft tissue mass that extends from the nasal cavity and paranasal sinuses into the pterygopalatine fossa and inferior orbital fissure and, posteriorly, into the left cavernous sinus encasing the left internal carotid artery (*white arrows in A–C*). This soft tissue mass is of low signal intensity on the T2-weighted images and enhances intensely after administration of gadolinium. Magnetic resonance angiography, (*D*) demonstrates to advantage the stenosis and irregularity of the lumen of the left internal carotid artery along the petrous and cavernous segments (*white arrows*).

imaging, the presence of extensive bone and cartilaginous destruction in excess of the amount of associated soft tissue in an adequate clinical setting suggests the diagnosis (**Fig. 30**).[9,12] Brain infarcts are a possible complication when the intracranial vessels is involved.[11,12,15]

Necrotizing otitis externa begins as an infection of the external auditory canal and may secondarily spread to the parotid space inferiorly, medially into the tympanic cavity, and, from there, anteriorly into the petrous apex and clivus and posteriorly into the jugular foramen. Internal jugular vein and dural sinus thromboses are common complications of this aggressive infection.[9,22]

SUMMARY

Cross-sectional imaging has a pivotal role in the evaluation of the CSB, which has limited clinical access. Lesions affecting this anatomic area may arise primarily from the skull base proper or from

neurovascular structures traveling through the skull base or may arise secondarily from lesions originating from the intracranial compartment or from the extracranial head and neck. Subdivision of the CSB into middle, off-midline, and lateral compartments and knowledge of the anatomic structures contained in each of these compartments are useful in limiting differential diagnoses. Putting together the clinical setting, location, and cross-sectional imaging features and playing with the statistics can provide a good approximation of the final diagnosis. Additionally, and most importantly, imaging is used to provide the exact mapping of the CSB and to plan surgical or focused radiation therapy with increasing accuracy.

ACKNOWLEDGMENTS

The author acknowledges Drs. David Coutinho, Fernando Torrinha, Sérgio Cardoso, Domingos Coiteiro, Robert Lufkin, Bert de Foer, and Jan Casselman for providing her with some of the images presented in this article and thanks the departments of ENT, Head and Neck Surgery, and Pathology of the Cancer Institute of Lisbon for their continuing support.

REFERENCES

1. Durden DD, Williams DW III. Radiology of skull base neoplasms. Otolaryngol Clin North Am 2001;34(6): 1043–64.
2. Som PM, Curtin HD. Head and neck imaging, skull base. 4th edition. St. Louis (MO): Mosby Year Book; 2003. p. 261–373, 783–863.
3. Curtin HD, Chavali R. Imaging the skull base. Radiol Clin North Am 1998;36(5):801–17.
4. Atlas SW. Magnetic resonance imaging of the brain and spine. 3rd edition. Philadelphia: Lippincott Williams & Wilkins; 2002.
5. Weber AL. Imaging of the skull base. Eur J Radiol 1996;22(1):68–81.
6. Pierot L, Boulin A, Guillaume A, et al. Imaging of skull base tumours in adults. J Radiol 2002;83: 1719–34.
7. Ehab Y, Hanna, DeMonte Franco. Comprehensive management of skull base tumours. 1st edition. New York, London: Informa healthcare; 2009.
8. Borges A. Skull base tumours part I: imaging technique, anatomy and anterior skull base tumours. Eur J Radiol 2008;66:338–47.
9. Borges A. Skull base tumours part II: central skull base tumours and intrinsic tumours of the bony skull base. Eur J Radiol 2008;66:348–62.
10. Chong VF, Fan YF, Tng CH. Pictorial review: radiology of the sphenoid bone. Clin Radiol 1998;53: 882–93.
11. Fishbein NJ, Kaplan MJ. Magnetic resonance imaging of the central skull base. Top Magn Reson Imaging 1999;10(5):325–46.
12. Casselman JW. The skull base: tumoral lesions. Eur Radiol 2005;15(3):534–42.
13. Borges A, Casselman J. Imaging the cranial nerves: part I: methodology, infection and inflammatory, traumatic and congenital lesions. Eur Radiol 2007; 17(8):2112–25.
14. Lufkin R, Borges A, Villablanca P. Teaching atlas of head and neck imaging. 1st edition. New York: Thieme; 2000. p. 3–31, 82–104, 303–36, 370–80.
15. Lufkin R, Borges A, Nguyen K, et al. MRI of the head and neck. 2nd edition. MRI Teaching File Series. Philadelphia: Lippincott Williams & Wilkins; 2001.
16. Tomura N, Hirano H, Sashi R, et al. Comparison of MR imaging and CT in discriminating tumour infiltration of cortex and bone marrow in the skull base. Comput Med Imaging Graph 1998;22(1):41–51.
17. Borges A, Lufkin R, Huang A, et al. Frequency-selective fat-suppression MR imaging: localized asymmetric failure of fat suppression mimicking orbital disease. J Neuroophthalmol 1997;17(1): 12–7.
18. Casselman J, Mermuys K, Delanote J, et al. MRI of the cranial nerves—more than meets the eye: technical considerations and advanced anatomy. Neuroimaging Clin N Am 2008;18(2):197–231.
19. Ishida H, Mohri M, Amatsu M. Invasion of the skull base by carcinomas: histopathologically evidenced findings with CT and MRI. Eur Arch Otorhinolaryngol 2002;259(10):535–9.
20. Patel SG, Singh B, Polluri A, et al. Craniofacial surgery for malignant skull base tumours: report of an international collaborative study. Cancer 2003; 98(6):1179–87.
21. Clayman GL, DeMonte F, Jaffe DM, et al. Outcome and complications of extended cranial-base resection requiring microvascular free-tissue transfer. Arch Otolaryngol Head Neck Surg 1995;121(11): 1253–7.
22. Chong FH, Khoo BK, Fan YF. Imaging of the nasopharynx and skull base. Magn Reson Imaging Clin N Am 2002;10:547–71.
23. Pamir MN, Ozduman K. Analysis of radiological features relative to histopathology in 42 skull base chordomas and chondrosarcomas. Eur J Radiol 2006;58(3):461–70.
24. Crockard A. Chordomas and chondrosarcomas of the cranial base: results and follow-up of 60 patients. Neurosurgery 1996;38(2):420–7.
25. Yu Q, Wang P, Shi H, et al. Central skull base invasion of maxillofacial tumours: computed tomography appearance. Oral Surg Oral Med Oral Pathol Oral Radiol Endod 2000;89(5):643–50.
26. Borges A, Casselman J. Imaging the cranial nerves: part II: primary and secondary neoplastic conditions and neurovascular conflicts. Eur Radiol 2007;17(9): 2332–44.
27. Majoie CB, Hulsmans FJ, Castelijns JA, et al. Primary nerve sheath tumours of the trigeminal nerve: clinical and MR findings. Neuroradiology 1999;41:100–8.
28. Borges A. Trigeminal neuralgia and facial nerve palsy. Eur Radiol 2005;15(3):511–33.
29. Williams LS. Advanced concepts in the imaging of perineural spread of tumour to the trigeminal nerve. Top Magn Reson Imaging 1999;10:376–83.
30. Neff B, Sataloff RT, Storey L, et al. Chondrosarcoma of the skull base. Laryngoscope 2002;112(1): 134–9.
31. Rosenberg AE, Nielsen GP, Keel SB, et al. Chondrosarcoma of the skull: a clinicopathologic study of 200 cases with emphasis on its distinction from chordoma. Am J Pathol 1999;23:1370–8.

32. Rosenberg AE, Brown GA, Bhan AK, et al. Chondroid chordoma—a variant of chordoma. A morphologic and immunohistochemical study. Am J Pathol 1994;101:36–41.

33. Chow LT, Kumta SM, King WW. Extra-articular pigmented villonodular synovitis of the temporomandibular joint. J Laryngol Otol 1998;112(2):182–5.

34. Tanaga K, Suzuki M, Nameki H, et al. Pigmented villonodular synovitis of the temporomandibular joint. Arch Otolaryngol Head Neck Surg 1997;123(5): 536–9.

35. Bui P, Ivan D, Olivier D, et al. Chondroblastoma of the temporomandibular joint: report of a case and literature review. J Oral Maxillofac Surg 2009;67(2):405–9.

36. Gaudet EL Jr, Nuss DW, Johnson DH Jr, et al. Chondroblastoma of the temporal bone involving the temporomandibular joint, mandibular condyle and middle cranial fossa: case report and review of the literature. Cranio 2004;22(2):160–8.

37. Connor SE, Umaria N, Chavda SV. Imaging of giant tumours involving the anterior skull base. Br J Radiol 2001;74:662–7.

38. Slootweg PJ. Maxillofacial fibro-osseous lesions: classification and differential diagnosis. Semin Diagn Pathol 1996;13:104–12.

39. Chong VF, Khoo JB, Fan YF. Fibrous dysplasia involving the base of the skull. AJR Am J Roentgenol 2002;178:717–20.

Index

Note: Page numbers of article titles are in **boldface** type.

A

Amino acid PET tracers, ^{18}F-labeled, in brain tumors, 636
  in brain tumor, 634
Anesthesia, tumor resection and, 600–601
Arculate fasciculus, MR tractography studies of, 586
Astrocytoma, low-grade, perfusion MR imaging in, 533, 536
Avastin, recurrent glioblastoma multiforme treated with, 546, 550, 552, 553

B

Bevacizumab, and irinotecan (CPT11), in glioblastoma, 650, 653
Bithalamic tumor, low-grade, axial FLAIR image of, 538
Brain, eloquent cortex of, direct electrical stimulation mapping of, 578
    mapping of, 578–579
  functions of, mapping of, historical perspective on, 573–574
  irradiation of, effects on normal brain parenchyma, and radiation injury, **657–668**
  language center of, 587
  plasticity of, and tumor resection in diffuse tumors, 608–609
    language-related hemispheric asymmetries and, and brain plasticity, 587–591
Brain injury, radiation-induced, clinical symptoms and signs of, 657–658
    histopathology of, 659–660
    neurobehavioral symptoms and signs of, 659
    radiologic signs of, 658–659
  radiation necrosis, and pseudoprogression, 660
Brain-mapping, technique of, 598–599
Brain tumor patients, plasticity in, 589–590
Brain tumor research, advanced MRI in, translation from animal to human, **517–526**
  diffusion MRI in, 519–522
  magnetic resonance spectroscopy in, 518–519
  perfusion MRI in, 522–524
Brain tumor(s), classification, epidemiology, management, and outcome of, 626
  diffusion imaging for therapy response assessment of, **559–571**
  magnetic resonance perfusion and permeability imaging in, **527–557**
  metastatic, PET imaging in, 641

molecular imaging (PET) of, **625–646**
  perfusion and vascular permeability, pathophysiology of, 527–528
  positron emission tomography in, 626–627
  presurgical mapping of verbal language in, with functional MR imaging and MR tractography, **573–596**
  residual/recurrent, differentiating post-therapy radiation necrosis from, 631–632

C

Cavernous sinus vascular malformations, 681
Chondroblastoma, 687
Chondromatous giant cell tumor, 687
Cortical language centers, 587
Craniotomy, awake, patient selection criteria for, 580–562

D

3-Deoxy-3-[18F]Fluorothymidine PET, in brain tumors, 639
DES mapping, during tumor resection, 602–603
Diffusion magnetic resonance tractography, 583–586
Diffusion MRI, coregistration with histology, in 9L gliosarcoma, 520, 522
  diffusion concepts in, 560–562
  for prognosis and treatment monitoring, 564–568
  for therapy response assessment of brain tumors, **559–571**
  in brain tumor research, 519–522
  in characterization of tumor, 562–563, 564
  in 9L gliosarcoma, 520, 521
  presurgical planning with, 583–586
  to grade tumor, 563–564, 565
Diffusion tensor imaging, as biomarker for neurotoxicity and radiation necrosis, 661–662
Diffusion tensor imaging color maps, 583, 584
DTI-FT, preoperative, for tumor resection, 606–607

E

EEG/ECOG, recording of, during tumor resection, 601–602, 605
EGFR, in glioblastoma, 649
Electrical stimulation mapping, intraoperative, for validation of functional MRI, 579–580, 581, 582–583

United States
Postal Service

Statement of Ownership, Management, and Circulation
(All Periodicals Publications Except Requestor Publications)

1. Publication Title
Neuroimaging Clinics of North America

2. Publication Number
0 1 0 - 5 4 8

3. Filing Date
9/15/09

4. Issue Frequency
Feb, May, Aug, Nov

5. Number of Issues Published Annually
4

6. Annual Subscription Price
$264.00

7. Complete Mailing Address of Known Office of Publication (Not printer) (Street, city, county, state, and ZIP+4®)

Elsevier Inc.
360 Park Avenue South
New York, NY 10010-1710

Contact Person
Stephen Bushing

Telephone (Include area code)
215-239-3688

8. Complete Mailing Address of Headquarters or General Business Office of Publisher (Not printer)

Elsevier Inc., 360 Park Avenue South, New York, NY 10010-1710

9. Full Names and Complete Mailing Addresses of Publisher, Editor, and Managing Editor (Do not leave blank)

Publisher (Name and complete mailing address)

John Schrefer, Elsevier, Inc., 1600 John F. Kennedy Blvd. Suite 1800, Philadelphia, PA 19103-2899

Editor (Name and complete mailing address)

Joanne Husovski, Elsevier Inc., 1600 John F. Kennedy Blvd. Suite 1800, Philadelphia, PA 19103-2899

Managing Editor (Name and complete mailing address)

Catherine Bewick, Elsevier, Inc., 1600 John F. Kennedy Blvd. Suite 1800, Philadelphia, PA 19103-2899

10. Owner (Do not leave blank. If the publication is owned by a corporation, give the name and address of the corporation immediately followed by the names and addresses of all stockholders owning or holding 1 percent or more of the total amount of stock. If not owned by a corporation, give the names and addresses of the individual owners. If owned by a partnership or other unincorporated firm, give its name and address as well as those of each individual owner. If the publication is published by a nonprofit organization, give its name and address.)

Full Name	Complete Mailing Address
Wholly owned subsidiary of	4520 East-West Highway
Reed/Elsevier, US holdings	Bethesda, MD 23814

11. Known Bondholders, Mortgagees, and Other Security Holders Owning or Holding 1 Percent or More of Total Amount of Bonds, Mortgages, or Other Securities. If none, check box ▸ None

Full Name	Complete Mailing Address
N/A	

12. Tax Status (For completion by nonprofit organizations authorized to mail at nonprofit rates) (Check one)
The purpose, function, and nonprofit status of this organization and the exempt status for federal income tax purposes
☐ Has Not Changed During Preceding 12 Months
☐ Has Changed During Preceding 12 Months (Publisher must submit explanation of change with this statement)

PS Form 3526, September 200? (Page 1 of 3 (Instructions Page 3)) PSN 7530-01-000-9931 PRIVACY NOTICE: See our Privacy policy in www.usps.com

---

13. Publication Title
Neuroimaging Clinics of North America

14. Issue Date for Circulation Data Below
May 2009

15. Extent and Nature of Circulation

		Average No. Copies Each Issue During Preceding 12 Months	No. Copies of Single Issue Published Nearest to Filing Date
a. Total Number of Copies (Net press run)		2475	2200
b. Paid Circulation (By Mail and Outside the Mail)	(1) Mailed Outside-County Paid Subscriptions Stated on PS Form 3541. (Include paid distribution above nominal rate, advertiser's proof copies, and exchange copies)	1255	1163
	(2) Mailed In-County Paid Subscriptions Stated on PS Form 3541 (Include paid distribution above nominal rate, advertiser's proof copies, and exchange copies)		
	(3) Paid Distribution Outside the Mails Including Sales Through Dealers and Carriers, Street Vendors, Counter Sales, and Other Paid Distribution Outside USPS®	429	403
	(4) Paid Distribution by Other Classes Mailed Through the USPS (e.g. First-Class Mail®)		
c. Total Paid Distribution (Sum of 15b (1), (2), (3), and (4)) ▸		1684	1566
d. Free or Nominal Rate Distribution (By Mail and Outside the Mail)	(1) Free or Nominal Rate Outside-County Copies Included on PS Form 3541	110	108
	(2) Free or Nominal Rate In-County Copies Included on PS Form 3541		
	(3) Free or Nominal Rate Copies Mailed at Other Classes Through the USPS (e.g. First-Class Mail)		
	(4) Free or Nominal Rate Distribution Outside the Mail (Carriers or other means)		
e. Total Free or Nominal Rate Distribution (Sum of 15d (1), (2), (3) and (4)) ▸		110	108
f. Total Distribution (Sum of 15c and 15e) ▸		1794	1674
g. Copies not Distributed (See instructions to publishers #4 (page #3)) ▸		681	526
h. Total (Sum of 15f and g) ▸		2475	2200
i. Percent Paid (15c divided by 15f times 100)		93.87%	93.55%

16. Publication of Statement of Ownership
If the publication is a general publication, publication of this statement is required. Will be printed ☐ Publication not required
in the November 2009 issue of this publication.

17. Signature and Title of Editor, Publisher, Business Manager, or Owner

Stephen R. Bushing

Stephen R. Bushing – Subscription Services Coordinator

Date September 15, 2009

I certify that all information furnished on this form is true and complete. I understand that anyone who furnishes false or misleading information on this form or who omits material or information requested on the form may be subject to criminal sanctions (including fines and imprisonment) and/or civil sanctions (including civil penalties).

PS Form 3526, September 2007 (Page 2 of 3)

Printed and bound by CPI Group (UK) Ltd, Croydon, CR0 4YY

03/10/2024

01040362-0019